Proceedings of the Sixth International Symposium on Olfaction and Taste

Held at Gif-sur-Yvette, Paris, France, 15-17th July, 1977.

Edited by
J. Le Magnen
P. Mac Leod

ISBN 0-904-14708-8
Published by Information Retrieval
London & Washington DC

Information Retrieval Ltd.,
1 Falconberg Court,
London W1V 5FG, England

Information Retrieval Inc.,
1911 Jefferson Davis Highway,
Arlington, Va, 22202, USA.

Printed in England by Information Printing Ltd. Eynsham.

Contents

Contents continued

Contents

Contents continued

Contents

Introduction

The Sixth International Symposium on Olfaction and Taste was held from July 15th to July 17th near Paris, prior to the 27th International Congress of Physiological Sciences. I.S.O.T. VI was, like the five preceeding symposia, sponsored by the International Commission " Olfaction and Taste " of the International Union of Physiological Sciences. It was placed under the special auspices of the European Chemoreception Research Organization.

Yngve Zotterman, fifteen years after organizing the First International Symposium " Olfaction and Taste " in Stockholm, was the General Chairman of the 1977 meeting.

In response to the ever growing income of new information, the scientific program underwent two modifications: on the one hand, ten oral sessions were devoted to the main topics presently under active investigation; each session involved four or five short lectures presented by invited speakers and, for the first time, two of them were devoted to applied chemosensory physiology; on the other hand, all the " hot " experimental material was presented in a large poster exhibition, instead of short oral communications. 102 posters were daily presented by their authors during four to five hours and were, like the preceding " Market place symposium " in Melbourne, a very successful and highly appreciated way of discovering new data and exchanging ideas.

The lectures were given by leading experts who stimulated the audience by mixing new and classic findings into a single critical overview. A common feeling of insufficient discussion of these talks will undoubtedly lead future I.S.O.T. organizers to consider whether more focused and less numerous contributions should be preferable, and to evaluate the respective advantages of plenary and simultaneous sessions.

Hopefully, the Proceedings of the meeting, with 46 full papers and 95 abstracts of poster presentations, will help others to give a second thought to so many facets of chemical senses research.

Not only the scientific programme but the social events too, contributed to cheerful and friendly contacts, be it the get together in Collége de France, the Bastille day dancing party, visiting Versailles or Cathedrale de Chartres or dining at Trianon hotel.

The local organizing committee[1] wishes to thank all the 220 participants who came from 18 countries for having contributed to the success of the Conference.

---

[1] Chairman: J. Le Magnen
Members: A. Holley, E.P. Köster, P. Laffort, P. Mac Leod, D. Ottoson.

Opening Address

Advances in chemoreception researches

J. Le Magnen

Laboratoire de Neurophysiologie Sensorielle et Comportementale, Collège de France,
11, place Marcelin Berthelot, 75231 - Paris Cedex 05, France

The Organizing Committee of this Symposium has asked me to give an opening address as a scientific welcome.

My intention is to give an appreciation of the present state of knowledge in our field of investigation, to evaluate the solid advances this Symposium will be hopefully proposing.

It is commonly agreed that 30 years ago, at the end of the second world war, the knowledge on OLFACTION AND TASTE, as compared to the other sensory modalities, was still extremely limited. The number of workers involved in the field was limited to perhaps ten to fifteen persons. The number of published works per year did not exceed ten... A fortunate time, in which investigators engaged in this field had the feeling of being explorers of a new world. To-day, the number of workers approximates six to eight hundred and the number of publications will soon reach one thousand per year.

Did this rapid growing-up result in a decisive progress of knowledge ? Certainly, yes. Many definite stages have been passed to which it is no longer needed to come back.Before saying further what these steps were, what definite and unrevisable knowledge has been acquired in recent years, I would like to say that one of the reasons for such successful advances is that investigators in our field have generally been preserved from various dangers, of biases which to-day universally affect the advance and the profitability of scientific research. The first bias is ... "la mode"... the "fashion". New lines of investigations, often based upon the appearance on the market of a new technique, of some technical device which may be used to obtain particular results, or of a new pharmacological agent, suddenly emerge. Immediately and without discrimination, everybody rushes to them. Such an increasing constraint of the fashion is due to the naive postulate, increasingly admitted, that all new things are necessarily better. An easy way to take advantage of this belief that the newest is the best, is to say and do the opposite of that which is no longer new. But, as has been said by a french writer :"Qu'est-ce que la mode ? C'est ce qui se demode" (What is Fashion ? It is that which is going out of Fashion)... and more and more rapidly somebody trapped by the current fashion is the victim of a new fashion.

Another difficulty is in the overflow of the literature, in the enormity of the current scientific production which may be considered as an overproduction, versus the capacity of consumption by the human brain. This overflow leads to a widespread ignorance of the literature. More dangerous than this excusable ignorance is the neglect of the literature and particularly of published works of the more distant past. As a result of the fascination of the up-to-dateness in some disciplines, only the literature of the past 2 or 3 years is now considered and cited.

One of the consequences is a constant repetition of the same findings by various investigators. In a field other than chemoreception, I know the case of a phenomenon which has been discovered and rediscovered four times within fifteen years by four different investigators, three of them belonging on the same country and of course ignoring their respective precursors. Again, this trend is not a matter of ignorance only. A tendency exists to consider that all data, all the acquired knowledge has to be permanently revised and reexamined, that nothing is ever definitely established and sure. Doubt is a necessary tool of the scientific mind ;but a universal scepticism is, instead, a negation of Science itself. Science per se, and ideally, is the opposite of the legend of the Sisyphean stone.

In our field, what is definitively established ? What have been, in the past decennium, the real and now unquestionable discoveries ?

A fascinating and decisive advance has been realized in the

basic field of neuro-anatomy. Largely, unknown twenty years ago, the fine structure of peripheral organs of olfaction and taste in vertebrates and invertebrates has been explored and disclosed thanks particularly to electron miscroscopic studies. The recently acquired knowledge on the neuronal architectonic of the olfactory bulb[11, 12, 13, 16] has permitted a study of the functional anatomy of this organ which is presently perhaps the most advanced study in existence of a brain structure. The tracing of olfactory and gustatory central projections has also benefited from new and efficient autoradiographic techniques, and recently of the use of ^{14}C, 2 D.G.... The important finding by Norgren[7] of direct gustatory projections to the limbic cortex and the hypothalamus has confirmed the previously proposed seperation between the thalamo-neocortical and the extra-thalamic-forebrain projections[6], now displayed in all sensory modalities. This finding also confirmed the prominent role in olfaction and taste of the extra-thalamic forebrain system which is likely linked with the role of chemoreception in regulatory behaviours.

In physiological studies a discrete but, nevertheless, basic progress was represented by the improvement of techniques permitting the management and the measurement of the peripheral delivery of odour and taste stimuli, in animals as well as in human beings. This exact assessment and control of stimuli was a prerequisite for new advances. The use of pure compounds, of defined natural odours such as isolated pheromones, or food odours, has also contributed essentially to our advances in the past years.

Thanks to convergent results yielded by single unit electrophysiological recordings by psychophysics and by studies on structure-activity relationships, some definitive conclusions have been drawn on the neural mechanism of olfactory and taste stimulation and discrimination. The "across-fiber pattern" hypothesis is no longer an hypothesis. Definitive evidence has now been provided supporting the idea that the spatial distribution of the activation of peripheral sensory cells, associated with topographical neuronal arrangements, is responsible for sending to the brain a specific neural message by each olfactory, as well as gustatory, stimulus. It is a striking confirmation of the pioneer works and assumptions of Adrian[1,2] and Pfaffmann[10], 30 years ago, of the similarity between olfaction and taste with other sensory modalities. Peripherally, odour and taste are analysed and coded in a neural fiber pattern, like the timbre of an instrument is analysed and coded by the cochlea or a picture by the retina.

From this step, two different perspectives are open for present and future investigations. First, there is the identification of the molecular basis for the specific differential activation of sensory cell membranes... the problem of the so-called "receptor sites". The rapid discovery by biochemists of hormonal and neurotransmitter protein receptors and their study of the mechanism of recognition of substrates by such molecules gives the hope of decisive analogous findings in the near future in external chemoreception systems.

The other perspective, so far hardly investigated, is the study of the central processing of information transmitted to the brain by peripheral organs. The discrimination or non-discrimination of odours and tastes, as revealed by animal behaviour and by subjective perceptions in man, is entirely dependent on this central processing of efferent signals which, peripherally, are largely redundant and overlap one another. The sensory organ makes potentially separable a very high number of stimuli. The brain only discriminates some of them rather than others. By analogy to other sensory modalities and on the basis of some pioneer works (Tanabe and Takagi)[17], it is presumed that the central processing leading to the discriminative performance is a graded selection along the central pathways of the differential characteristics of peripheral patterns. This selection leads to a specific response of a central neuron to a particular stimulus only at the terminal level. Specialist receptors, found peripherally in invertebrates, are found in the hypothalamus in vertebrates.

What are the stimuli so analysed and separated by the brain from the overflow of peripheral information ? They are not pure molecular components from their mixtures, as defined by the chemist. Only the nose and the brain of a chemist (because he is interested) discriminate pure molecules and components of a mixture of molecules. Stimuli recognized and separated by the brain, under the pressure of behaviour, are those (pure compounds of specific mixtures) emanating from environmental sources : a food object, a sex object, a warning signal and so on. I discriminate the coffee odour, not the five hundred compounds it contains. Likewise in taste, it is presumed that the peripheral information provided by sweet or bitter substances could allow the discrimination of several types of sweetness and bitterness. However, this is not the case, because the efferent neuronal arrangement is genetically programmed in such a manner that only the common characteristics of the sweet-like afferent information are separated from the common characteristics of bitter-like messages.

Such a central selection of specific characteristics of afferent messages and their separation from others, as well as the implied neuronal arrangement, are obviously flexible. They are, in each species and each individual, determined by the pressure of behaviour. Through natural selection and under the pressure of the primary survival value for the species of feeding, defensive and sexual behaviours, the basic structures and functions of sensory organs have either been selected and genetically transmitted, or not. Individually, the process of natural selection continues. In perceptual learning of sensory discrimination, as in the case of phylogenetic evolution, non-useful discriminations are eliminated while the behaviourally significant patterns are reinforced and their neuronal background organized accordingly..

One of the important steps in the progress of chemoreception studies was to consider that a sensory system is not a closed apparatus but instead is included in control systems and brain pathways subserving regulatory behaviours. The recent finding by various investigators[3, 4, 5, 8, 9, 14, 15] of state dependent (hunger or thirst) responses of hypothalamic and bulbar neurons of food objects are, in this line, very important and promising discoveries.

Hopefully, this VIth International Symposium on Olfaction and Taste will contribute further to these fascinating advances in Chemoreception Research.

REFERENCES.

1. Adrian, E.D. (1942), J. Physiol., 100, 459-473.
2. Adrian, E.D. (1950), Electroenceph. Clin. Neurophysiol., 2, 377-378
3. Aleksanyan, Z.A. Buresova, O. and Bures, J. (1976), Physiol. and Behav., 17 (2), 173-181.
4. Chaput, M. (1975), Distension stomacale et activité du bulbe olfactif chez le rat, Thesis, Lyon.
5. Glenn, J.F. and Erikson, R.P. (1976), Physiol. and Behav., 16 (5), 561-569.
6. Le Magnen, J. (1975), in "Olfaction and Taste V", Denton, D.A. and Coghlan, J.P. ed., Academic Press, (N.Y.), 381-388.
7. Norgren, R. (1976), J. Comp. Neur., 166, 17-30.
8. Pager, J., Giachetti, I., Holley, A. and Le Magnen, J. (1972), Physiol. and Behav., 9, 573-579.
9. Pager, J. (1974), Physiol. and Behav., 13, 523-526.
10. Pfaffmann, C. (1941), J. Cell. Comp. Physiol., 17, 243-258.
11. Pinching, A.J. and Powell, T.P.S. (1971), J. of Cell Science, 9 (2), 305-346.
12. Pinching, A.J. and Powell, T.P.S. (1971), J. of Cell Science, 9 (2), 347-378.
13. Pinching, A,J. and Powell, T.P.S. (1971), J. of Cell Science, 9 (2), 379-410.
14. Rolls, E.T., Burton, M.J. and Mora, F (1976), Brain Res., 111, 53-67.
15. Sharma, K.N., Dua-Sharma, S., Gopal, V. and Jacobs, H.L. (1971), Proc. of the XXV International Union of Physiological Sciences, Vol. IX, Abstr. 1517, p.510.
16. Shepherd, G.M. (1972), Physiol. Rev., 52, 864-917.
17. Tanabe, T., Yarita, H., Iino, M., Ooshima, Y. and Takagi, S.F. (1975), J. Neurophysiol., 38 (5), 1269-1281.

MOLECULAR BASIS OF CHEMORECEPTION

Abstracts of Poster Presentations

Structure of odour molecules and multiple activities of receptor cells

Karl-Ernst Kaissling

Max-Planck-Institut für Verhaltensphysiologie, 8131 Seewiesen, GFR

ABSTRACT

   Several dynamic and static parameters of receptor potentials show different structure-activity relationships and suggest that several molecular processes with different chemical specificity contribute to the cell response. This is demonstrated with single cell recordings from pheromone receptor cells of Bombyx mori, Antheraea polyphemus and A. pernyi.

   We hope to learn something about a chemosensitive system if we study the relationship between the molecular structures of chemical agents and the activities released by these agents. One difficulty with this approach is that biological systems usually have several chemodetectors with different chemical specificities or, in other words, different types of chemical filters. The word filter is used here for any functional link which produces a chemically specific response of the investigated system. With more than one type of filter any structure-activity relationship depends upon the way these filters are combined and act together. These filters may be arranged in parallel or in series which would, respectively, broaden or narrow the range of compounds to which the system is able to respond.

   In the case of gustatory and olfactory organs we have parallel filters if we consider the receptor cell as a filter unit. It is perhaps less obvious that we are also confronted with the problem of filter interaction if we study single receptor cells. We would deal with parallel filters, if a cell has several types of detectors, i.e. receptor molecules, as has frequently been discussed, for instance for the cells of the generalist type[1]. Even if a cell type would bear only one species of receptor molecule we could have several filters, however, in a serial array.

   One group of filters could be generated by the stimulus adsorbing and conducting structures, such as mucus layer, cuticle, etc.. Adsorption, however, seems to be relatively unspecific in moth antennae[2]. Another filter effect could be generated by "early inactivation" of the odor molecules. We postulate inactivation in systems like moth antennae which accumulate the odor molecules during the stimulus and show, nevertheless, a constant receptor potential amplitude as long as we stimulate and a decline of the receptor potential after the end of stimulation[3]. In the following, however, we assume a relatively fast and unspecific inactivation process which, therefore, will be neglected in our considerations.

Probably the most important group of serial filters would be represented by the various chemical reaction steps occurring at the receptor molecule itself. This means that, for instance, binding between odor and receptor molecule and the activation of the receptor molecule, i.e. a conformational alteration of the molecule leading to membrane depolarization, could depend on different structural properties of the stimulus compound. In principle, each reaction step could have its own chemical specificity. Recordings from single bombykol receptor cells have been interpreted accordingly[3,4,5]. In this paper we will summarize these findings and add results obtained in pheromone receptor cells of <u>Bombyx mori</u> and also of saturniid moths.

The basic observation is that several parameters of the receptor potential, the primary cell response, depend in a different manner upon the stimulus compounds. We evaluate <u>static</u> parameters such as i) the saturation amplitude of the receptor potential, and ii) the stimulus concentration which is necessary to reach the half-saturation amplitude of the receptor potential ($S_{1/2 \text{ response}}$). Both parameters are derived from the dose response curve, which shows the steady amplitude of the receptor potential (Fig.1) versus the stimulus concentration. As <u>dynamic</u> parameters we use iii) the half-time of the rise (τ_{rise}) and iv) the half-time of the decline of the receptor potential ($\tau_{decline}$). In addition we use a further dynamic parameter, namely the degree of v) receptor potential fluctuations. So far we distinguish only two extremes, fluctuating and smooth receptor potentials (iii-v see fig.1).

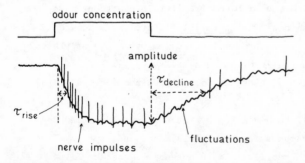

Figure 1

Sometimes we use further static parameters as, for instance vi) the relative stimulus concentration needed for a standard response amplitude or vii) the relative amplitude of receptor potential at a given stimulus concentration. These parameters are, however, less useful because they vary considerably with the standard amplitude or the stimulus concentration which we choose for the comparison.

In the following we will demonstrate that each response parameter may have its own chemical specificity and that it is often impossible to say compound A is more effective than compound B. The upper diagram of fig.2 shows dose response curves of the steady receptor potential (here electroantennogram, EAG) amplitude[3,4]. All of the tested compounds act on the bombykol receptor cell of male moth of <u>Bombyx mori</u>. The lower part of fig.2 gives the corresponding decline times ($\tau_{decline}$). The decline times of E10, E12-bombykol (not shown) are indistiguishable from those of bombykol. The following table shows the rank orders of four compounds of fig.2 according to the parameters I), II) or IV).

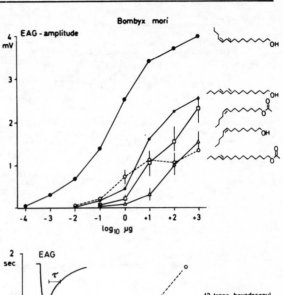

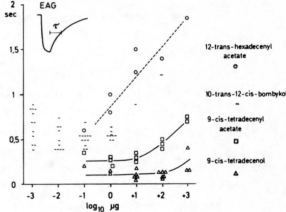

Figure 2

$S_{1/2}$ response	Saturation amplitude	decline time
low	high	short
1. bombykol	bombykol	Z9-14C ol
2. E12-16C ac	E10,E12-bombykol	bombykol
3. E10,E12-bombykol	(Z9-14C ol)	E10,E12-bombykol
4. Z9-14C ol	E12-16C ac	E12-16C ac
high	low	long

Fig.3 shows electroantennogram responses of about equal amplitude produced by bombykol and 5 related double unsaturated alcohols with varying chain length. It is obvious that the amounts of odor (given in µg) on the sources

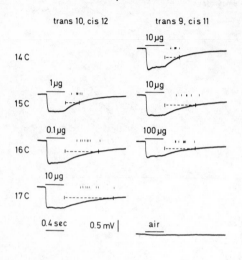

Bombyx mori, EAG

trans 10, cis 12   trans 9, cis 11

14 C   10 μg

15 C   1 μg   10 μg

16 C   0.1 μg   100 μg

17 C   10 μg

0.4 sec   0.5 mV | air

Figure 3[15]

do not correlate with the decline times (indicated by the length of the hatched lines). The points of half return of the EAG's of 6-8 further antennae are indicated by small lines above each dashed line.

It is not yet possible to make reliable predictions about the type of effect which will be induced by a new compound. So far any molecules with a chain of 14 Carbon atoms induced relatively short decline times (Fig.2,3). This is true also for all mono-unsaturated alcohols with cis or trans configurations of the double bonds in positions 6 to 12. Interestingly, also Z9-tetradecenyl acetate has a shorter decline time although it has altogether 16 carbon atoms (Fig.2). Primary mono-unsaturated alcohols with 16 carbon atoms generate declines similar to those of bombykol responses with but one exception: Z10-hexadecenal leads to a three times shorter decline time. This shows that a faster decline is not induced only by shorter molecules.

The rule that shorter molecules induce shorter decline times holds true also for pheromone receptor cells of male saturniid moths Antheraea polyphemus and Antheraea pernyi. Each of the long olfactory hairs has two cells, one of which responds to E6,Z11-hexadecadienyl acetate, the other to E6,Z11-hexadecadienal[3,6]. Both compounds have been found in the female abdominal glands of A. polyphemus[6]. These cells respond to all tested compounds with 14 carbon atoms with relatively short decline times as described for Bombyx. This is also true for the mono-unsaturated compounds with 16 carbon atoms, contrary to the situation in Bombyx (see above). The effect of leaving out the E6 double bond can be seen in recordings from a single aldehyde receptor cell (Fig.4) and from a single acetate receptor cell (Fig.5). Fig.5 shows a faster decline even if a second double bond is present but in a completely wrong position (E14). The decline time is more similar to the one after pheromone stimulation if the second double bond is at Z5 or Z7, i.e. near to the E6 double bond of the pheromone.

We shall not discuss here the rise time of the receptor potential which depends strongly on the stimulus strength and also on the stimulus compound (Fig.4)[7].

Rather we want to consider the <u>fluctuations of the receptor potential</u>. They were discovered in bombykol receptor cells [3,4] but are obvious also in the saturniid pheromone receptors, especially in the "acetate cells" (Fig.5). Fluctuating receptor potentials are induced by the pheromone compounds and by some derivatives. Other related compounds induce smooth receptor potentials. Fluctuating receptor potentials always elicit irregular impulse firing which also continues during the decline phase. Smooth receptor potentials lead to more regular impulse firing and do not induce impulses during the decline phase (Fig.5). The parameter "fluctuation" is not correlated with the effectiveness of compounds if ranked according to the receptor potential amplitudes. Z11 and Z7, Z11-hexadecadienyl acetate show similar amplitudes with 1 µg stimuli but differ strongly in the degree of fluctuations (Fig.5). It seems that smooth receptor potentials and short decline times often occur together.

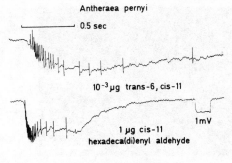

Antheraea pernyi

0.5 sec

10^{-3} µg trans-6, cis-11

1 µg cis-11 hexadeca(di)enyl aldehyde

1mV

Figure 4[16]

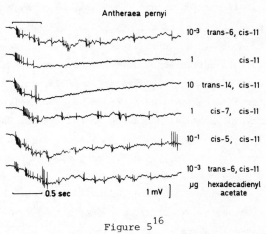

Antheraea pernyi

10^{-3} trans-6, cis-11

1 cis-11

10 trans-14, cis-11

1 cis-7, cis-11

10^{-1} cis-5, cis-11

10^{-3} trans-6, cis-11

µg hexadecadienyl acetate

0.5 sec 1 mV

Figure 5[16]

How could fluctuating and smooth receptor potentials be generated? It has been suggested earlier[3,4] that the fluctuating potentials are composed of a few and relatively large "elementary receptor potentials" whereas the smooth potentials consist of many superimposed small elementary responses. Elementary receptor potentials[3,4,8] precede and probably elicit single nerve impulses (Fig.6). Such transient potential steps could be produced by opening of a single ion channel of a conductance of about 10^{-10} mho [3]. This value is similar to that of ion channels found in muscle cell membranes at the motor endplate. They have a conductance of about $3 \cdot 10^{-11}$ mho [9,10] and are opened if two acetyl-

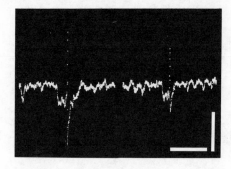

Fig.6: Elementary receptor potential and nerve impulse, recorded from a bombykol receptor cell (left) and from a second receptor cell (right) which responds to E10, Z12-hexadecadienal ("bombykal"). Calibration 100msec, 0,5 mV.
Both receptor cells occur in every ol- factory hair (Sensillum trichodeum) of the male moth. Bombykal seems to be a second pheromone component of the fe- male[14].

choline molecules bind to one acetycholine receptor molecule[19,20]. Correspon- dingly, an ion channel could be opened by a hypothetical pheromone receptor molecule if it is activated due to binding of an odor molecule. One odor mole- cule should be sufficient because it has been shown that one bombykol mole- cule is sufficient to elicit one nerve impulse[11,12]. Our explanation of the smooth receptor potentials - superimposition of many but small elementary responses - would mean that a receptor molecule can undergo different confor- mational changes depending on the ligand. One change or "activation" would lead to a large, another to a small average ion conductance $\bar{g}$ per open chan- nel. Interestingly, the opening time of acetylcholine induced ion channels depends on the agonist[18].

Earlier[4,5,12] we discussed a hypothetical model which was originally proposed by DEL CASTILLO and KATZ 1956[13] for the acetylcholine reception at motor endplates:

$$ S \ + \ R \ \underset{k_{-1}}{\overset{k_1}{\rightleftharpoons}} \ RS \ \underset{k_{-2}}{\overset{k_2}{\rightleftharpoons}} \ R'S \qquad \Delta G_{membrane} = \bar{g} \cdot R'S $$

It includes binding of the agonist S to a receptor molecule R and the forma- tion of a complex RS which can change into a "depolarizing form" R'S. One activated complex R'S induces an increase of membrane conductance $\bar{g}$, possibly by opening an "ion channel"[9,10,17]. This simple model could account for the observed changes of all parameters discussed so far[4,5] (Fig.7). For instance a shift of $S_{1/2}$ response to higher concentrations could be produced by an in- creased binding constant $K = R \cdot S/RS = k_{-1}/k_1$, by an increased activation constant $M = RS/R'S = k_{-2}/k_2$ or by a decreased membrane conductance $\bar{g} = \Delta G_{membrane}/R'S$ per activated receptor molecule (ΔG = increase of membrane conductance). A decreased saturation level of the dose response curve $\Delta V'_{max}$ could be due to a larger M or smaller $\bar{g}$ but not to a change of K. The degree of fluctuations would depend on $\bar{g}$, i.e. the width of the ion channel, or on M if the lifetime of the open channel varies. The decline time should tell us something about velocity constants of the model. Presumably the decline time reflects the velocity constant k_{-1} rather than k_{-2}. The

$$R + S \xrightleftharpoons{K} RS \xrightleftharpoons{M} R'S \qquad \Delta G = \bar{g} \cdot R'S$$

$$\frac{R'S}{R_{(tot)}} = \frac{1}{\dfrac{K \cdot M}{S} + M + 1} \qquad \frac{\Delta V}{\Delta V_{(\Delta G = \infty)}} = \frac{1}{\dfrac{G}{\Delta G} + 1}$$

$$\frac{\Delta V(R'S)}{\Delta V_{(\Delta G = \infty)}} = \frac{1}{\dfrac{K \cdot M \cdot Q}{S} + M \cdot Q + Q + 1}$$

$$\frac{\Delta V_{R'Smax}}{\Delta V_{\Delta G = \infty}} = \frac{1}{M \cdot Q + Q + 1} = \Delta V'_{max}$$

$$S_{\frac{1}{2}} resp. = \frac{K \cdot M \cdot Q}{M \cdot Q + Q + 1} = \Delta V'_{max} \cdot K \cdot M \cdot Q$$

$$S_{\frac{1}{2}} occ. = \frac{K}{1 + \dfrac{1}{M}} = S_{\frac{1}{2}} resp. \frac{1}{1 - \Delta V'_{max}}$$

$$K = \frac{S \cdot R}{RS}$$

$$M = \frac{RS}{R'S}$$

$$Q = \frac{G}{\bar{g} \cdot R_{tot}}$$

Figure 7[5]: The figure shows the three assumed reaction steps at the top. The two formulae in the second row give R'S as a function of S and ΔV as a function of the increase of membrane conductance ΔG. The constant G includes the resting conductance of the cell membrane as well as other conductances of an equivalent circuit diagram of the receptor cell. Both these functions are hyperbolic, and can be combined via the assumption $\Delta G = \bar{g} \cdot R'S$. The result is a hyperbolic dependence of the receptor potential ΔV on the stimulus concentration S, as given in the third row of the figure. The three variables K, M and $\bar{g}$ affect the function $\Delta V = f(S)$ in different ways. An increase of K would shift the dose-response curves towards higher concentrations but would leave their shape unchanged in a semilog plot. The same effect can be obtained by an increase of M or a decrease of $\bar{g}$. However, the saturation amplitude $\Delta V'_{max}$ starts decreasing as soon as the sum of the terms $M \cdot Q + Q$ becomes larger than about 0.1. In addition, the shift of the curves towards higher stimulus concentrations approaches a limit since the concentration $S_{1/2}$ response causing half-maximum response response cannot exceed K. – $S_{1/2}$ response corresponds to the K_b-value used by Morita[17] who proposed an alternative model. $S_{1/2}$ occ. is the stimulus concentration at which half of the receptor molecules are occupied by the stimulus ($RS + R'S = 1/2 R_{tot}$).

latter constant should determine the average duration of the elementary receptor potentials (<100 msec) and not appreciably influence the much longer decline time.

In principle, each velocity constant of the discussed model or of any equivalent alternative model may depend on different properties of the ligand and would, therefore, indicate separate structure-activity relationships for each reaction step. Careful evaluation of the various observed response parameters might eventually lead to a determination of the reaction constants and to a better understanding of the molecular processes involved in chemoreceptor excitation.

I thank Mrs. C. Zack for valuable comments and Miss U. Rager for technical assistance.

REFERENCES

1) D. Schneider, V. Lacher, and K.E. Kaissling (1964) Z. Vergl. Physiol. 48, 632-662.
2) G. Kasang and K.E. Kaissling (1972) Int. Symp. Olfaction & Taste IV, D. Schneider, ed., Wiss. Verlagsgesellsch. Stuttgart, 200-206.
3) K.E. Kaissling (1974) In Biochemistry of Sensory Functions. L. Jaenicke, ed., 25th Colloq. Ges. Biol. Chemie, Mosbach. Springer-Verlag, Heidelberg, 243-273.
4) K.E. Kaissling (1974) Verh. Dtsch. Zool. Ges. 67, 1-11.
5) K.E. Kaissling (1976) In Structure-Activity Relationships in Chemoreception, ECRO-Symposium Wädenswil. Ed.: G. Benz, Information Retrieval, London, 137-148.
6) J. Kochansky, J. Tette, E.F. Taschenberg, R.T. Cardé, K.E. Kaissling, and W.L. Roelofs (1975) J. Insect Physiol. 21, 1977-1983.
7) K.E. Kaissling (1969) Int. Symp. Olfaction & Taste III, C. Pfaffmann, ed., Rockefeller University Press, New York, 52-70.
8) K.E. Kaissling (1974) Mitt. Max-Planck-Gesellsch., 400-423.
9) B. Katz and R. Miledi (1972) J. Physiol. 224, 665-699.
10) C.R. Anderson and C.F. Stevens (1973) J. Physiol. 235, 655-691.
11) K.E. Kaissling and E. Priesner (1970) Naturwissenschaften 57, 23-28.
12) K.E. Kaissling (1971) In Handbook of Sensory Physiology, IV, 1, ed. L.M. Beidler, Springer-Verlag, Berlin, 351-431.
13) J. Del Castillo and B. Katz (1956) Proc. Roy. Soc. B 146, 369-381.
14) K.E. Kaissling, H.J. Bestmann and G. Kasang, Nature, in press.
15) The compounds were kindly provided by H.J. Bestmann, Erlangen.
16) The compounds were kindly provided by W. Roelofs, H.E. Hummel and M. Jacobson.
17) H. Morita (1969). Int. Symp. Olfaction & Taste III, ed. C. Pfaffmann, Rockefeller Univ. Press, New York, 370-381.
18) B. Katz and R. Miledi (1972) J. Physiol. 230, 707-717
19) V. E. Dionne and C. F. Stevens (1975) J. Physiol. 251, 245-270
20) F. Dreyer, K.-D. Müller, K. Peper and R. Sterz (1976) Pflügers Arch. 367, 115-122

Some aspects of molecular recognition by chemoreceptors

Paul Laffort

Physiologie de la Chimioréception, C.N.R.S., 91190 Gif-sur-Yvette, France

ABSTRACT
         Chemoreception involves, as is often asserted, three types
of rather diversified sensory modalities, which are, respectively, Olfaction by generalist receptors, Olfaction by specialist
receptors and Taste. While anatomic and functional differences
are sometimes evident, it seems that these three modalities can
be characterized by their particular effectiveness functions in
reference to physico-chemical continua. Several examples will be
considered. The three chemosensory modalities raise the same two
fundamental questions in relation to molecular coding :
         1°) Is there one or several types of molecular receptor for
each neuro-receptor ?
         2°) What, in the molecular structure of the stimulus can be
independently significant for different molecular receptors, thus
allowing for a basic discrimination process ?
         Some answer elements to these two questions are offered for
consideration. Concerning the second one, the study will be focused on factor ε, one of those proposed by LAFFORT and LAFFORT
et al., for several years.

1 - EFFECTIVENESS FUNCTIONS IN CHEMORECEPTION AS REFERRED TO PHYSICO-CHEMICAL CONTINUA

The most usual continuum is the number of CH_2 of an homologous series. Figure 1 reproduces comparative olfactory effectiveness[27] of normal carboxylic acids for man and for specialist receptors of *Locusta migratoria* as a function of carbon atoms number[27]. The differences between the two curves are the higher effectiveness for the specialist receptors, as well as the symetrical and almost gaussian shape. The specifity, however, does not seem narrower in one or the other case.

There is an equally great difference between gustatory and olfactory responses as between olfactory specialists and generalists. They are similarly bound, however, to suddenly evolving phenomena seemingly relevant to the "catastrophe theory"[26]. The word "catastrophe" must be taken in its etymological meaning of upsetting, i.e., an accident in a previously continuous variation of a system.

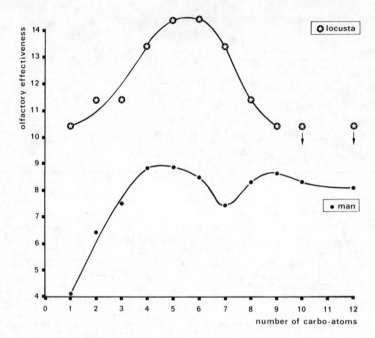

Figure 1. - Comparison between olfactory effectiveness of normal carboxylic acids for man and for *Locusta migratoria* as a function of carbon atoms number[7, 21].

Though imperfectly, Figures 2 and 3 illustrate this concept. Figure 2 shows the variation of sapidity[28] of phenylalanine as a function of specific rotation, chosen, in this case, as an appropriate continuum. A disruption of the effectiveness curve is observed concomitantly with a sudden change of quality. It may be, of course, objected that, in this case, we have not five pure components, but two components and three mixtures. Figure 3 shows an index of sweetness of seven hexoses[24] as a function of a "composite continuum", empirically associating specific rotation and melting point. Bitterness appears suddenly for βD-mannose. The validity of this particular continuum is obviously not proved by these examples.

II - NUMBER OF MOLECULAR RECEPTOR TYPES IN A GIVEN NEURORECEPTOR

We have shown, in 1966, that dose-response curves can generally be well represented by a hyperbola in log.-log. coordinates, with a horizontal branch, and with an oblique one with a slope ranging from 0 to 1. The equation proposed is :

$$I = \frac{I_1}{\left[C/_C + \left(I_1/I_M \right)^{1/n} \right]^n}$$

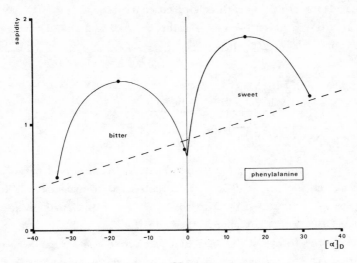

Figure 2. – Variation of sapidity[28] of phenylalanine for man, as a function of its specific rotation.

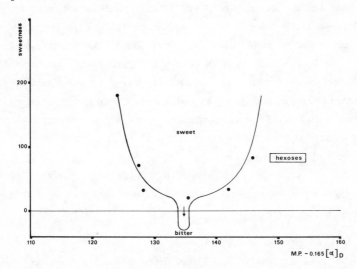

Figure 3. – Sweetness for man of seven hexoses, versus a "composite continuum", empirically associating melting point and specific rotation. From left to right, they are : β D-fructose, α D-glucose, α D-mannose, β D-mannose, β D-galactose, α D-galactose and β D-glucose. A singularity appears for β D-mannose[24].

in which n is the steepness (or exponent value), I is the sensory (or electrical) response, I_1 is the lower response significantly different from the background noise, I_M is the highest response, C is the stimulus concentration, and

C_1 is the concentration for I_1 (or threshold concentration).

When n = 1, this equation becomes similar to that of BEIDLER, under the condition of writing : $K = I_1/(C_1 I_M)$:

$$ I = \frac{\left(\dfrac{I_1}{C_1\,I_M}\right) C\,I_M}{1 + \left(\dfrac{I_1}{C_1\,I_M}\right) C} \equiv \frac{KC\,I_M}{1 + KC} $$

Figure 4 shows, for example, that this equation, with only 4 parameters, takes into account, as well in log.-log. coordinates as in semi-log., EAG values of *Bombyx mori*, stimulated by Bombycol[8, 9, 29]. This figure reveals clearly that BEIDLER'S law is not appropriate for the case.

PATTE[20] suggested to apply the LAFFORT equation to the single cell response in order to evaluate the number of molecular receptor types involved in a given neuroreceptor. If the slope value nears 1, BEIDLER's law becomes valid and it can be concluded that only one type of molecular receptor is involved in the considered cell. A case in point is that of the single receptor cell of *Bombyx mori*, stimulated by Bombycol[8, 9] : n = 1.06. If the slope is significantly inferior to 1, BEIDLER's law is no longer appropriate, which implies that more than one type of macro-molecules is involved in the chemoreception of the considered cell. Such is the case of the single neuroreceptor of *Locusta migratoria*[7] : n = 0.41. It would probably be quite interesting to develop this kind of measurements on vertebrates, as well as to refine the full meaning of slope and plateau values.

Let us note the important difference in steepness for Bombycol either obtained from EAG or from single cell recording, probably due to a recruitment phenomenon in the former.

III - THE ε MOLECULAR FACTOR.

Since 1968, several sets of molecular properties have been proposed, as probably implied in the recognition mechanism of olfactory receptors[2, 13, 14, 15, 16, 17, 18]. These sets formerly included three properties derived from the structure. Now 6 relevant molecular properties have been identified, all experimentally measured by Gas Chromatography.

Some coherence is found between these several versions of molecular properties. Thus, Figure 5 shows mutual correlations between the ε values of these six versions, concerning 75 substances, this factor was previously called P[13]. Since it is the less classic of those we have proposed, we will

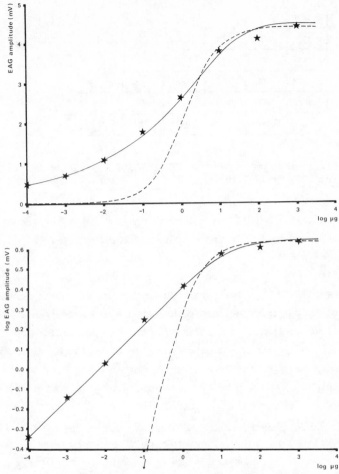

Figure 4. - Electroantennogram (EAG) of *Bombyx mori* stimulated by Bombycol[8, 9] in semi-logarithmic coordinates (top half) and in log.-log. coordinates (bottom half), dotted line from BEIDLER's equation, continuous line from LAFFORT's equation[11].

focus the present study on this ε factor which stands for "local voluminal polarizability" in pharmacology as well as in physical chemistry. We have selected the definition of LAFFORT et al[17], because the values obtained according to this definition are presently known for 228 substances[20].

1°) Importance of the ε factor in Olfaction

Four examples allow us to evaluate this importance :

- Human olfactory thresholds. A regression-correlation for the olfactory thresholds of 103 substances versus four terms (the four molecular factors

E 1970	1				
E 1971	0.78	0.78			
E 1972	0.82	0.82	0.99		
E 1973	0.84	0.84	0.88	0.94	
E 1976	0.83	0.83	0.89	0.92	0.98
	E 1968	E 1970	E 1971	E 1972	E 1973

Figure 5. – Correlation matrix (after PEARSON) of six versions of ε factor, proposed by LAFFORT, or LAFFORT et al.[12, 14, 18] for 75 substances.

of LAFFORT et al. in their 1973 version) shows that ε has the second range after α and before π and ρ, in the weight of the global correlation obtained, which is here of 0.67[20].

– Qualitative discrimination in man. Susan SCHIFFMAN et al. established by psychophysics in 1977, a similarity odour triangular matrix for 19 substances. For 17 of those, these authors established a distance triangular matrix based on our 1973 version of molecular factors. The decreasing order of the weight in the global correlation obtained between the two matrices was :ε, α, ρ and π. Using Raman spectra, these authors obtain a slightly better correlation :0.69 instead of 0.40. However, the meaning of this correlation is not yet clear in terms of molecular structure.

– Olfactory discrimination of optical isomers in man. JONES and ELLIOT published in 1975 a very interesting study on this topic, showing that among ten pairs of odorous optical isomeric substances, some are clearly discriminated and some are not. Results are given in this publication after a quite sophisticated statistical processing. In 1972, the same study was verbally presented without this processing and with slightly different results :discrimination for six pairs of substances having a ring structure, absence of discrimination for four flexible pairs of substances having the secondary alcohol function. With reference to this first presentation, the hypothesis was made in 1975, that discrimination appears only when ε is high. The value of ε in its 1973 version has been established for six of the ten pairs of substances studied by these authors. Table 1 reproduces the values found. It would be interesting to know if the discrimination is effective for substances with high values of ε and without ring (presence of S, I or Br for example).

SUBSTANCES	ε 73	SUBSTANCES	ε 73
CARVONE	+ 0.87	2 – HEXANOL	– 0.06
α–PINENE	+ 0.44	2 – HEPTANOL	– 0.07
2 –BUTANOL	+ 0.11	2 – OCTANOL	– 0.21

Table 1. – Values of ε (1973 version) for six of the ten substances studied by JONES and ELLIOT (1972, 1975) in decreasing order (see text).

–Peripheral discrimination in frog. Single unit activity of frog olfactory receptors stimulated successively by 20 different substances was recorded. From mathematical processing of the responses (correlation matrix after PEARSON and BENZECRI'S "correspondences analysis"), some similarity emerges between six of the 20 substances studied, characterized by an arylic nucleus. Table II reproduces the 1973 ε values for 13 of the 20 substances used by

SUBSTANCES	ε 73	SUBSTANCES	ε 73
ACETOPHENONE	1.10	DECANOL	0.24
BENZENE	0.92	PROPANOL	0.19
ANISOL	0.62	BUTANOL	0.07
NITROBENZENE	0.55	PENTANOL	– 0.17
PYRIDINE	0.42	ISOAMYL ACETATE	– 0.23
BENZALDEHYDE	0.30	HEPTANOL	– 0.28
		BUTYRIC ACID	– 0.94

Table II. – ε values (1973 version) for 13 of the 20 substances studied by HOLLEY (1974) and DUCHAMP et al. (1974), in decreasing order. Two olfactory clusters are set off.

these authors : on the left side appears the "arylic group" including Pyridine[30], on the right side a second group of substances is found as an other small cluster (three alcohols and isoamylacetate)[3].

2°) ε factor implication in physical-chemistry of solutions

Two examples are proposed :

– SNYDER et al. theory of an expanded solubility parameter. According to this theory[25], all phenomena of solution and adsorption can be explained by the five partial solubility parameters of solutes and of solvents and by the molvolume of solutes. As attested by these authors, the five partial solubility parameters are the parameters of dispersion (δ_d), orientation (δ_o), induction (δ_{in}), acidity (δ_a), and basicity (δ_b). They can be established from the molecular structure, from physico-chemical properties and from spectrographic data. A critical study of this theory has been done[18] on an experimental chromatographic basis, from which three conclusions emerged. The first one was that a good correspondence is found between α, ρ and π and $V\delta_d$, $V\delta_o$ and $V\delta_a$, respectively. The second one was that a fifth factor must be taken in account, namely β, equivalent to $V\delta_b$. The third conclusion was that the SNYDER et al. theory applied to chromatography agrees well with experimental data for the four quoted terms, not for $V\delta_{in}$, which can be replaced by the factor ε, identified to $(V_{20}/V_b)\delta d^{31}$.

– Importance in gas chromatography of molecular weight of the stationary phase

E. KOVATS showed in 1977, that, other things being equal, retention indices in G.L.C. depend on molecular weight of the stationary phase. This entirely new result must be added to the SNYDER et al. theory for a better understanding of stationary phases. On the other hand, this "KOVATS effect" depends of the solute nature. It appeared that, to the exclusion of any other property, the ε factor accounts for this "solute nature". More precisely, we have[19, 22] :

$$I \ (C87) - I \ (\text{squalane})_{\text{at } 120^\circ C} = 25\varepsilon_{73} \quad (N = 28, \ r = 0.84)$$

CONCLUSION

One might draw a double conclusion about these different facets of the recognition mechanism in chemoreception. In the first place, dose–response functions of single units should be a useful tool to learn more about the number of macromolecular receptor types involved in each neuroreceptor. In the second place, definition and experimental measurements of continua involved in chemoreception should be developed and improved. Among those proposed by several authors, it seems that factor ε, or factor of "local voluminal polarizability", according to LAFFORT et al.[17] should be considered as quite robust.

REFERENCES

1. BEIDLER, L.M. (1954) – J. Gen. Physiol., 38, 133–139.
2. DRAVNIEKS, A. and LAFFORT, P. (1973) – J. Theoret. Biol., 38, 335–342.
3. DUCHAMP, A., REVIAL, M.F., HOLLEY, A. and MAC LEOD, P. (1974) Chemical Senses and Flavor, 1, 213–233.
4. HOLLEY, A. (1974) in Transduction Mechanism in Chemoreception. pp.275–293, T.M. POYNDER, ed., Information Retrieval Ltd., London.
5. JONES, F.N. (1972) – VIIe Symposium Mediterranéen sur l'Odorat, Cannes, May 1972, (unpublished).
6. JONES, F.N. and ELLIOT, D. (1975) – Chemical Senses and Flavor, 1, 317–321.
7. KAFKA, W.A. (1970) – Z. Vergl. Physiol., 70, 105–143.
8. KAISSLING, K.E. (1971) in Handbook of Sensory Physiology, Vol. IV/1, pp. 351–431, L.M. Beidler, ed., Springer-Verlag, Berlin – Heidelberg – New-York.

9. KAISSLING, K.E. (1974) in Biochemistry of Sensory Funcitons, pp. 243-273, L. Jaenicke, ed., Springer-Verlag, Berlin - Heidelberg - New - York.
10. KOVATS, E. sz. (1977) - Pers. Communic., Ecole Polytechnique Federale de Lausanne (Switzerland).
11. LAFFORT, P. (1966) - J. Physiol. Paris, 58, 551.
12. LAFFORT, P. (1968) - Olfactologia, 1, 95-104 (Suppl. Cahiers d'Oto-Rhino-Laryngologie, 3, n°5).
13. LAFFORT, P. (1969) in Olfaction and Taste III, pp. 150-157, C. Pfaffman ed., Rockefeller University Press, New-York.
14. LAFFORT, P. (1972) - VIIe Symposium Mediterranéen sur l'Odorat, Cannes, May 1972 (unpublished)
15. LAFFORT, P. (1975) in Structure-Activity Relationships in Chemoreception, pp. 185-195, G. Benz, ed., Information Retrieval Ltd., London.
16. LAFFORT, P. and DRAVNIEKS, A. (1972) in Olfaction and Taste IV, pp.142-148, D. Schneider, ed., Wiss.-Verlagsges, MBH., Stuttgart.
17. LAFFORT, P., PATTE, F. and ETCHETO, M. (1974) - Ann. N.Y. Acad. Sci., 237, 193-208.
18. LAFFORT, P. and PATTE, F. (1976) - J. Chromatog., 126, 625-639.
19. McREYNOLDS, W.O. (1970) - Personal communication.
20. PATTE, F. (1977) - Thesis, (in press), Lyon, France.
21. PATTE, F., ETCHETO, M. and LAFFORT, P. (1975) - Chemical Senses and Flavour, 1, 283-305.
22. RIEDO, F. FRITZ, D., TARJAN, G. and KOVATS, E. sz. (1976) - J. Chromatog., 126, 63-83.
23. SCHIFFMAN, S.S., ROBINSON, D.E. and ERICKSON, R.P. (1977) - Chemical Senses and Flavor, 2, 375-390.
24. SCHALLENBERGER, R.S. and ACREE, T.E. (1971) in Handbook of Sensory Physiology, Vol. IV/2, pp. 221-277, L.M. Beidler, ed., Springer-Verlag. Berlin - Heidelberg - New - York.
25. SNYDER, L.R., KARGER, B.L. and EON, C.H. (1976) - Anal. Chem.(submitted for publication).
26. THOM, R. (1972) - Stabilité Structurelle et Morphogénèse, W.A. Benjamin, Inc., Reading (Massachussets).
27. Effectiveness is taken as the negative $\log_2$ of molar fraction needed to obtain : the minimum of perception for man[21], and an increasing of 30 impulses by second on cells of *Sensilla caeloconica* for *Locusta migratoria*[7],
28. Sapidity is taken as the reverse of human gustatory threshold expressed in $g/1^{12}$. The phenylalanine isomers have been supplied by CALBIOCHEM.
29. Derived parameters from experimental data are :
    BEIDLER's equation : I_M = 4.39 mV, K = 0.784 μg^{-1}
    LAFFORT's equation : C_1 = 10 μg I_1 = 0.45 mV I_M = 4.48 mV, n = 0.191.
30. Pyridine is not included in the cluster found by DUCHAMP et al., but it is the only substance among 20 having a highly basic character (represented by our β factor in the 1976 version). On the other hand Benzaldehyde is included in the olfactory cluster, but as a border line case.
31. V_{20} being the molvolume at 20° C and V_b the molvolume at boiling point.

Taste properties of sugar molecules

Gordon G. Birch

National College of Food Technology, University of Reading, Weybridge, Surrey, UK

ABSTRACT

Sugar molecules are probably the simplest entities in which basic tastes may be correlated with absolute stereochemical features, and hydrogen bonding mechanisms seem to underlie their interaction with receptor sites. It is a logical consequence of such hydrogen bonding that sugar molecules should be considered as "polarised" on taste receptors, and structural features which elicit basic tastes may now be tentatively identified in sugars as well as related classes of compounds. Sugars and their derivatives are almost always sweet, bitter or bitter/sweet and gustatory response is clearly related to size as well as shape in these and other simple molecules.   Recent evidence that sweet and bitter receptor sites may be situated in close proximity is re-examined with a view to elucidating the manner in which sugar molecules are presented and "polarised" on the receptor site.

INTRODUCTION

In any fundamental study of taste it is an attractive prospect if a single basic taste can be examined in depth, free from complications of flavour and odour. The prospect becomes doubly attractive when the stimulus molecules all belong to a single chemical class in which simple parameters of configuration and conformation may be absolutely defined. The sugars are probably the simplest molecules in which the relationship between basic taste and structure may be examined in great detail. There is now[1] a wealth of information available in carbohydrate chemistry and sugar molecules are ideal for studying the relationships between steric, polar and lipophilic features which are clearly responsible for their taste properties.

THE SHALLENBERGER HYPOTHESIS

After a number of earlier[2] publications by various authors concerning the relationship between polyhydroxy character and sweetness in sugars, it was not until 1963 that Shallenberger[3] first propounded a simple yet elegant hypothesis relating sweetness to hydrogen bonding. Ultimately sweetness could be due to reciprocally hydrogen bonded complexes involving AH,B systems in sapid molecules and receptors. Intramolecular hydrogen bonds in sugar molecules rendered hydroxyl groups on sugars unavailable for complexing with receptors and hence diminished sweetness. Thus the geometry of the AH,B system, along with the stereogeometry of the entire molecule, governed its 'fit' with the receptor, and its taste properties. Subsequently, as knowledge of carbohydrate chemistry has increased, Shallenberger[4] has modified his original hypothesis (a) to accept that intramolecular hydrogen bonding may in some cases enhance sweetness by increasing the acidity of the AH proton (Fig.1)[5] and (b) to include Kier's γ dispersion site within the sweet pharmacophore (Fig.2). Inspection of molecular models reveals that the tripartite pharmacophore is identical in enantiomers. Hence D- and L-sugars, which exhibit multiple chirality, have the same taste. In amino acids on the other hand, which possess only one asymmetric carbon atom, one enantiomer is usually sweet and the other bitter.

MAPPING OF SAPOPHORIC FUNCTIONS IN SUGAR MOLECULES

Stepwise chemical modification of sugar molecules by substitution or elimination of hydroxyl groups is a logical way to search for AH,B systems and other sapophoric features in sugar molecules. In practice this approach may easily be complicated (a) by different conformational possibilities in the molecules selected and (b) by multiple isomerism. Generally gluco-pyranoside types of molecule exist overwhelmingly in the favoured $^4C_1$ conformation and are ideal analogues in which to study effects on taste of chemical modification, because their absolute stereostructures are defined. Extensive chemical manipulation in these molecules has established that the third and fourth hydroxyl groups are involved in the sweetness response

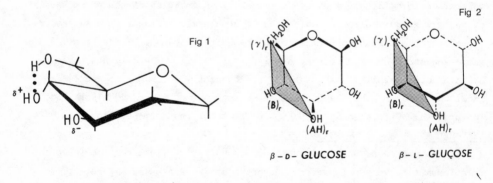

Fig 1   Fig 2

β - D - GLUCOSE β - L - GLUCOSE

Fig.1. Hydrogen bonding of the primary alcohol group to the AH proton of glucopyranoside structures, enhancing sweetness (Shallenberger, 1977)

Fig.2. Identical sweet pharmacophores in D and L enantiomers of sugars (Shallenberger, 1977)

whereas the first, second, sixth hydroxyls and the ring oxygen atom do not
seem to be necessary (Fig.3).   Strikingly, this latter group of functions are
all involved in bitterness.   Thus the molecules all seem to be "polarised"
with potentially sweet "ends" and potentially bitter "ends".   The bitter "end"
surrounds the anomeric centre which is chemically the most reactive part of
the molecule.

ASSOCIATION OF SWEETNESS AND BITTERNESS

Chemical modification of sugars almost always results[6] in products which
are sweet or bitter or bitter/sweet.   Tastelessness only seems to occur in
those derivatives which are insoluble.   Alteration of only one molecular
feature (e.g. substitution of one hydroxyl group, change in configuration at
only one chiral centre) appears to be sufficient to change the taste from
purely sweet to purely bitter or <u>vice versa</u>.   Relatively few cases exist
in which the molecule is both bitter and sweet, and an experiment[7] with one
of these, methyl α-D-mannopyranoside, already indicates that the molecule
may span both types of receptor site simultaneously.   This shows that at
least some of the sweet and bitter receptor sites may be in close proximity
(Fig.4), which is consistent with many of the common features of sweet and
bitter compounds, e.g. their dependence on stereochemical, polar and
lipophilic factors.   It is also consistent with the current concept of
"polarisation" of sapid molecules on receptor sites and it is interesting
that the extremely rare cases in which sweetness as well as bitterness are
completely (or nearly completely) absent are usually confined to symmetrical
analogues of the sugars (e.g. 1,2:4,5-cyclohexane tetrol and the dimerised
forms of dihydroxy acetone and DL-glyceraldehyde).

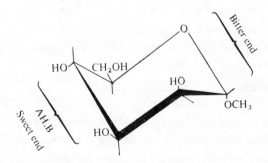

Fig.3.   "Polarisation"of bitter/sweet sugar analogues on taste
    receptors

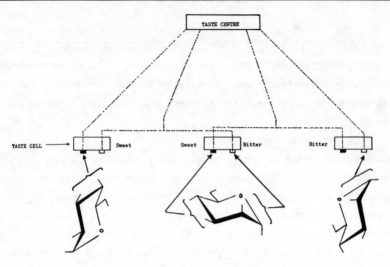

Fig.4. Proximity of some sweet and bitter receptor sites for
sugar types of molecule.

EFFECTS OF MOLECULAR SIZE AND SHAPE ON TASTE

It has already been established[2] in a taste comparison between methyl
α-D-glucopyranoside and α,α-trehalose and other analogues, that only one
sugar residue in an oligosaccharide may actually elicit the sweetness
response. More recently[8] this molar proportionality of sweetness has been
demonstrated for the entire homologous series of maltodextrins present in
glucose syrups, which implies that, at least for oligosaccharides containing
the 1,4 α-D-glucopyranoside linkage, considerable "free space" must exist in
a particular direction alongside the sweet receptor site. Similar
considerations may also apply to the bitter receptor site.

The singular effect of modified sugar residues on taste is also clearly
illustrated by comparing the responses to chlorodeoxy derivatives. In Fig.5
the trehalose analogue which is completely bitter differs only in one sugar
residue from the sucrose analogue which has recently been reported as
intensely sweet by Hough and Phadnis[9].

ONSET TIME, INTENSITY AND PERSISTENCE OF TASTE

Differences in onset time, intensity and persistence of taste among
related sapid structures obviously may affect taste panel comparisons so
that falsely high or low taste scores may be reported. The relationship
between these three effects depends on molecular structure, and their very
existence suggests that the mechanisms responsible for onset time and
persistence in sapid molecules may differ from the intensity-governing

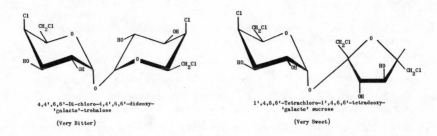

4,4',6,6'-Di-chloro-4,4',6,6'-dideoxy-
'galacto'-trehalose

(Very Bitter)

1',4,6,6'-Tetrachloro-1',4,6,6'-tetradeoxy-
'galacto' sucrose

(Very Sweet)

Fig.5. Sweetness or bitterness of single modified sugar residues
in related chlorodeoxy sugar analogues

mechanism at the level of the ion-channel. In other words an interaction
between the stimulus molecule and the receptor must precede interaction
with the ion-channel. However, if this is true, the initial reaction with
the receptor must be related in some way with the interaction at the ion-
channel and implies some sort of "orderly queue" of molecules approaching
the ionophor. In a related field of chemoreception Kaissling[10] has
recently pointed out that the receptor molecule and the ionophor may be a
single molecular entity. Experiments are now needed to substantiate the
existence of these separate mechanisms which would certainly serve to
explain onset time, persistence and intensity as well as synergism and
the orientation of sapid molecules on receptors. Furthermore, the localised
persistence of molecules implicit in this idea is consistent with the sub-
threshold concentrations of sugar residually detectable in saliva.

CONCLUSIONS

By studying single basic taste responses to a single class of simple
stereochemically defined molecules it seems possible to identify certain
features of these molecules which are most likely involved with a particular
taste[11]. Basically, asymmetric molecules may be "polarised" on taste
receptors with one part of the molecule responsible for sweetness and the
other part bitterness. The two basic tastes are thus stereochemically,
as well as spatially, associated. Further analysis indicates that time and
intensity relationships of the basic tastes also depend on chemical
structure and hence should be separately measured in psychophysical
experiments. This type of subdivision of basic tastes into elemental
factors may be a necessary preliminary to further understanding of the
orientation properties of sugar molecules at each stage of stimulus
interaction with receptor site.

REFERENCES

1. Shallenberger, R.S. and Birch, G.G. (1975) Sugar Chemistry. AVI. Westport, Connecticut

2. Birch, G.G. (1976) Crit. Rev. Food Sci.Nutr. 8, 57-95

3. Shallenberger, R.S. (1963) J. Fd. Sci. 28, 584-589

4. Shallenberger, R.S. (1977) in Sensory Properties of Foods (Birch, G.G., Brennan, J.G. and Parker, K.J. eds) Applied Science. London

5. Kier, L.M. (1976) in Structure Activity Relationships in Chemoreception (Benz, G. ed.) IRL. London and Washington

6. Birch, G.G. (1976) in Structure Activity Relationships in Chemoreception (Benz, G. ed.) IRL. London and Washington

7. Birch, G.G. and Mylvaganam, A.R. (1976) Nature 260, 632-634

8. Kearsley, M.W., Birch, G.G. and Djedzic, S. (1978) Lebensmit. Wiss. u. Technol. In press.

9. Hough, L. and Phadnis, S.P. (1976) Nature 263, 800

10. Kaissling, K.E. (1976) in Structure Activity Relationships in Chemoreception (Benz, G. ed.) IRL. London and Washington

11. Lee, C.K. and Birch, G.G. (1975) J.Sci. Fd. Agric. 26, 1513-1521

A subsite model on the sweet-taste reception mechanism of the rat

Yasutake Hiji, T. Imoto, S. Kuraoka and M. Sugiyama

*Department of Physiology, Tottori Univ. Med. Sch., Yonago 683, **Department of Physiology, Kumamoto Univ. Med. Sch., Kumamoto 860, and Ginkyo College of Med. Technol., Shimizu, Kumamoto 860, Japan

ABSTRACT
        The data of the integrated responses obtained from the chorda tympani nerve of the rat as well as monkey were analysed theoretically, assuming that the neural response to sugars could be produced by a certain type of the complex combination between sugar molecules and receptor.Two different types of sugar reception exist depending on the sugar. The first type is the formation of a complex involving two stimulus molecules for mono-saccharides, the second one, the formation of a complex involving only one stimulus molecule for disaccharides and probably for trisaccharides as well.

INTRODUCTION

        Traditionally, relative sweetness has been defined as the ratio of concentrations of sweeteners corresponding with sucrose in sweetness. Otherwise, threshold concentrations are compared to each other as a relative sweetness. However, it has been said that threshold concentrations give no information of suprathreshold sweetness because the relative sweetness often varies with concentration. For example, the sweetness of 10 % sucrose is equivalent to that of 15.5 % glucose while 40 % sucrose is equivalent to 48.1 % glucose in the sweet sensation of man[1]. The same is said in the neural responses to sweeteners. It is interesting to elucidate the reason why each dose-response curve shows such a different pattern among different sugars. For this purpose, we theoretically analysed the electrophysiological data of the integrated responses of the chorda tympani nerve of the rat (Wistar strain)[2] and of the monkey (*Macaca fuscata*)[3] assuming that the neural responses to sugars could be produced by a certain type of complex formation between sugar molecules and receptors.

RESULTS AND DISCUSSION

If one molecular reaction, such as S (sugar molecule) + P (receptor molecule) $\rightleftharpoons$ SP, continues to n molecular complexing, an equation (1) is given from each of the dissociation constants ($K_1 \cdot K_2 \ldots \ldots K_n$).

$$K_1 \cdot K_2 \ldots \ldots K_n = \frac{[S]^n[P]}{[S_nP]} \quad \text{------(1)}$$

On the assumption that the neural response magnitude (R) is proportional to concentration of n molecular complex formation $[S_nP]$, the equation (1) is converted into an equation (2).

$$R \propto [S_nP] = \frac{[S]^n[P]}{K_1 \cdot K_2 \ldots \ldots K_n} \quad \text{----(2)}$$

In low concentration of stimuli, the total number of receptors [P] almost remains, because of a few number of receptors occupied by sugar molecules. Then an equation (3) is obtained.

$$\log R \propto n \log S \quad \text{----------------(3)}$$

When magnitudes of the neural responses to sugars are plotted on the double logarithmic coordinate, straight lines are obtainable, as shown in Fig. 1, in low concentrations of each sugar. Values of n calculated from each of the slopes are about 2 for monosaccharides such as glucose or fructose and 1 for disaccharides, sucrose or maltose, respectively. The present result may indicate that two molecular reactions are necessary for the molecule of monosaccharide to induce the sweetness.

In the case of the two molecular complex formation, dissociation constants of K_1 and K_2 may represent as follows:

$$K_1 = \frac{C([P] - [SP] - [S_2P])}{[SP]} \quad \text{-------(4)}$$

$$K_2 = \frac{C[SP]}{[S_2P]} \quad \text{--------------------(5)}$$

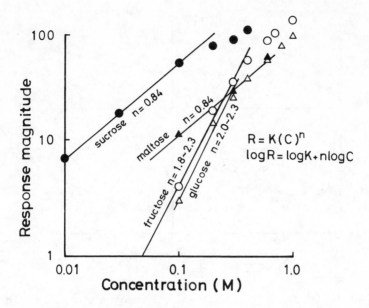

Fig. 1. A linear relationship in low concentration (C), plotting magnitude of the neural responses (R) on the double logarithmic scale.

Then, by assuming that magnitude of the maximum response (Rm) in the taste nerve is proportional to the number of the total bound sugar receptors, and if the condition [S] = C>> [P] is true, a taste equation (6) for the two molecular complex formation is obtained from both constants of (4) and (5).

$$C/R = \frac{K_1 \cdot K_2 + K_2 \cdot C + C^2}{R_m \cdot C} \quad ------(6)$$

While an equation (7), which is known as the Beidler's equation[4] may be employed, provided that the sweetness is induced by one molecular complex formation

$$C/R = \frac{C + K}{R_m} \quad --------------(7)$$

Two different types of relationships such as linear and hyperbolic plots are obtained for mono- and disaccharides, respectively, by plotting C/R against C as shown in Fig. 2.

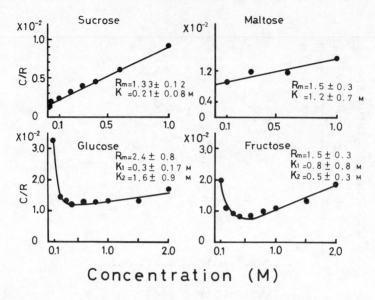

Fig.2. Two different types such as straight and hyperbolic relationships for mono- or disaccharide, plotting magnitude of the
neural responses (R) on the coordinate   C/R and C (concentration).

The existence of these two types of plots indicates that while
one molecule of disaccharide only is sufficient to elicit a neural response, it may be necessary that two molecules of a monosaccharide combine to the sugar receptor to elicit a neural response, because the hyperbola obtained with monosaccharides is
based on two molecular reaction (equation 6). Each value for R_m
and dissociation constant was calculated from each equation by
means of the least square method and presented in Figure 2. The
same result is obtained in the monkey : neural responses show
an hyperbolic relationship for monosaccharides and a linear one
for disaccharides when plotting C/R against C.

It has been said that trisaccharides or bigger polysaccha-
rides formed with sweet oligosaccharides are tasteless. For
example, it has been reported that maltose, which is a disaccharide of glucose, produces sweet taste in man, while maltotriose
(trisaccharide) is very slightly sweet and maltotetraose (tetra-
saccharide of glucose) tasteless[5]. In the rats, the chorda tympani nerve responds well to maltotriose and a measurable response appears in a concentration range from 0.01 to 0.05M.

A linear relation is also obtained when C/R is plotted against C for maltotriose, suggesting that the formation of a complex with one molecule of trisaccharide is likely to occur. In other words, two glucose moieties in the trisaccharide molecule might take part in the complex formation, indicating that there are possibly two sub-sites in the sugar receptor site.

On the basis of experimental evidence so far available, it is suggested that two types of sugar reception is a common feature among different species. One type is the formation of a complex with two stimulus molecules for monosaccharides, the other one the formation of a complex with one stimulus molecule for disaccharides and probably trisaccharides. A similar model was already proposed for the fly by Morita and Shiraishi[6] who have reported that the sugar receptor site is composed of two subunits which can be occupied either by one molecule of disaccharide or by two molecules of monosaccharide.

These results indicate that the subsite model previously proposed in the case of an enzyme reaction[7] might be also valid for the sweet taste reception mechanism. The differences between different animal species could then merely consist in different values of the dissociation constants as it is shown in Table 1.

Further experiments are presently being carried on to try and disclose whether one and the same dual receptor site can be occupied by various sugar molecules.

Sugars			Fly *		Rat		Monkey	
Glucose	K_1		0.1	M	0.3	M	3.1 6	M
	K_2		0.1	M	1.6	M	0.07	M
Fructose	K_1		0.015	M	0.8	M		
	K_2		0.06	M	0.5	M		
Sucrose	K		0.06	M	0.2	M	0.06	M
Maltose	K		0.1	M	1.2	M		
Maltotriose	K				2.4	M		

(left vertical labels: Saccharides — mono — di — tri)

* Data taken from Morita and Shiraishi (1968)

Table 1. Dissociation constants for various sugars summarized in each case of several animals.

REFERENCES

1. Lichtenstein,P.E.(1948) J.Exp.Physiol.38,578-582
2. Noma,A.,Goto,J. and Sato, M.(1971) Kumamoto Med.J.24,1-7
3. unpublished data
4. Beidler,L.M.(1954) J. Gen.Physiol.38,133-139
5. Birch, G.G.,Lee,C.K. and Rolfe,E.J.(1970) J.Sci.Fd Agric.21, 650-653
6. Morita,H. and Shiraishi,A.(1968) J.Gen.Physiol.52,559-583
7. Hiromi,K.(1970) Biochem.Biophys.Res.Commun.40,1-6

The receptor sites for sugars in chemoreception of the fleshfly and blowfly

Hiromichi Morita, Koh-Ichi Enomoto, Michio Nakashima, Ichiro Shimada* and Hiromasa Kijima

Department of Biology, Faculty of Science, Kyushu University 33, Hakozaki, Fukuoka 812, Japan

ABSTRACT
      Looking for inhibitors specific for the glucose-binding site or for the fructose-binding one in single labellar sugar receptor cells of the fleshfly, Boettcherisca peregrina, effects of alkyl glycosides, aryl glycosides, and their related compounds were examined. No completely specific inhibitors were found, but p-nitrophenyl α-D-mannopyranoside strongly inhibited the responses to fructose compared with those to sucrose and to glucose.
      Nojirimycin strongly inhibited the enzyme activity of PII-D type of the blowfly, Phormia regina, and its K_i was in a range of $10^{-5} \sim 10^{-6}$ M. Its effects on the sugar receptor cell, however, were detected only above $10^{-1} \sim 10^{-2}$ M. Examination of its effects by ultramicro assay showed that the glucosidase located at the tip of the intact chemosensory hair was much more resistant to nojirimycin than the α-glucosidase of PII-D type.

INTRODUCTION

From the results of behavioral studies by Dethier, Evans and Rhoades (1956)[1] and Evans (1961)[2], Evans (1963)[3] postulated that there were two types of receptor sites in a single sugar receptor cell of the blowfly, one being the glucose-binding site and the other the fructose-binding site. Morita and Shiraishi (1968)[4] studied the responses of single labellar sugar receptor cells of the fleshfly to wide ranges of concentrations of several sugars and to their mixtures. The responses to mixtures of 0.05 M glucose plus various concentrations of fructose could be regarded as the same of the responses to separately given stimuli, i.e., the responses to mixture of 0.05 M glucose and fructose were higher than those to plain fructose solutions roughly by the amplitude of response to 0.05 M glucose. Nevertheless, the responses to mixtures of 1 M glucose and various concentrations of fructose were the same as those to 1 M glucose. This means that there is a strong interaction between stimulations by glucose and by fructose. On the other hand, Shimada et al. (1974)[5] functionally separated two receptor sites in single labellar sugar receptor cells of the fleshfly by treatment with p-chloromercuribenzoate (pCMB). Since the response to fructose was not changed by the

treatment with 1 to 2 mM pCMB for 3 min while that to glucose was lost completely, it is natural to conclude that the binding sites for glucose and for
fructose are different entities.

An apparent contradiction between the above two results is resolved if
we assume an interaction in electrogenesis of the receptor potentials. Fig. 1
illustrates the situation as an electric circuit diagram of the receptor mem-

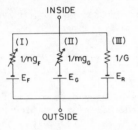

Fig. 1. Electric circuit diagram of the receptor membrane.

brane. Fructose and glucose may independently
open the ion gates (represented by channels I
and II, respectively) by binding with their own
receptor sites. When the conductances, ng_F and
mg_G, are both low, the amplitude of the receptor potential is roughly proportional to the
sum of ng_F and mg_G. When one of the conductances, e.g., mg_G, is sufficiently high, however,
contribution of ng_F to the receptor potential
will be negligible. If mg_G took a special value so that the membrane potential resulting from channels II and III was the same as E_F, the receptor membrane would be kept at this potential level at any values of ng_F. Thus, fructose and glucose can independently activate channels I and II, respectively,
but there will be a strong interaction between channels I and II.

It is unlikely, however, that glucose does not compete with fructose at
all for the fructose-binding site. The result shown by Fig. 2 suggests the

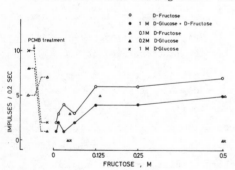

Fig. 2. Competition between glucose
and fructose after treatment with
pCMB[13].

existence of this competition between
glucose and fructose. After the tip of
the labellar chemosensory hair of the
fleshfly was treated with pCMB, the
sugar receptor within the chemosensory
hair did not respond to glucose stimulation, namely, responded neither to 0.2
M (filled triangles) nor to 1 M glucose
(crosses). Responses to 0.1 M fructose
(empty triangles) are seen approximately normal after the treatment. The re-
sponses to plain fructose solutions (empty circles) were always higher in
magnitude than those to the mixtures with 1 M glucose at the same concentration of fructose (filled circles). The simplest explanation of this result
may be to assume that glucose does not stimulate but compete with fructose
for the fructose-binding site to some extent.

Thus, there is no difficulty to assume that the single labellar sugar receptor cell of the blowfly and fleshfly contains two different binding sites for glucose and for fructose, though their differentiations for stimulants are not complete. The present paper shows our results recently obtained in looking for any strong inhibitors specific for glucose or fructose stimulation.

MATERIAL AND METHODS

Imagoes of 4 to 6 day-old of the fleshfly, Boettcherisca peregrina, were used. Impulses were recorded from the side-wall of the chemosensory hair of the labellum. All experiments were performed at temperatures $23 \pm 1°C$ and relative humidities 70 to 80%. Under these circumstances, the impulse frequency in the sugar receptor responding to mixtures of a sugar and an inhibitor could be regarded to be constant from 0.15 to 0.4 sec after the beginning of the stimulus. Therefore, we adopted the number of impulses during this period as the amplitude of response as usual[4].

Some of the chemicals used were synthesized in our laboratory. Among them, βMeMP, βMeMF, βEtGP, and βMe(3D)GP were not obtained as crystalline form but as syrup. The purity was checked by thin-layer chromatography and NMR spectroscopy. They showed that βMeMP and βMeMF were more than 80% pure and that βEtGP and βMe(3D)GP were chromatographically pure.

RESULTS AND DISCUSSION

Table I lists up the results of a survey of the inhibitory effects of several alkyl glycosides and related compounds on 0.1 M sucrose, 0.2 M glucose and 0.1 M fructose stimulations. The concentrations of the above three sugars were approximately mid point concentrations $(a_{V_\infty/2})$, which give rise to the half-maximum responses to the sugars, respectively. All these glycosides and related compounds inhibited the responses to the sugars of given concentrations almost to the same extent at relatively high concentrations.

The effects of some aryl glycosides were surveyed in the same way as above, and were found to be somewhat different among stimulations by different sugars.

Abbreviations βEtGP, ethyl β-D-glucopyranoside; βMe(3D)GP, methyl β-D-3-deoxy-glucopyranoside; 3OMeG, 3-O-methyl-D-glucose; αMeMP, methyl α-D-mannopyranoside; βMeMP, methyl β-D-mannopyranoside; αMeMF, methyl α-D-mannofuranoside; βMeMF, methyl β-D-mannofuranoside; styracitol, 1,5-anhydro-D-mannitol; mannitan, 1,4-anhydro-D-mannitol; βThioG·Na, β-thioglucose Na salt; βpNPGP, p-nitrophenyl β-D-glucopyranoside; βPGP, phenyl β-D-glucopyranoside; salicin, saligenin β-D-glucopyranoside; βpNPMP, p-nitrophenyl β-D-mannopyranoside; αpNPMP, p-nitrophenyl α-D-mannopyranoside; pNPOH, p-nitrophenol.

Table I. Inhibition of responses to sugars by alkyl glycosides and related compounds[6].

INHIBITOR	CONCENTRATION OF INHIBITOR, M	STIMULANT	CONCENTRATION OF STIMULANT, M	INHIBITION, %	NUMBER OF TESTS
βEtGP	0.5	SUCROSE	0.1	33.8 ± 13.2	
		GLUCOSE	0.2	35.5 ± 16.0	5
		FRUCTOSE	0.1	23.5 ± 20.9	
βMe(3D)GP	1.0	SUCROSE	0.1	66.5 ± 2.5	
		GLUCOSE	0.2	83.9 ± 15.6	5
		FRUCTOSE	0.1	79.3 ± 14.3	
30MeG	2.0	SUCROSE	0.1	18.3 ± 26.7	
		GLUCOSE	0.2	15.4 ± 15.2	10
		FRUCTOSE	0.1	27.0 ± 17.6	
αMeMP	1.0	SUCROSE	0.1	42.4 ± 19.2	
		GLUCOSE	0.2	53.6 ± 16.7	13
		FRUCTOSE	0.1	65.5 ± 18.4	
βMeMP	1.0	SUCROSE	0.1	2.8 ± 14.7	
		GLUCOSE	0.2	10.2 ± 25.6	7
		FRUCTOSE	0.1	8.7 ± 15.6	
αMeMF	1.0	SUCROSE	0.1	66.6 ± 6.8	
		GLUCOSE	0.2	58.6 ± 13.5	7
		FRUCTOSE	0.1	54.1 ± 11.7	
βMeMF	1.0	SUCROSE	0.1	52.7 ± 8.8	
		GLUCOSE	0.2	62.3 ± 13.5	5
		FRUCTOSE	0.1	51.9 ± 17.1	
STYRACITOL	2.0	SUCROSE	0.1	22.0 ± 13.3	
		GLUCOSE	0.2	24.5 ± 22.8	7
		FRUCTOSE	0.1	26.4 ± 13.9	
MANNITAN	2.0	SUCROSE	0.1	38.3 ± 17.8	
		GLUCOSE	0.2	30.0 ± 27.5	9
		FRUCTOSE	0.1	29.6 ± 23.6	
βThioG·Na (pH 7.1)	0.1	SUCROSE	0.1	2.9 ± 9.5	
		GLUCOSE	0.2	1.6 ± 11.5	16
		FRUCTOSE	0.1	2.8 ± 9.2	

Therefore, the effects were inspected a little bit more precisely on these compounds, i.e., we studied concentration effects of the inhibitors on the responses to sugars of fixed concentrations, and obtained the concentration of 50% inhibition (K_{50}^{I}), at which the response was reduced to 50%. The results were listed in Table II. Except for αpNPMP, K_{50}^{I} was almost the same for responses to the three sugars of given concentrations. Close examinations as to these inhibitors are illustrated by Figs. 3, 4 and 5. In these figures, the concentrations of sugars are normalized so that the mid point concentration ($a_{V_{\infty}/2}$) for each plain sugar is unity, and the amplitude of response is also normalized so that the maximal response to each plain sugar is unity;

Table II. Inhibition of responses to sugars by aryl glycosides and other compounds[6].

INHIBITOR	STIMULANT	CONCEN-TRATION OF STIMULANT, M	K^{I}_{50}, mM	NUMBER OF TESTS
βpNPGP	SUCROSE	0.1	12.2 ± 5.5	
	GLUCOSE	0.2	9.9 ± 5.2	7
	FRUCTOSE	0.1	12.7 ± 4.8	
βPGP	SUCROSE	0.1	18.8 ± 4.4	
	GLUCOSE	0.2	26.3 ± 4.0	5
	FRUCTOSE	0.1	24.7 ± 4.7	
SALICIN	SUCROSE	0.1	83.5 ± 28.9	
	GLUCOSE	0.2	97.3 ± 29.6	4
	FRUCTOSE	0.1	85.0 ± 37.0	
βpNPMP	SUCROSE	0.1	8.3 ± 1.1	
	GLUCOSE	0.2	6.4 ± 0.5	3
	FRUCTOSE	0.1	8.3 ± 0.8	
αpNPMP	SUCROSE	0.1	17.3 ± 6.2	
		0.2	16.7 ± 6.6	
	GLUCOSE	0.2	4.9 ± 2.7	6
		0.6	23.1 ± 11.5	
	FRUCTOSE	0.1	2.0 ± 0.5	
		0.4	3.6 ± 1.5	
QUNININE·HCl	SUCROSE	0.1	18.0 ± 1.4 ⎫	
	GLUCOSE	0.2	13.9 ± 5.1 ⎬ × 10^{-3}	6
	FRUCTOSE	0.1	15.3 ± 4.4 ⎭	
pNPOH	SUCROSE	0.1	7.8 ± 2.2	
	GLUCOSE	0.2	8.0 ± 2.6	3
	FRUCTOSE	0.1	6.8 ± 0.4	

empty circles and triangles represent the responses to plain sucrose and fructose solutions, respectively, and the same filled ones those to mixtures with an inhibitor. Fig. 3 shows that 10 mM αpNPMP shifted the response curve to the right, suggesting the competition between this inhibitor and sucrose or fructose. In contrast to this inhibitor, βpNPGP changed the shape of response curve especially for sucrose stimulation as shown by Fig. 4, i.e., it greatly increased the steepness in the response curve for sucrose stimula-

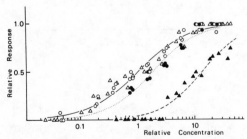

Fig. 3. Effect of 10 mM αpNPMP on responses to sucrose (circles) and to fructose (triangles). Responses to plain sugar is represented by empty symbols, and those to mixtures with αpNPMP by filles ones[6].

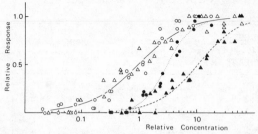

Fig. 4. Effects of 40 mM βpNPGP on responses to sucrose and to fructose. Symbols the same as in Fig. 3[6].

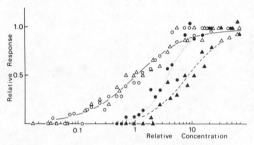

Fig. 5. Effects of 20 μM quinine·HCl on response. Symbols the same as in Fig. 3[6].

tion. Almost the same results were obtained with quinine hydrochloride, which is completely different in chemical structure from any sugars and their derivatives, as shown by Fig. 5. All results of these inhibitors show that the maximum response is the same, independently of existence of the inhibitors, for stimulation either by sucrose, by glucose or by fructose. Therefore, the characteristics of the response curve modified by the inhibitors are its steepness (measured by the Hill coefficient, n_H) and the mid point concentration ($a_{V\infty/2}$). Table III shows the results of such analyses. The last but one column represents the shift of the mid point concentration of the response-curve by the inhibitor. It has been known that quinine inhibits the response of the salt receptor as well as the sugar receptor. Such is the case for βpNPGP, as shown by Fig. 6, where filled and empty circles represent the

Table III. Effects of some inhibitors on characteristics in responses to sugars [6].

INHIB-ITOR	CONCEN-TRATION OF INHIBITOR	STIM-ULANT	$a_{V\infty/2}$	n_H	$\dfrac{a^I_{V\infty/2}}{a_{V\infty/2}}$	NUMBER OF TESTS
- - -	- - -	SUCROSE	0.089 ± 0.036	1.1 ± 0.2	- - -	27
		GLUCOSE	0.33 ± 0.08	1.6 ± 0.2	- - -	23
		FRUCTOSE	0.070 ± 0.031	0.9 ± 0.1	- - -	36
βpNPGP	40 mM	SUCROSE	0.40 ± 0.10	2.1 ± 0.3	4.5 ± 1.3	8
		GLUCOSE	1.01 ± 0.06	2.1 ± 0.3	3.0 ± 0.8	6
		FRUCTOSE	0.75 ± 0.14	1.2 ± 0.2	9.3 ± 1.6	15
QUININE·HCl	20 μM	SUCROSE	0.33 ± 0.09	2.2 ± 0.3	4.2 ± 0.7	8
		GLUCOSE	1.09 ± 0.29	2.6 ± 0.6	4.1 ± 0.9	6
		FRUCTOSE	0.61 ± 0.20	1.3 ± 0.1	9.1 ± 3.5	11
αpNPMP	10 mM	SUCROSE	0.20 ± 0.07	1.3 ± 0.1	2.3 ± 0.5	11
		GLUCOSE	0.86 ± 0.11	2.0 ± 0.2	2.5 ± 0.5	11
		FRUCTOSE	0.70 ± 0.18	1.2 ± 0.1	15.7 ± 6.9	10

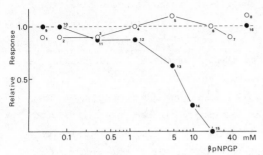

Fig. 6. Inhibition of the salt receptor response by βpNPGP. Responses numbered as 1, 8, 9 and 16 are the control[6].

responses of the salt and water receptors, respectively. Although the response of the water receptor was not affected, that of the salt receptor to 0.5 M NaCl was completely inhibited by βpNPGP at 20 mM. The similarity in action between quinine and βpNPGP suggests that βpNPGP might act on the sugar receptor membrane not as a glucoside toward the glucose-binding site, but as a hydrophobic reagent toward the lipid phase of the membrane. The effects of αpNPMP are similar to those of mannose which strongly competes with fructose but weakly with sucrose and glucose[4].

The last group of substances we tested are those which are known as specific inhibitors for glycosidase of different sources from blowfly or fleshfly.

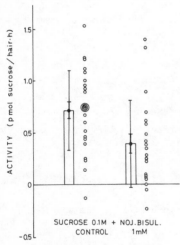

Fig. 7. Effects of nojirimicin bisulfite on glucosidase activity at the tip of the intact chemosensory hair. Long bar is standard deviation of measurements (δ), and short bar the standard deviation of means (δ/√n; n : number of measurements).

Among them nojirimycin is the strongest inhibitor for glucosidase, its working concentration being as low as $10^{-5} \sim 10^{-6}$ M[7,8]. The results of examination on the effects of nojirimycin* were unexpected. This substance was not effective at all immediately after it was dissolved, but it stimulated the sugar receptor at concentration above 0.2 M more than 1 hr after dissolution. Nojirimycin bisulfite* exhibited inhibition above 40 mM at neutral pH, though its inhibition was observed at 10^{-5} M for α-glucosidase of other sources. Nakashima et al.[9] in our laboratory worked on inhibitory effects of these substances on solubilized preparation of α-glucosidase of PII-D type in the blowfly, <u>Phormia regina</u>, which has been thought as the most probable candidate for the receptor molecule[10,11]. They found that the inhibition constants (K_i) of such substances for PII-D type of α-glucosidase were also in a range of $10^{-5} \sim 10^{-6}$ M.

* A kind gift from Dr. S. Inoue, Meiji Seika Co. Yokohama.

Kijima et al. are now studying the effects of nojirimycin bisulfite on α-glucosidase activity at the tip of the intact chemosensory hair of the blowfly. One of the results is shown by Fig. 7. The methods of ultramicro assay for glucosidase activity are described elesewhere[12]. Glucosidase activity (the control is shown by the column on the left side) was reduced to about 50% by 1 mM nojirimycin bisulfite (column on the right side). The values of measurements, which are shown by empty circles, are distributed over a wide range, and therefore it is difficult to conclude definitely. We can say, however, that the glucosidase at the tip of the intact hair is much more resistant to nojirimycin, compared with the solubilized preparation.

As to the problem of whether or not the α-glucosidase is the receptor molecule, the answer will be given by experiments of isolation of several good receptor mutants and those of reconstruction, which are now under progress in our laboratory and elsewhere.

*Present address: Department of Biological Science, Tohoku University, Kawauchi, Sendai 980, Japan

REFERENCES

1) Dethier, V. G., Evans, D. R. and Rhoades, M. V. (1956) Biol. Bull. 111, 204-224

2) Evans, D. R. (1961) Science 133, 327

3) Evans, D. R. (1963) Olfaction and Taste (Y. Zotterman, Ed.) pp.165-176, Machmillan Co. New York

4) Morita, H. and Shiraishi, A. (1968) J. Gen. Physiol. 52, 559-583

5) Shimada, I., Shiraishi, A., Kijima, H. and Morita, H. (1974) J. Insect Physiol. 20, 605-621

6) Enomoto, K. and Morita, H.   In preparation

7) Reese, E. T., Parrish, F. W. and Ettlinger, M. (1971) Carbohyd. Res. 18, 381-388

8) Lai, H. L. and Axelrod, B. (1973) Biochem. Biophys. Res. Commun. 54, 463-468

9) Nakashima, M. et al.   In preparation

10) Amakawa, T., Kijima, H. and Morita, H. (1975) J. Insect Physiol. 21, 1419-1425

11) Kijima, H., Amakawa, T., Nakashima, M. and Morita, H. (1977) J. Insect Physiol. 23, 469-479

12) Kijima, H., Koizumi, O. and Morita, H. (1973) J. Insect Physiol. 19, 1351-1362

13) Unpublished data obtained by I. Shimada

Specific aspects of chemoreception in bacteria

Gerald L. Hazelbauer

Wallenberg Laboratory, University of Uppsala, Box 562, S-751 22 Uppsala, Sweden

ABSTRACT

The chemoreceptors that mediate chemotaxis in enteric bacteria are discussed from the point of view of general questions that might be asked of any sensory receptor system. Three queries relate to the general problem of correlating in vivo sensitivity and in vitro affinity. Determination of sensitivity of an intact sensory system by affinity of receptor for ligand is documented for the maltose receptor of Escherichia coli. Reduction of sensitivity of a sensory system by a morphological barrier between receptor and environment is described for the maltose receptor. Chemotaxis toward glucose is discussed as an example of multiple receptors for a single attractant. Finally signal transduction is considered and the development of a new chemoreceptor, for arabinose, is described as a possible example of a mutationally induced interaction of a binding protein and a signal transducing component.

INTRODUCTION

The chemoreceptors that mediate chemotaxis in the enteric bacteria Escherichia coli and Salmonella typhimurium are the most extensively characterized and best understood sensory receptors. Most participants in this symposium are concerned with sensory systems that are less well understood at the biochemical level and, perhaps, more complex than bacterial chemoreceptors. It seems appropriate to use this opportunity to summarize information about bacterial chemoreceptors that provides direct answers to questions which could be asked about any sensory receptor. It would be a bit presumptuous to claim a wide generality for these specific examples. However I would venture to note that the recent dramatic expansion in information available about bacterial chemotaxis has increased rather than diminished the number of analogies with receptor systems in higher organisms. My own inclination is to think that basic mechanistic principles should be common to most chemoreceptors. That opinion is not uncommon among workers in the field [1,2].

After a very brief summary of bacterial motility and chemotaxis I will consider four aspects of chemoreception, three of which are related to the general problem of correlating in vivo sensitivity and in vitro affinity.

BACTERIAL MOTILITY AND CHEMOTAXIS

Enteric bacteria exhibit chemotaxis towards a number of sugars and amino acids[3,4]. Chemoreceptor mediated recognition of changes in the concentration of these compounds[5] results in a transitory alteration in the pattern of rotation of bacterial flagella [6,7]. These left-handed protein helicies power cell movement by rotating counterclockwise [8,9], forming a coordinated bundle of several flagella that pushes the cell forward[10]. Clockwise rotation results in opposing, uncoordinated forces pulling the cell, causing a "tumble"[11] which results in the reorientation of the bacterium in a new, randomly chosen direction[12]. In an isotropic environment, cells tumble about once a second[12], and the path of a swimming cell resembles a three-dimensional random walk[2,12]. Favorable changes in concentration of a chemotactically active compound (i.e. increase in attractant concentration or decrease in repellant) supress clockwise flagella rotation [6,7] and thus tumbles [12,13,14]. The time spent swimming in a favorable direction is increased relative to neutral or unfavorable directions, making the path in a gradient a "biased random walk" resulting in net migration along the gradient [2,12]. The bacteria respond to temporal as well as spatial gradients[13,16].

Over twenty-five different receptors have been identified in enteric bacteria. It appears that signals reporting percent occupancy of each receptor[7,5,17] are channeled to a common point where changes in occupancy are determined and summed algebraically[7,14,18], resulting in supression or induction of tumbles.

IS SENSITIVITY OF THE INTACT SENSORY SYSTEM DETERMINED BY AFFINITY OF RECEPTOR BINDING SITE FOR LIGAND ?

The chemoreceptors for galactose[19,20], ribose[21] and maltose[22,23] are available as pure proteins. In the case of all three receptors, binding of sugar to pure protein in vitro is exactly reflected in the chemotactic response of whole cells[20,21,24]. This relationship is illustrated in Fig.1, in which binding of maltose to pure receptor, the maltose-binding protein, is compared to chemotactic response of E. coli to maltose, as assayed by two separate techniques. The rotation assay records response of individual cells to temporal changes in concentration from zero to the value plotted on the abscissa. Such drastic temporal gradients result in complete supression of clockwise rotation of flagella, thus of tumbles[6,7]. Flagellar rotation is observed by using cells "tethered" to microscope slides by antibody attached specifically to a flagellum and nonspecifically to the glass[6,7,9]. In such a condition, it is the cell, rather than the flagellum that rotates, predominantly in a counterclockwise

direction interspersed with reversals to clockwise rotation. Maximum response
to a temporal gradient of maltose is approximately 350 seconds.

The capillary assay records response of a population of bacteria to a
spatial gradient formed as attractant diffuses from the mouth of a microcapill-
ary into a suspension of free-swimming cells[25]. In Fig. 1, number of cells mi-
grating up the gradient into the capillary is plotted versus concentration
around the capillary mouth, as determined by Adler's extrapolation[25] of an
equation describing the gradient[26]. That concentration, 1/100 of the initial
level in the capillary, is probably a reasonable approximation of the stimulus
to which cells are exposed. Metabolic destruction of the attractant gradient
is probably not important in these experimental conditions, since drastic reduction in bacterial concentration does not shift the response curve[23].

CAN SENSITIVITY OF THE INTACT SENSORY SYSTEM BE MODIFIED BY A MORPHOLOGICAL
BARRIER BETWEEN THE SURROUNDING ENVIRONMENT AND RECEPTOR?

Chemoreceptor organs of many organisms are anatomically complex, and
access of ligand to receptor sites may be limited. In such situations, it is
not unreasonable to be concerned that concentration of ligand at the receptor
site is not identical to concentration in the surrounding environment. Thus
dose-response relationships determined for a whole organism or an intact sensory organ may not correspond to the actual binding affinity of receptor for
ligand. This discrepancy is particularly serious if an apparent affinity

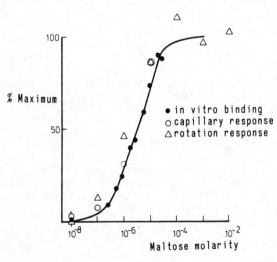

Fig.1: Interaction of pure receptor and ligand compared to
chemotactic response of intact
organisms. Cells of strain pop
1048 were grown and assayed
for response as described in
the text and previously[23]. Maltose-binding protein was purified[22] from the same strain
and binding to maltose determined by equilibrium dialysis[23] at 25° with a total binding site concentration of 7.4
μM. Response in the capillary
assay is expressed as percent
of an extrapolated maximum of
$3.8 \cdot 10^4$ cells accumulated
above background and is plotted versus maltose concentration around the capillary
mouth (see text). Rotation response is expressed as percent
of an averaged maximum response
of 350 s at 25°.

constant as estimated from in vivo and in situ studies is one of the few criteria available for identification of putative isolated or solubilized receptors.

The study of taxis of E.coli toward the disaccharide maltose provides an example of the effect of an accessibility barrier on sensitivity of the organism to a chemoattractant. As illustrated in Fig. 1, the behavioral response of normal E.coli K12 to maltose corresponds very closely to the binding of that sugar to pure receptor protein. Yet even in these cells the cytoplasmic membrane and its associated chemoreceptors are separated from direct contact with the environment by an outer membrane. This structure is in some ways analogous to outer membrane of a mitochondrion or to nuclear membrane in that it limits passage of large molecules, but allows passage of small ones[27]. It is probable that small molecules traverse outer membrane by diffusion through protein-lined pores[27,28]. Maltose and related higher polymers (malto-triose etc.) require the presence of a specific outer membrane protein, of about 45,000 molecular weight, for optimal passage into the cell[29,30,31]. Mutant strains missing the protein are easy to obtain, since bacteriophage lambda infects E.coli by attaching to this protein[32]. Maltose enters these mutant cells only when it is present at high concentrations, presumably utilizing another pore, less specific for its size and shape. Maltose-binding protein purified from a mutant strain exhibits the same affinity for maltose as protein from normal cells[30,31], yet the apparent affinity of the maltose chemoreceptor in mutant cells, as deduced from the response of whole cells, if fifty-fold weaker than normal (Fig. 2 and ref. 30). For cells lacking the specific outer membrane protein, the behavioral response to maltose does not correspond to

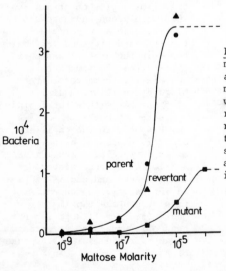

Fig.2: Response in the capillary assay to maltose by wild-type E. coli pop 1048 (o) a "barrier-defective" strain carrying mutation lamB 204 (■) and a strain in which the mutation has reverted lamB 204 r2 (▲). Data is adapted from Fig. 2 of reference 30 plotted as described in the text. Reduced accumulations obtained at sugar concentrations above saturation are not shown, but instead saturation is indicated as a dashed line.

binding of sugar to its isolated, pure receptor protein. The outer membrane
protein is again produced by cells in which the mutation has reverted back to
normal, and these bacteria respond normally to maltose (Fig. 2 and ref. 30).

CAN A COMPOUND BE RECOGNIZED BY MORE THAN ONE RECEPTOR ?

A cell or an organism might contain multiple receptors for a single chemical. The sensitivity to that compound would be determined by a combination
of the individual receptors, and it might be expected that no isolated, individual receptor would exhibit the same properties as the intact system. For
most chemoattractants of E.coli, including those discussed above, the relationship is "one attractant - one receptor". The best documented exception is
glucose. That sugar is recognized by three independent receptors, one which
binds primarily glucose[33], one which binds glucose and galactose[20], and one
which binds mannose and glucose[33]. The unambiguous description of this multi-
receptor situation required characterization of independent mutant strains
defective in a single receptor as well as strains carrying combinations of mutations[3,33].

Fig. 3 shows glucose response of strains possessing various combinations of
the three glucose receptors. Elimination of the high affinity glucose-galactose receptor results in a distinct reduction in sensitivity toward glucose,
but further reduction occurs only when all three receptors are lacking and
response to glucose is eliminated.

The pattern of responses of mutant strains is paralleled in patterns of

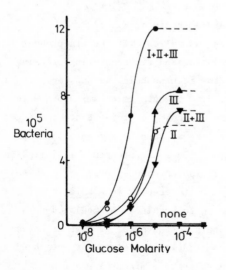

Fig.3: Response in the capillary
assay to glucose by E.coli strains
carrying various combinations of
receptors that recognize glucose.The
glucose-galactose receptor is designated as I, the mannose-glucose as II,
and the glucose as III. The data is
adapted from references 3 and 33,
plotted as described for Fig. 2. The
larger accumulations are the result
of higher cell densities used[25].

inhibition among the ligands of the three glucose receptors. Glucose completely inhibits response to galactose, but galactose only partially inhibits response to glucose[3]. Mannose only marginally inhibits glucose response of wild type cells and significantly inhibits response of mutants missing glucose-galactose receptor, while glucose completely eliminates response to mannose[3]. Galactose and mannose do not inhibit each other[3].

HOW ARE SIGNALS TRANSDUCED FROM RECEPTOR TO EFFECTOR ?

The answer is not yet apparent for bacterial chemoreceptors, but an emerging principle appears to be focusing of tactic signals into pathways shared by more than one receptor[24,34]. The best documented case of a pathway shared by signals from two independent receptors is the galactose and ribose receptor pair. These two sugars are recognized by different receptors[3]. Binding studies with pure proteins demonstrate that galactose-binding protein does not bind ribose, nor does ribose-binding protein bind galactose[35]. Yet high, isotropic concentrations of ribose partially inhibit response to galactose[3], and when cells contain a ten-fold excess of ribose receptor over galactose receptor, saturating levels of ribose eliminate sensitivity to a gradient of galactose[35]. The inhibition disappears in the absence of ribose receptor[35]. The phenotype conferred by a mutation called trg suggests a simple model for this inhibition [35,36]. These mutations affect taxis towards both ribose and galactose, but are not located in the structural genes of either receptor for those sugars[36]. It may be that both ribose-binding and galactose-binding proteins interact with the product of the trg gene, and in that interaction send chemotactic signals to the flagellar motor.

These ideas led me to attempt to obtain a strain of E.coli that had developed a new chemoreceptor. The logic was as follows. If the trg product interacts physically with both galactose-binding and ribose-binding proteins[35], then the product must have a binding site for each protein, perhaps one site that recognized a domain on each receptor. E.coli contains a family of peripherial membrane proteins, termed periplasmic binding proteins that bind specific sugars and amino acids[37]. All of them are apparently recognition components for specific active transport systems[38]. Only the proteins binding galactose, maltose and ribose, respectively, are also chemoreceptors[3,20]. Arabinose-binding protein[39,40] does not function as a chemoreceptor in E.coli.

The bacteria exhibit a marginal response to arabinose[41], mediated by a very weak binding of galactose-binding protein to the sugar[20]. However galactose-binding and arabinose-binding proteins are closely related as evidenced by shared antigenic determinants[42]. Thus a relatively minor alteration in

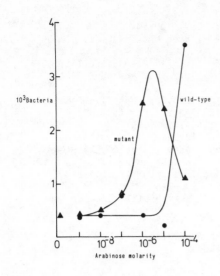

Fig.4: Response in the capillary assay to arabinose by wild-type E.coli, pop 1048 (o) and a mutant (▲) that has acquired increased sensitivity to arabinose. Both strains produce arabinose-binding protein constitutively (araC) and were grown with glycerol as the carbon source, and assayed as described previously[23]. The data is plotted as described in the text. Reduced accumulations obtained at sugar concentrations above saturation are included.

arabinose-binding protein, or in trg product might allow arabinose protein to fit into the trg protein site usually reserved for galactose protein. If these assumptions are valid, then a mutant strain with such an alteration would exhibit new, improved taxis towards arabinose.

Mutagenesis and imposition of a strong selection pressure for ability to swim up a gradient of arabinose, have allowed isolation of mutant strains that have increased chemotactic sensitivity towards arabinose (Fig. 4). Preliminary evidence indicates that the new sensitivity is mediated by arabinose-binding protein. Further characterization of these mutants may well provide new information about the mechanism of signal transduction.

ACKNOWLEDGEMENTS

Unpublished work described here was supported by USPHS Grant AI 12858 and grants from the Swedish Natural Sciences Research Council. I thank Birgitta Berneholm for technical assistance.

REFERENCES

1. Adler,J. (1975) Ann.Rev.Biochem. 44, 341-356
2. Koshland,D.E., Jr. (1974) FEBS Letters 40 (suppl), S3-S9
3. Adler,J., Hazelbauer,G.L., and Dahl,M.M. (1973) J. Bacteriol. 115,824-847
4. Mesibov,R. and Adler,J. (1972) J. Bacteriol. 112, 315-326
5. Adler,J. (1969) Science 166, 1588-1597
6. Larsen,S.H., Reader,R.W., Kort,E.M., Tso,W.-W. and Adler,J. (1974) Nature 249, 74-77
7. Berg,H.C. and Tedesco,P.M. (1975) Proc.Nat.Acad.Sci. USA 72, 3235-3239
8. Berg,H.C. and Anderson,R.A. (1973) Nature 245, 380-382
9. Silverman,M. and Simon,M. (1974) Nature 249, 73-74
10. Macnab,R.M. (1977) Proc.Nat.Acad.Sci. USA 74, 221-225

11. Macnab,R.M. and Ornstein,M.K. (1977) J.Mol.Biol. 112, 1-30
12. Berg,H.C., and Brown,D.A. (1972) Nature 239, 500-504
13. Macnab,R.M. and Koshland,D.E., J., (1972) Proc.Nat.Acad.Sci. USA 69, 2509-2512
14. Tsang,N., Macnab,R.M. and Koshland,D.E., Jr, (1973) Science 181, 60-63
15. Spudich,J.L. and Koshland,D.E.,Jr. (1975) Proc.Nat.Acad.Sci. USA 72,710-713
16. Brown,D.A. and Berg,H.C. (1974) Proc.Nat.Acad.Sci. USA 71, 1388-1392
17. Mesibov,R., Ordal,G.W. and Adler,J. (1973) J.Gen.Physiol. 62,203-223
18. Adler,J. and Tso,W.-W. (1974) Science 184, 1292-1294
19. Anraku,Y. (1968) J.Biol.Chem. 243, 3116-3122
20. Hazelbauer,G.L. and Adler,J. (1971) Nature New Biol. 230, 101-104
21. Aksamit,R.R. and Koshland,D.E.,Jr. (1974) Biochemistry 13, 4473-4478
22. Kellerman,O. and Szmelcman,S. (1974) Eur.J.Biochem. 47, 139-149
23. Hazelbauer,G.L. (1975) J.Bacteriol. 122, 206-214
24. Hazelbauer,G.L. and Parkinson,J.S. (1977) Microbiolial Interactions, Reissig,J., ed. Chapman & Hall. In press.
25. Adler,J. (1973) J.Gen.Microbiol. 74, 77-91
26. Futurelle,R.P. and Berg,H.C. (1972) Nature 239,517-518
27. Nakae,T. and Nikaido,H. (1975) J.Biol.Chem. 250, 7359-7366
28. Nakae,T. (1975) Biochem.Biophys.Res.Commun. 64, 1224-1230
29. Szmelcman,S. and Hofnung,M. (1975) J.Bacteriol. 124, 112-118
30. Hazelbauer,G.L. (1975) J. Bacteriol. 124, 119-126
31. Szmelcman,S., Schwartz,M., Silhavy,T.J., and Boos,W. (1976) Eur.J.Biochem. 65, 13-19
32. Randall-Hazelbauer,L.L. and Schwartz,M. (1973) J.Bacteriol. 116, 1436-1466
33. Adler,J. and Epstein,W. (1974) Proc.Nat.Acad.Sci. USA 71, 2895-2899
34. Parkinson,J.S. (1977) Ann.Rev.Genetics. In press.
35. Strange,P.G. and Koshland,D.E.,Jr. (1976) Proc.Nat.Acad.Sci. 73, 762-766
36. Ordal,G.W. and Adler,J. (1974) J. Bacteriol.117, 517-526
37. Rosen,B.P. and Heppel,L.A. (1973) Bacterial Membranes and Walls. Levie,L., Ed. pp. 209-239, Marcel Dekker, New York
38. Boos,W. (1974) Ann.Rev.Biochem. 43, 123-246
39. Hogg, R.W. and Englesberg,E. (1969) J. Bacteriol. 100, 423-432
40. Schleif,R. (1969) J.Mol.Biol. 46, 185-196
41. Hazelbauer,G.L., Mesibov,R.E. and Adler,J. (1969). Proc.Nat.Acad.Sci. USA 64, 1300-1307
42. Parsons,R.G. and Hogg,R.W. (1974) J.Biol.Chem. 249, 3608-3614

Abstracts of Poster Presentations

Structure and taste of amino acids and related compounds Hans-Dieter Belitz,
Herbert Wieser and Rudolf Treleano (Institut für Lebensmittelchemie der TU
and Deutsche Forschungsanstalt für Lebensmittelchemie, 8000 München, GFR)

The sweet and bitter thresholds of amino acids and of some related compounds
were determined. The occurence of sweet taste depends on amino and carboxyl
groups, the occurence of bitter taste depends only on the amino group,which
can be substituted. Sweet taste decreases strongly on transition from α-
amino acids to ß-amino acids; γ-amino acids are not sweet. N-Acylation or
esterification abolish the sweet taste, but increase the bitter taste.
The length, shape and polarity of the side chain R are important both for
the quality and for the intensity of taste. Up to R = C_2H_5 L- and D-amino
acids are sweet. R > C_2H_5 causes bitter taste of increasing intensity in
the L-series and increasing sweet taste in the D-series. The influence of
shape is seen from the threshold values (mM/1) of isomeric compounds, e.g.
D-nor leucin (5-8), D-leucine (2-5), D-isoleucine (8-12) and tert-leucine
(tasteless). Very bulky side chains seem to abolish any taste sensation.
The influence of polar substituents in the side chain is strongly dependent
upon their nature and position. Cyclic compounds are especially useful tools
for the elucidation of steric requirements for taste. Taste quality and
intensity of 1-aza-cycloalkane-2-carboxylic acids and 1-amino-cycloalkane-
1-carboxylic acids are dependent on size (n) and substitution of the rings.
The threshold values of the latter compounds pass through a minimum at n=
6 for sweet and at n=8 for bitter taste. All together in the series of
amino acids and related compounds sweet taste requires electrophilic and
nucleophilic and hydrophobic groups, while bitter taste requires only
electrophilic and hydrophobic groups. Superposition of the structures
of some compounds tested, shows the positions allowed and forbidden for
sweet taste and may give an idea of the shape of the sweet receptor.

Electron spin resonance spin label studies of the mouse olfactory epithelium, and a cooperative model for olfactory transduction

A.D. Clark, L.J. Dunne, S.J. Wyard, & L.H. Bannister (Divison of Biological Sciences, Guy's Hospital Medical School, London Bridge S.E.1. England)

The intermolecular interactions of odorous molecules with mouse olfactory epithelium have been investigated using electron spin resonance spectroscopy (ESR). A series of nitroxide spin labels, chosen to provide a variety of odours, were synthesized and solutions of these were introduced into the nasal chamber of the mouse. The olfactory tissue was removed and the motional constraint of the spin label in the epithelium measured by ESR spectroscopy. A direct correlation was found between the olfactory potency of a compound and its degree of motional constraint which reflects the inter-molecular interactions associated with olfaction. However, comparisons made with other membranes used as control tissue do not reveal any special feature of the ol-factory epithelium. The fluidity of the olfactory membrane was also investigated us-ing a series of non-odorous lipid spin labels and from some of these spectra order parameters was calculated. The olfactory membrane is shown to have a highly fluid centre and compact outer surface. A model for olfactory transduction was also in-troduced. It is based upon a cooperative transition between two conformational states of a receptor protein, and it applies the equations of Changeux et al[1], to the olfactory system. This theory has been modified to consider the partitioning of an odour bet-ween the olfactory mucus, and the membrane. The model supports our interpretation of our experimental electron spin resonance spin label results[2]. By numerical solu-tion we show the predicted response of the system, as a function of odour dose. Graphs to show the effect of (1) the partition coefficient between membranes and mucus, (2) the strength of the cooperative coupling and (3) the difference in the strength of odour binding to the two protein conformation states, were presented.

1. Changeux, J.P., Thiery, J., Tung, Y., Kittel, C. (1967)
    Proc. Nat. Acad. Sci. USA 57 335-341
2. Bannister L.H., Clark, A.D., Dunne, L.J. & Wyard, S.J. (1975)
    Nature 256 517-8

Molecular aspects of sweet taste Guy A. Crosby, Grant E. DuBois and
Robert E. Wingard, Jr. (Chemical Synthesis Laboratories, Dynapol
1454 Page Mill Rd., Palo Alto, California, 94304, U.S.A.)

A number of new nonglycosidic dihydrochalcones (DHC's) have been
prepared and many found to be intensely sweet (1,2). However, all
DHC's reported thus far display some degree of delayed taste onset
and lingering aftertaste. Several of the simple sulfoalkyl analogs
discussed here, such as I, appear to have the most desirable taste-
timing qualities of all reported dihydrochalcone sweeteners (2).
Both the hydrophobic nature and phenolic character of the DHC's
are believed to be a major cause of the undesirable temporal qualities
characteristic of these sweeteners. A model of the DHC molecule ,
containing two hydrogen donor-acceptor units within a "bent" conformation, has been proposed as the most plausible counterpart for
the sweet taste receptor (2). The lingering aftertaste may also be
explained, in part, with this model (3).

$$KO_3S(CH_2)_nO$$

I

References:

1. DuBois, G. E., Crosby, G. A. and Saffron, P. (1977) Science, 195:397.
2. DuBois, G. E., Crosby, G. A., Stephenson, R. A. and Wingard, R. E.
   (1977) J. Agric. Food Chem. 25 in press.
3. Crosby, G. A., DuBois, G. E. and Wingard, R. E. (1977) In: S.
   Held (ed), Flavor: Its Chemical, Behavioral, and Commercial
   Aspects, Westview Press, Boston.

A model for transduction in gustatory receptors J.A. DeSimone,
J.D. Bond and S. Price, (Department of Physiology, Medical College of
Virginia, Virginia Commonwealth University, Richmond, Virginia 23298,
U.S.A.)

Substances capable of eliciting gustatory responses are in most
instances impermeable to cell membranes and are often nonionic. This
suggests that depolarization of taste cells occurs by an indirect
mechanism. The speed with which the afferent nerves respond to a
sapid substance on the tongue argues further against a mechanism
involving cation diffusion from receptor sites of microvilli to the
basal regions of the cells. This suggests that transformation of the
chemical stimulus to electrical events below the tight junction involves traveling waves of activity along the cell membranes. The
current view of cell membranes stresses their fluidity. Thus, pressure
waves should be able to be propagated in the fluid phospholipid phase.
Lipids spread at oil/water interfaces respond to changes in salt and
acid concentrations with proportional changes in surface pressure.
Surface pressure responses of mixed phosphatidic acid-lecithin films
to changes in salt concentration suggest that water taste may be a
response to changes in local pH. Accordingly, we propose the following
transduction mechanism: (1) nonionic sapid substances interact with
bound receptors in the microvilli, ionic substances interact directly
with membrane phospholipids; (2) local changes in the membrane induce
surface pressure changes which propagate to below the tight junctions;
(3) this results in a change in the density of charged sites, thus, in
a change in surface potential; (4) the altered surface potential alters
the ion permeability; 5) ion exchange results in depolarization or
hyperpolarization of the receptor cell. This model can account for
responses to each taste modality, including water taste.

The Allosteric-Membrane-Enzyme Hypothesis for Coding and Transduction in the Primary Olfactory Neurones G.H.Dodd, A.Menevse and T.M.Poynder, (Department of Molecular Sciences, University of Warwick, Coventry, U.K.)

INTRODUCTION   The hypothesis presented here is based on biochemical studies of olfactory mechanisms. It suggests that the initial events in olfaction do not require esoteric physical mechanisms of the kind postulated in several olfactory hypotheses. As we have previously suggested, olfaction can be viewed as belonging to one of the possible classes of ligand-membrane interactions.

HYPOTHESIS   We imagine that odorants act as regulatory ligands of a receptor enzyme system in the plasma membrane of the olfactory neurones. The catalytic subunits of the enzyme are probably intrinsic membrane proteins located on the inner surface of the plasma membrane. The regulatory subunits, located on the outer surface of the membrane, may be linked to the catalytic moiety of the enzyme either through protein-protein interactions or through protein-phospholipid interactions. The latter type of interaction, in conjunction with the liquid crystalline properties of the phospholipids, might enable one catalytic subunit to share several types of regulatory subunits. The catalytic subunits of the enzyme would provide amplification in the transduction step, whilst the regulatory subunits would provide specific binding sites which would form the basis of the coding in the primary neurones. Some odorants may activate the membrane enzymes through binding to the phospholipid region of the membrane. The proteins involved in the generation of receptor potentials are probably common to all neurones, including the primary olfactory cells.

EXPERIMENTAL EVIDENCE   The evidence from three types of experiments support the hypothesis. Enzyme studies have identified adenylate cyclase as a possible candidate enzyme. The enzyme occurs in olfactory mucosa and is involved in the generation of the EOG. Chemical modification studies provide evidence for the occurrence of olfactory receptor proteins with defined specificities. Binding studies on fraction obtained from olfactory mucosa confirm the presence of receptor proteins.

This work was supported by the Medical Research Council , U.K.

<u>Experimental evidence for several receptor sites involved in</u>
<u>sweet taste chemoreception</u> A. Faurion, S. Saito, P. Mac Leod,
(Laboratoire de Neurobiologie Sensorielle, EPHE, CNRS, (ERA 623).
CEN/FAR, BP n° 6, 92260 Fontenay-aux-Roses.)

In order to test the hypothesis that sweet taste in mediated by
more than one type of receptor site, we have measured intensity
functions of 12 sweet tasting chemicals for 9 subjects.
Subjects were 4 males and 5 females from 20 to 30 years old.
Stimuli were Aspartame, Chloroform, Cyclamate, Dulcin, Fructose,
Glucose, Leucine, Monellin, Saccharin, Stevioside, Thaumatin and
Sucrose. The reference scale for intensity matching was a series
of 7 sucrose solutions from 8g/l to 134g/l in a geometric progression of x1.6 steps. A similar series of 7 solutions with the same
ratio was prepared for each stimulus : concentrations were adjusted so that all Nr.4 solutions were judged equally sweet in a
preliminary paired comparison test. Stimuli were presented in
random order and subjects were asked to match the perceived
sweetness intensity against the sucrose scale.
A linear regression slope was calculated from about 90 responses
for each subject to each sweetener. The resulting matrix of 9 x
12 slopes was reduced through factor analysis and 4 independent
factors were then extracted, accounting for 94 % of the total
variance. Pearson's r coefficient confirms the factor analysis
display of 4 groups of covariant stimuli i.e. :

1   Aspartame, Monellin, Cyclamate, Sucrose, Saccharin, Dulcin,
    Fructose, Glucose.

2   Chloroform.

3   Thaumatin, Stevioside.

4   Leucine.

Blocking of Heliothis virescens sex pheromone reception by protein specific
reagents James L. Frazier and James R. Heitz, (Departments of Entomology
and Biochemistry, Mississippi Agricultural and Forestry Experiment Station,
and Mississippi State University, Mississippi State, Mississippi 39762
U.S.A.)

A combined behavioral and electrophysiological study was undertaken to
compare the blocking effect of several protein specific reagents on sex
pheromone reception. Treatment of male antennae for 10 minutes with 2.5 x
10^{-5}M. inhibitors in sodium phosphate buffer (pH 7.4) resulted in blockage
of both the EAG and of pheromone activated behavior. Reagents binding
with sulfhydryl, hydroxyl, amino, and indole, groups exhibit varying
amounts of blockage. Behavioral blockage at 24 hrs. posttreatment was
independent of pheromone habituation and resulted from a combination of
buffer and inhibitor effects. Behavioral blockage from the sulfhydryl
inhibitor, FMA, could be reversed with cysteine. Attempts at site-
specific protection from FMA by sex pheromone pretreatment yielded
questionable results.

Electroolfactograms in normal and specifically anosmic mice   Stephen J.
Goldberg and Steven Price, (Depts. of Anatomy and Physiology, Med. Col.
of Va.-VCU, Richmond, VA. 23298, USA)

Olfactory receptor potentials corresponding to the electroolfactogram
(EOG) were recorded in normal and specifically anosmic male mice in order
to develop electrophysiological criteria for differentiating the normal
from the anosmic mice. Hundreds of mice were individually screened by
training them to escape a shock associated with the delivery of four
odorants (benzaldehyde, salicylaldehyde, geraniol, menthol). Some animals
exhibited specific anosmias by their inability to escape the shock in the
presence of one (sometimes two) of the odors, but could escape when the
other odors were individually presented. We have isolated strains of mice
which show these genetic specific anosmias.

An air-dilution olfactometer was used to deliver 1 second blocks of
odor, at known concentrations, to the animals nose. A tracheal tube for
respiration and another tube ascending to the posterior naris were inserted
under pentobarbital anesthesia. Controlled suction could be applied to
the ascending tube to produce an artifical sniff during odor presentations.
The olfactory bulbs were removed and a potassium citrate (1.6M) filled
pipette was inserted in a canal of the cribriform plate to record the EOG.

Our preliminary results indicated that recordings made from dorso-
medial areas of the cribriform plate show EOGs of equivalent amplitude
(0.5-1.0 mV) and duration (1 sec.) to all four odorants when presented in
equivalent concentrations. Results from the anosmic mice have tentatively
shown that the EOG amplitude is reduced to all four odorants when compared
to the response in normal mice and that the odorant to which the animal is
behaviorally anosmic shows the greatest response reduction.

It appears likely that at least some component of the genetic specific
anosmia is due to a defect at the receptor level.

This work was supported by grants PHS DE-04271 and NSF BNS76-02153.

Preliminary data suggesting alteration of odorant molecules by interaction
with receptors David E. Hornung, (Biology Department, St. Lawrence University,
Canton, New York 13617) and Maxwell M. Mozell, (Physiology Department,
Upstate Medical Center, Syracuse, New York 13210)

To provide insight into the olfactory receptor-odorant molecule interaction,
radioisotope techniques using a flow dilution olfactometer provided a
tritiated odorant stimulus controlled for flow rate, volume, and partial
pressure. This stimulus was presented to the intact olfactory sac of the
bullfrog through a cannula placed in the external naris. Labelled molecules
leaving the olfactory sac were collected in a trap placed at the end of an
internal naris cannula. Following a tritiated odorant presentation, non-
radioactive room air was drawn through the sac at a rate of 16 ml/min. The
trap containing a total of 20 ml, half being benzene and half being distilled
water, was changed every 10 seconds for 2 minutes following stimulation.
The radioactivity of each of these trap phases was determined by liquid
scintillation counting techniques. When, in three controls, the frog was
bypassed by connecting the internal and external naris cannulas, less than
0.02% of the tritiated octane was recovered from the water fraction of the
trap. However, when the octane was presented into the olfactory sac, the
absolute amount of the radioactivity recovered from the water fraction
increased about 15 fold (replicated in three animals). Furthermore, if prior
to octane presentation the olfactory sac were treated with N-ethylmaleimide,
a blocker of receptor activity (Getchell, M. and R. Gesteland, Proc. Nat.
Acad. Sci. 69:1494, 1972), the water soluble fraction was reduced to that of
the control (also replicated in three animals). Can it be, then, that in
the interaction between the olfactory molecule and the olfactory receptor the
molecule is somehow transformed?

<u>Sweet and bitter taste of some monosaccharides</u>* W. Jakinovich, Jr.,
(Procter and Gamble Company, Miami Valley Laboratories, Cincinnati, Ohio,
U.S.A.)

The relationship between sweet and bitter taste and molecular structure
was examined in a group of monosaccharides (solutions were tasted). I
found that methyl α-D-glucopyranoside was not just sweet as previously
believed. When the intense sweetness of this compound was reduced by the
sweet taste inhibitor, gymnemic acid, bitterness was observed. Compounds
with structures similar to that of the methyl sugar as α-D-glucopyranose
and β-D-glucopyranose that lack the methyl group are not bitter even
after gymnemic acid treatment. Furthermore, the importance of the C-2
hydroxyl was demonstrated when I compared the taste of methyl α-D-
mannopyranoside with the taste of methyl α-D-glucopyranoside. The
compound methyl α-D-glucopyranoside has an equatorial C-2 hydroxyl. In
the tests it was very sweet and weakly bitter. The compound methyl α-D-
mannopyranoside has an axial C-2 hydroxyl. It was weakly sweet and
strongly bitter. Methyl β-D-mannopyranoside, which possesses both the
equatorial methyl substituent at C-1 and the axial hydroxyl, was extremely
bitter and devoid of sweetness. That bitterness in these <u>manno-</u> compounds
resulted from the axial hydroxyl at C-2, was clearly demonstrated when I
compared the tastes of compounds which lack the C-1 -OCH$_3$ group, such as
1,5-<u>anhydro</u>-D-mannitol, which has an axial hydroxyl at C-2 and was sweet
and bitter, and 1,5-<u>anhydro</u>-D-glucitol, which has an equatorial hydroxyl
at C-2 and was sweet and not bitter. Therefore, bitterness of these
compounds resulted from (1) a methoxy at C-1, (2) orientation of the C-1
methoxy, and (3) the presence of an axial hydroxyl at C-2.

*Work done at the Department of Zoology, The University of Michigan,
 Ann Arbor, U.S.A.

Model acceptor simulates receptor cell specifity Wolf. A. Kafka,
(Max·Planck-Institut für Verhaltensphysiologie, D 8131 Seewiesen)

Steric and electronic properties of stimulant molecules are related to electrophysiological data which reflect the specificity
of acceptor interaction and activation in single olfactory receptor cells of insects. It can be concluded that consecutive
testing of different submolecular features during the transduction processes   cannot account for the observed specificity of
cell response; rather, at least once, an overall recognition of
the stimulant molecule must have occurred. This process can be
simulated by a physico-mathematical model of "cooperative multiposition interaction". The hypothetical acceptor which deter -
mines the chemical specificity of a given type of receptor cell
is defined by number, geometrical arrangement, polarisabilities,
dipole moments, and steric access-abilities of binding positions.
Although the transferred energies are in the range of thermal
fluctuations (10^{-23}kcal/molecule), the selective binding to, and
the activation of the model acceptor is achieved when the energy
of interaction is appropriately distributed amongst 3 to 5 interaction positions;   models of 3 or 5 positions however did not
count for the known discriminating capacities of the sensory
cells. The magnitude of binding and/or activation energy can be
reflected by the time course of bioelectrical events during receptor cell excitation. The model acceptor can be gradually modified to accommodate stepwise changes in cell specificity as can
be observed in comparative studies in insects: (i) By differently
arranging electronically equivalent acceptor positions, specificities can be generated resembling the responses of receptors for
different homologous   key compounds; (ii) Specificity differences
between receptors for the same key compound are simulated by keeping constant geometrical arrangement of the interacting positions whilst changing the electronic properties for at least 1 of
them. However, the mathematical model does not yet indicate whether this change reflects an alteration in the electronic setup
of the actual acceptor, or merely one in the steric access to the
interaction positions. Recent electrophysiological results support the latter.

Possible role of "functional units" involved in conformers of odorants

T. Kikuchi, (Department of Biological Science, Tohoku University, Kawauchi, Sendai 980, Japan)

In the past few years some development have been seen in the structure activity relationships in insect pheromones, applying an idea of "functional unit" which indicates the odor perception is produced by a pair of functional groups occupying a particular interval. However, to estimate probabilities of "functional unit" formation with the use of chemical model, severe difficulties will be encountered. The problems include the extremely laborious work to build up conformers and complex procedures to eliminate conformers in which interatomic repulsions are involved. But the problems are now largely solved by the use of a computer program. For the specificities of 18 sweaty odors for iso-valeric acid anosmia (Amoore et al., 1968) and those of 14 malty odors for iso-butyraldehyde anosmia (Amoore et al., 1976), I now present demonstrations that the specificities for iso-valeric acid anosmia might be produced by a "proton acceptor-methyl unit" with an average interval of about 5 Å (r = 0.97) and that those for iso-butyraldehyde anosmia is produced by two "proton acceptor-methyl units" with average intervals of about 4 and 7 Å, respectively, being modified by steric hindrance between odor molecules and receptor sites (r = 0.90).

Kikuchi, T. and Fukazawa, Y. Molecular features of sweaty odors specific to iso-valeric acid anosmia: A conformational analysis by digital computer. Proc. Nat. Acad. Sci. (submitted).
Kikuchi, T. and Fukazawa, Y. Correlation of specificities in iso-butyraldehyde anosmia with molecular characteristics involved in conformers of aliphatic aldehydes and related compounds. Chem. Sens. Flav. (submitted).

<u>Role of Membrane-Bound Ca^{2+} in Taste Reception of the Frog</u> Kenzo Kurihara, Tadashi Kashiwagura and Naoki Kamo, (Faculty of Pharmaceutical Sciences, Hokkaido University, Sapporo, Japan)

(1) The frog gustatory responses to various salts and distilled water were greatly enhanced after the tongue was treated with an alkaline solution above pH 7.5 containing salts of low concentration. The incubation of the alkali-treated tongue in the solution of pH 6.0 containing Ca^{2+} restored reversibly the function of the gustatory receptor to that before the treatment, while Mg^{2+} had no ability to restore the function. (2) Similar enhancement of the salt responses was brought about by the treatment of the tongue with ANS. The ANS-treatment modified the specificity of the receptor to various monovalent cations. (3) The alkali- or ANS-treatment modified the temperature dependence of the salt responses. (4) The tongue incubated in Ringer solution of pH 5.5 brought about a great decrease of the responses to salts and distilled water. The function of the tongue thus modified was restored to that before the modification by incubating the tongue in Ringer of pH 7.0. (5) It was concluded that Ca^{2+} bound to the receptor membrane is released by the alkali- or ANS-treatment and that the incubation of the tongue in the acidic Ringer lets Ca^{2+} bind tightly to the membrane. Ease of a conformational change of the acceptor domains in response to adsorption or desorption of chemicals depends on the amount of the membrane-bound Ca^{2+}. (6) The presence of trace of the transition metal ions in salt stimuli also brought about a great enhancement of the responses. During continuous application of stimulating solutions, a tonic response increased abruptly about 2 min after the appearence of a phasic response. This enhancement was not brought about by a release of the membrane-bound Ca^{2+} but the mechanism of the enhancement seemed to be similar to that by the Ca^{2+}-removal. We emphasize that a conformational change of the acceptor domains plays an important role in the transduction process of the gustatory response.

Interactions between repellent quinones and purified receptor lipoprotein from Periplaneta americana sensory neurons D. M. Norris, Michael F. Ryan, Joseph J. Piotrowski and Judith Hagemen, (University of Wisconsin, Madison, Wisconsin 53706, USA)

Olfactory molecules which serve as defensive (allomonic) agents are a major component of chemical communication among organisms. If man is to utilize such olfactory molecules to maximal advantage, knowledge of physicochemical mechanisms involved in the sensory perception of such substances is needed. A sulfhydryl-rich receptor lipoprotein for repellent 1, 4-naphthoquinones was isolated from membranes of primary sensory neurons in the antennae of Periplaneta americana. Genetically controlled differences in the physicochemical properties of this energy-transducing receptor have been demonstrated. Such differences correlate closely with the behavioral sensitivities of various strains of the cockroach to the naphthoquinones. Kinetic analysis of the in vitro interactions between the receptor and several repellent 1, 4-naphthoquinones indicated that the order of their association constants (K_{EQ}) matched the order of their relative in vivo repellency. The receptor was purified 56.9 fold, in terms of µg of naphthoquinone bound per µg of receptor protein, by affinity chromatography using a p-chloromercuricbenzoic acid (PCMB) ligand on a 16-carbon sidearm attached to Sepharose 4B. This level of purification compares very favorably with that of Schmidt and Raferty for the acetylcholine receptor. Amino acid analysis has allowed identification of 16 acids; cysteine, or cystine, constitute by far the major amino acid. A definitive molecular weight is dependent on identification of 3 or 4 yet unidentified amino acids. The isolation of such receptors has been reduced to a routine, but in vitro maintenance of their ability to bind the olfactory molecules remains a fine art. (Research supported by U. S. National Science Foundation grants No. GB-41868 and BNS 74-00953 to D.M.N.).

An alternative model of olfactory quantitative interaction in binary mixtures

F. Patte, (Physiologie de la Chimioréception - C.N.R.S. - 91190 GIF-SUR-YVETTE, France).

The vectorial model of olfactory quantitative interaction proposed in 1971 by BERGLUND et al. constitutes certainly an important progress in this field. According to these authors a single value can characterize each pair of substances. Therefore it would be possible to build triangular matrices as it is done for qualitative similarities. As we know this single value is the cos α of the following equation : $\Psi_{AB} = \sqrt{\Psi_A^2 + \Psi_B^2 + 2\Psi_A \Psi_B \cos \alpha}$
in which A and B represent the two substances of the mixture.

Two concepts are suggested to test this model as well as any other model based on perceived odorous intensity and not on concentrations :

$\sigma = \Psi_{AB}/(\Psi_A + \Psi_B)$ which is the synergy taken in its general meaning. When $\sigma > 1$, there is exaltation and when $\sigma < 1$, there is inhibition.

$\tau = \Psi_{AB}/(\Psi_A + \Psi_B)$ which is the "percentage" of perceived odorous intensity.

The curves of σ versus τ, according to the vectorial model for several values of cos α show that we have a family of curves similar to "catenary curves". Two other models generating respectively families of "V curves" and "U curves" are suggested. Experimental data from CAIN and DREXLER (1974) and CAIN (1975) concerning 4 pairs of substances seem to indicate that the "U curves" are the most suitable, the less suitable being the "V curves" and the "pseudo catenary curves" are found between the two. Correlation coefficients between the different experimental Ψ_{AB} and the calculated ones for these 4 pairs of substances are better according to the "U model" than with the vectorial model.

References : BERGLUND et al. (Acta Psychol. 1971, 35, 255-268)

CAIN and DREXLER (Ann. N.Y. Acad. Sci., 1974, 237, 427-439)

CAIN (Chem. Senses and Flav., 1975, 1, 339-352).

Specific anosmia to camphoraceous odorants P. Pelosi (Istituto di Industrie Agrarie, Università degli Studi di Pisa)

Thresholds to 1,8-cineole do not fit a gaussian curve, but exhibit a bimodal distribution. The subjects can be segregated into two groups, normal smeller with an average threshold of 0.02 p.p.m. and anosmics with a threshold about 60 times higher. This difference corresponds to almost 6 binary dilution steps. The occurrence of such anosmia in the population resulted of about 33%. The extent of the anosmia to 1,8-cineole was investigated testing two panels of people, anosmics and normals, with several compounds related to cineole by similarity of odour or molecular shape. Among them, camphor, fenchone and borneol showed anosmics' defects between 1.2 and 2.5 binary steps, whereas other compounds such as α-pinene, β-pinene and adamantane gave values within the experimental error. Other molecules, apparently not related to cineole, gave significant differences between the normal and anosmics' thresholds. These were 2,2,4-trimethyl-3-pentanol with an anosmics' defect of 2.6 and two cyclic ketals, 1,2-diisopropyl-1,3-dioxolane and 2,2,4,4,5,5-hexamethyl-1,3-dioxolane with defects of 1.6 and 1.5 respectively. The series of macrocyclic ketones from cyclo octanone to cyclododecanone showed some specificity with the C_9-C_{11} terms. These observations lead to conclude that the camphor odour is associated with compounds of about 10 carbon atoms and of rather spherical molecular shape, and that 1,8-cineole, which is the best representative of this class, can be regarded as the "camphor" primary odorant. Failure to smell it may be related to the absence of a specific receptor site. A comparison with the minty odorants shows that, although both odours are exhibited by 10 carbon molecules, the minty odour, epitomized by 1-carvone, requires a rather flat molecular shape in contrast to the almost round shape of 1.8-cineole. Moreover subjects anosmic to 1-carvone are normal to cineole and viceversa, showing that the minty and the camphor odours constitute two distinct classes.

The intensity slopes of the n-aliphatic alcohols P.H. Punter
and E.P. Köster (Psychol.Lab., State Univ. of Utrecht,
Varkenmarkt 2, Utrecht, Holland)

The decrease in slope of the n-aliphatic alcohols with increase
in chainlength, found by several authors using sniff-bottle
methods, may be due to anomalies in the head-space because of the
liquid dilution methods used. This would especially affect the
higher alcohols. Since, in relation to artificial membranes,
physico-chemical properties of the alcohols show a sharp change
at about C7-C8, it is regrettable that reliable olfactometric
data on these higher alcohols are lacking. In this study two
different air-dilution olfactometers are used to obtain psychophysical data on the alcohols from C3 to C12 (except C11). The
results are consistent for both olfactometers and show a strong
similarity with physico-chemical (1) data: there is a decrease
in slope from C3 (0.49) to C7 (0.28) after which the slope
increases (C12: 0.49). This pattern is similar to that found by
RATHNAMMA(1) who measured the slopes of the curves of log conc.
vs. the interfacial tension (oil/water) at log conc.= -2.3
(Moles/1, aqueous). Threshold measurements of the same alcohols
also showed good agreement with physico-chemical data(1), i.e.
with the equilibrium conc. of alcohol to produce a reduction in
interfacial tension of 1 dyne/cm. There is a decrease in
threshold from C3 (1,900 ppb) to C7 (53 ppb) after which there
is an increase (C12: 166 ppb). Plotting log threshold vs. the
slope shows a decrease in threshold and slope from C3 to C7 and
an increase from C7 to C12, in the former case the threshold
decreases faster than the slope, in the latter case the opposite
holds. From these data it seems that two processes play a role:
alcohols with decreasing chain length (from C7) become more water
soluble which decreases their stimulatory efficiency, alcohols
with increasing chain length (from C7) become more lipid soluble
which also decreases their stimulatory efficiency although less
than for the water soluble alcohols. C7 orients itself at the
membranous interface and shows the highest stimulatory efficiency
i.e. the lowest threshold and slope. These data suggest that the
membrane phospholipids, at least for the n-aliphatic alcohols,
may play an important role in odor reception.
(1) RATHNAMMA D.V. 1974, In: Adsorption at interfaces by K.L.
MITTAL Symposium series.

Structural investigation of Thaumatin I, a sweet tasting protein from Thaumatococcus Daniellii Benth H. van der Wel, (Unilever Research, NL-3133 AT Vlaardingen, The Netherlands)

Thaumatin is a basic protein with a sweetness intensity 10^5 times that of sucrose on a molar basis. Since proteins are charged molecules having characteristic numbers of both anionic and cationic side chains we focussed our interest in the first place on the selective chemical modification of these amino acid-side chains which may affect the total net charge of the molecule.

Modification of the NH_3^+ group of the lysine residues by methylation, a modification causing practically no change in the charge, has no influence on the sweetness intensity. Modification of the same side groups by acetylation, which results in a decrease in the total net charge, runs parallel with a decrease in the sweetness intensity. Modification of the cationic guanidino group of the arginine residues with 1,2-cyclohexanedione, which is also accompanied by a remarkable decrease in the net charge, has practically no influence on the sweetness intensity. Another selective chemical modification influencing the total net charge, is the iodination of the tyrosine residues. Two or three iodine atoms can be incorporated into the molecule while much of the sweetness is retained. Incorporation of more than three iodine atoms drastically diminishes the sweetness intensity.

For the present the conclusion might be drawn that most probably some of the lysine residues are involved in eliciting the sweet taste sensation. Besides this AH, B system, a third binding site (γ-interaction) is necessary to explain the sweet taste sensation. Perhaps some tyrosine residues are involved in this.

OLFACTION

Some freeze-etching data on the olfactory epithelium

Dontscho Kerjaschki

Dept. Pathology, EM Unit, University of Vienna, Spitalgasse 4, A1090 Vienna, Austria

ABSTRACT
Cell membranes of olfactory vesicles and cilia harbour about 1000 intramembranous particles (IMPs) per μ^2. This is significantly more than may be found in nonreceptor membranes of respiratory cilia indicating a high protein/lipid ratio for receptor membranes. On their surface receptor membranes carry negatively charged, neuraminidase sensitive groups which bind cationic ferritin (CF). Four different stages of development of olfactory vesicles are characterized by their cell junctions: A-state: The tip of the outgrowing dendrite produces few discontinuous tight junction ridges in its membrane. B-state: The dendrite has reached the pre-existing tight junction belt of the supporting cells (6-8 ridges), and the ridges start to fuse. C-state: An olfactory vesicle has developed, its tight junction comprising up to 25 ridges. D-state: A mature olfactory vesicle with numerous cilia and a tight junction made up of 6-8 rows of ridges.

INTRODUCTION
Three major cell types compose the olfactory epithelium in vertebrates: (i) The sensory cells, the perikarya of which reside in the middle zone of the pseudostratified epithelium, terminating in small varicosities with numerous specialized cilia in the epithelial surface (the olfactory vesicles)., (ii) The basal cells, a reservoir for newly outgrowing sensory cells during normal cell turnover, or after lesion of mature sensory cells., (iii) The supporting cells, which are intercalated between sensory dendrites and provide a thick carpet of microvilli engulfing the sensory cilia in adult animals. The membranes of sensory cells, especially of vesicles and cilia, are thought to harbour receptor sites for olfactory stimuli. Judging by their organelle content, supporting cells appear metabolically very active, their precise functional capacities, however, are essentially unknown to date.

Our study focuses on two points: (1) The presumptive olfactory receptor membranes with a view to finding morphological differences to non-sensory membranes, and (2) cell junctions, especially tight junctions, during outgrowth of sensory dendrites between preexisting supporting cells, a situation requiring dynamic changes in the structure of cell contacts in order to maintain the physiological properties of the whole epithelium.

A powerful morphological tool for the study of biological membranes is freeze etching technique. This method visualizes the interior aspect of cell membranes by splitting the lipid bilayer at the interior level of hydrophobic bonding thereby exposing intramembranous proteins in the form of intramembranous particles (IMPs)[1,2]. In the olfactory epithelium we demonstrate that membranes of sensory cilia and vesicles contain significantly more intramembranous protein than non-sensory cilia. Tight junctions, visualized as ridges predominating in the cytoplasmic fracture face of the membrane (P-face)[3], are formed at the tip of outgrowing dendrites, fuse with the preexistent meshwork of 6-8 ridges of supporting cells and subsequently regroup in a less complex 'adult' pattern. The number of IMPs increases during outgrowth of dendrites, displaying a burst as the forming vesicle is integrated into the olfactory surface. Some IMPs form rosette-like arrays, thought to precede the necklace of outgrown cilia. Gap junctions, considered as sites of intercellular electrical and metabolical coupling, are found only between supporting cells, yet are absent from sensory dendrites.[4]

The surfaces of vesicle membranes and of cilia contain negatively charged sessile groups, as indicated by their capacity to bind cationic ferritin (CF) in a diffuse pattern, when membrane proteins are immobilized by glutaraldehyde cross-linking. They are sensitive to digestion with neuraminidase, indicating that neuraminic acid imposes an electrostatic barrier on the receptor membrane surface.

MATERIALS AND METHODS

This study is based on the examination of 60 mice of different age. Details of preparation have been published earlier[4]. Freeze-etching was carried out in a Leybold-Heräeus EPA 100 machine. In the CF binding studies, nasal septa were fixed with 2,5% glutaraldehyde, washed overnight in buffer and then exposed to CF for 30 min. Some of the fixed specimens were exposed to neutral ferritin others treated with neuraminidase for 6 hours preceding   CF exposure.

RESULTS
     For convenience of description, four states in the development of an olfactory vesicle will arbitrarily be characterized as follows (Fig. 1):
A-state: The dendrite still lies within the intercellular space and its tip is distant from the supporting cell   junctional complex.
B-state: The dendrite tip has reached the supporting cells's tight junction belt. In an earlier publication this and the following situation were referred to as 'complex junction state[4]'.
C-state: A young olfactory vesicle is formed, characterized in thin sections by its light cytoplasm, clusters of centrioles and lack or paucity of cilia.
D-state: The adult olfactory vesicle has developed, with numerous cilia and few, if any, free centrioles. (Fig. 2)

Junctions and IMP variations during development
     In thin sections, tight junctions or zonulae occludentes are characterized in the olfactory epithelium and in all other epithelia as focal fusions of the outer leaflets of the cell mem-

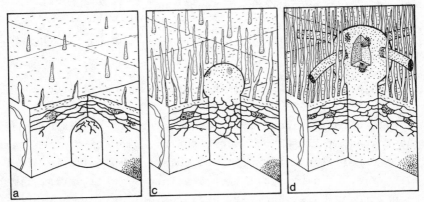

Fig. 1 Schematic   drawing of different stages of development of olfactory vesicles. The states are termed A,B,C,D, by criteria defined in the text.

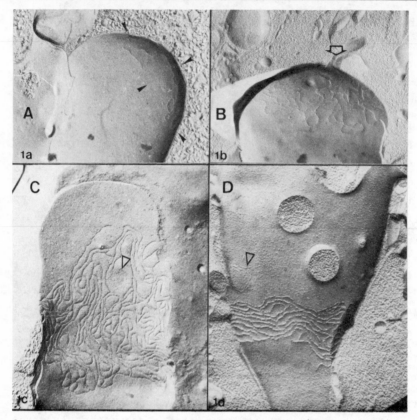

Fig. 2   Different states in olfactory vesicle outgrowth.
1a: A-state, the dendrite lies between supporting cells,
junctional ridges are prominent in the area de-
marcated by arrowheads. 1b: B-state, the dendrite has
reached the tight junction belt of supporting cells (arrow)
1c: C-state,a complex pattern of junctional ridges separates the newly formed vesicle from the interstitial
space. Arrow indicates a rosette of IMPs.   1d: D-state,
an adult vesicle with 7-8 junctional ridges, and two rosettes
(arrows). All figures x 40 000

branes of adjacent cells[5]. In mature olfactory epithelium (D-
state), supporting cells form 6-8 contacts with one another as
well as with olfactory dendrites. In accordance, this area exhibits 6-8 rows of ridges and complementary grooves at the intramembranous level. There is a typical polarity as found in other
epithelia, i.e. an almost straight continuous juxtaluminal fibril-
at the junctional base, however, a predominating meshwork of
open-ended ridges. This latter zone is supposed to be the site
of appositional growth of tight junctions in other epithelia by

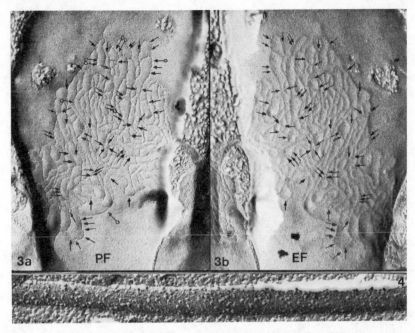

Fig. 3   Vesicle in C-state, matching replicas. Arrows
indicate interruptions of the tight junction ridges which
are complemented by particles left on the opposite fracture
face. Arrows labelled with an O represent true interruptions
in which no matching particle can be found. X 50 000

Fig. 4   Distal segment of an olfactory cilium, displaying
numerous IMPs. X 160 000

aggregation of globular subunits[6], as is displayed by our system
also. A part of the ridges in the mature pattern seems to be contributed by olfactory dendrites, because in the A-state, leading
tips of outgrowing sensory cells are covered by few ridges,form-
ing scallops and patterns lacking any polarity. The most impressive morphological changes to the tight junction take place in
the B- and C-states. (Fig. 3) In these situations, tight junctions are
formed by a complicated maze comprised of 15-20 rows of ridges,
a situation termed 'complex junction' and derived probably by fusion of junction from supporting cells and dendrites. As the
vesicle develops, the number of ridges is reduced to the D-state.
This mechanism may be similar to insect gut cells, which modulate
the geometry of their tight junctions by mechanical stretching,
induced by cyclic changes in the filling state of the cells[7].

The number of IMPs changes dramatically during dendrite maturation. (Fig. 5). There is an abrupt change from a membrane very poor in IMPs in state A, to a IMP-rich membrane between states B and C., definitely involving a burst of membrane protein synthesis and insertion into the membrane. Similar counts exist for maturation of cultured nerve cells and developing fibroblasts.

It should be pointed out that the number of IMPs in olfactory cilia and vesicle membranes is high in comparison to non-receptor cilia in respiratory epithelium (about 1000 IMP/μ^2 in the olfactory mucosa, 200 IMP/μ^2 in respiratory cilia). Similar results have been obtained for rat, frog and cow.[8,9] (Fig. 4)

The number of IMPs is somewhat lower on the sensory cell perikarya although the biochemical quality of particles may vary considerably for membrane areas separated by a tight junction belt.

Apart from randomly dispersed IMPs in the vesicles, clusters of IMPs are found forming concentric rings and overlaying centrioles [10]. These particles remain attached in almost equal amounts to both fracture faces of the membrane, in contrast to other IMPs which prefer the P-face after fixation. Rosette particles share this ability with IMPs forming the necklaces of cilia from various sources.

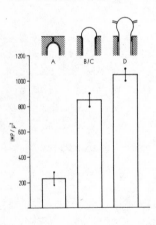

Fig. 5 Counts of intramembranous particles (IMP) in dendrite membranes in different stages of development.

Cilia

The whiplike olfactory cilia are certainly the most curious structure on the olfactory surface. Arising from the vesicle surface as common cilia with a typical 9+2 microtubular pattern in

connection with centrioles, they display a short, presumably ac-
tively mobile thick proximal segment, and subsequently continue
into long processes with elliptic transection   and two remaining
central microtubuli in the elliptic foci. As seen in TAG[11] fixed
material, tubuli contain 13 subunits (Fig. 6) and lack dynein
bridges. They appear connected to submembranous material by broad
bridges of poor electron density. A thin 30Å coat is visible on
the membrane surface. In freeze-fracture preparations this membrane is rich in IMPs.Towards the vesicle membrane they are separated by 5-7 rows of IMPs in typical necklace arrangment. IMPs
may form small clusters when glutaraldehyde treatment is omitted
before glycerinisation, as may also be found in lymphocyte[12] and
red cell membranes after damage of the submembranous fibrillar
proteins[13].

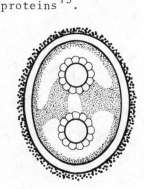

Fig. 6 Drawing of a transsected thin
segment of an olfactory cilium as seen
in tannic acid — glutaraldehyde fixed material.

Binding of cationic ferritin

After fixation with glutaraldehyde, cationic ferritin (CF)[14]
is bound diffusely to the membranes of olfactory and respiratory
mucosa, whereas neutral ferritin particles are not attached. Surprisingly, there is no significant labelling of the mucus in the
olfactory region and the ferritin particles are directly bound
to the membrane surface, thus excluding the possibility that con-
densed mucus coats membranes. The number of CF particles fairly
equals IMP counts, i.e.less than e.g. on endothelial cells in the
kidney where the tracer is arranged in a two-dimensional lattice.(Fig. 7)

Supporting cells

The surface of supporting cells is characterized by microvilli, varying in number with the animal age, fetal supporting
cells being virtually devoid of microvilli, whereas mature cells

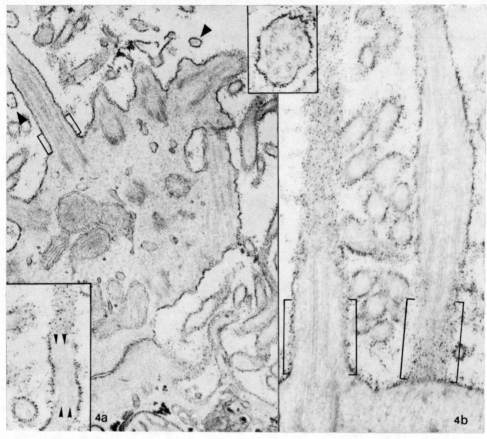

Fig. 7 Olfactory surface, prefixed with glutaraldehyde and exposed to cationic ferritin. 4a: Survey of an olfactory vesicle. The tracer sticks exclusively to the cell membranes, and not to the mucus. 4b: Thick segments of olfactory cilia, partially cut tangentially. The cationic tracer is evenly distributed on the membrane surface. Brackets indicate neck-regions of cilia. Inserts: Proximal and distal segments of olfactory cilia. 4a:x65 000, 4b:x150 000, Inserts:x160 000

extend several of these into the mucus. Not regarding the state of maturation, cell membranes facing the surface contain a particular type of IMP which is rodshaped in contrast to common globular particles- and appears to be the predominating type of IMP. Globular IMPs are found in microvilli membranes, and below the tight junction belt. In addition, small clusters of 60 A IMPs in rectangular arrangment have been found in this latter region.

In contrast to sensory neurons, supporting cells are coupled by gap junctions. These areas, identified by tightly packed IMPs are found either within the meshwork of junctional ridges, or as discrete patches near the cell apices as macular junctions.

DISCUSSION

Several attempts have been made for correlating the morphology of tight junctions with their functional 'tightness' as expressed e.g. by transepithelial electrical resistance. The study of Claude and Goodenough[15] suggests a parallel between these parameters: A one- or two-ridge tight junction indicating a low ($10\,\Omega$ cm^{-2}) transepithelial resistance, a 6-8 ridge tight junction, as in our case, should signal a resistance of a few thousands of $\Omega\,cm^{-2}$ at least. However, recent reports of exceptions from this tentative rule have cast some incertainty on these predictions[16]. Permeability may also be controlled by factors not visible in the electronmicroscope, as charge of strands, etc. We disagree with the interpretation that small interruptions which may be frequently seen in tight junction ridges, are transjunctional lanes for bulk solute transport. This view calls for support by matching replicas, in that defects of ridges are not complemented by particles remaining in the opposite fracture face[17]. Under these aspects tight junctions of the olfactory epithelium remain morphologically tight, even during outgrowth of new dendrites, and it should not be surprising to find high transepithelial resistance, although this cannot be directly concluded from morphological data.

Olfactory dendrites lack gap junctions which have been convincingly implicated in bulk metabolic and electrical coupling of various epithelial cells[18]. This assumption is in agreement with physiological data on the salamander olfactory mucosa[19]. By analogy, sensory cells of the inner ear lack gap junctions also[20]. Again, some caution seems indicated in these morphologically based conclusions, since it cannot be ruled out that single isolated IMPs serve a coupling function. However, in this case also the amount of coupling would be rather small in comparison to genuine gap junctions. In supporting cells, coupling by gap junctions is concentrated on cell apices.

The high amount of IMPs in receptor membranes of olfactory vesicles and cilia in comparison to respiratory cilia

may indicate some functional specialization.   IMPs are of course
not to be considered a homogenous type of proteins. In red cell
membranes[21], IMPs have been suspected to carry hydrophilic channels, and they may serve a similar purpose in the olfactory epithelium. A carbohydrate-rich protein in the cell membrane (glyco-
phorin) spans the membrane with a single helix only, which cannot be visualized by freeze etching. Presently we are trying
to discover whether aggregation of CF is paralleled by redistribution of IMPs in vesicle and ciliary membranes. Obviously, no
direct evidence for the nature of olfactory receptors may be deduced from our findings. They may reside in the lipid and/or
protein phase of membranes. Inhibition experiments with n-ethylmaleimide[22]   point to the proteinaceous moiety. However, these
problems clearly call for a biochemical analysis of purified
cilia and vesicle membranes.

REFERENCES

1.   Tillack,T.W. and Marchesi,V.T (1970)
     J.Cell Biol. 45,649
2.   Pinto da Silva,P and Branton,D. (1970)
     J.Cell Biol. 45,598
3.   Branton,D., Bullivant,S., Gilula,N.B., Karnovsky,M.J.,
     Moor,H., Mühlethaler,K. Northcote,D.H., Packer,L., Satir,P.,
     Speth,V., Staehelin,L.A., Steere,R.L., and Weinstein,R.S.
     (1975)
     Science 190,54
4.   Kerjaschki,D. and Hörandner H., (1976)
     J.Ultrastruct.Res. 54,420
5.   Farquhar,M.G. and Palade,G.E. (1963)
     J.Cell Biol. 17,375
6.   Montesano,R., Friend,D.S., Perrelet,A. and Orci,L. (1975)
     J.Cell Biol. 67,310
7.   Hull,B.E. and Staehelin,L.A. (1976)
     J.Cell Biol. 68,688
8.   Menco,B.P.,Dodd,G.H., Davey,M. and Bannister,L.H. (1976)
     Nature 263,597
9.   Menco,B., personal communication
10. Kerjaschki,D., Sleytr,U. and Stockinger,L. (1972)
     Naturwissenschaften 59,314
11. Futesaku,Y., Mizuhira,V. and Nakamura,H. (1972)
     J.Histochem.Cytochem. 20,155
12. McIntyre,J.A., Karnovsky,M.J. and Gilula,N.B. (1973)
     Nature New Biol. 245,147
13. Elsgaeter,A. and Branton,D., (1974)
     J.Cell Biol. 63, 1018
14. Danon,D., Goldstein,L., Marikovsky,Y., Skutelsky,E., (1972)
     J.Ultrastruct.Res. 38,500
15. Claude,P. and Goodenough,D.A. (1973)
     J.Cell Biol. 58,390

16. Martinez-Palomo,A. and Erlij,D. (1975)
    Proc.Natl.Acad.Sci.(USA) 72,4487
17. Kerjaschki,D. (1977)
    Microvascular Res., in press
18. Loewenstein,W.R. (1976)
    Cold Spring Harbor Symp.Quant.Biol. 40, 49
19. Getchell, T.V., personal communication
20. Jahnke,K., personal communication
21. Steck,T.L., (1974)
    J.Cell.Biol. 62,1
22. Getchell,M.L. and Gesteland,R.C. (1972)
    Proc.Natl.Acad.Sci. (USA) 69,1494

Structural organization of the olfactory pathways

Joseph L. Price

Department of Anatomy and Neurobiology, Washington University School of Medicine, 660 South Euclid Avenue, St. Louis, Missouri 63110, USA

ABSTRACT

This paper briefly reviews the organization of the olfactory system. The first part deals with the synaptic organization of the olfactory bulb, especially the reciprocal synapses between the mitral and tufted cells, and the granule and periglomerular cells. The second part describes the axonal projection of the mitral and tufted cells onto the olfactory cortex, and the organization of the association fiber system within the cortex. In the third part, the extrinsic projections of the cortex are discussed.

OLFACTORY BULB

As Cajal[1] clearly showed, olfactory stimuli entering the olfactory bulb along the olfactory nerves are relayed to the olfactory cortex by two similar types of neurons, the mitral and tufted cells. These cells are very much alike in the configuration and ultrastructural characteristics[2,3], and differ only in their laminar distribution within the olfactory bulb, and in the smaller size of the tufted cells. Activity in the mitral and tufted cells is modulated through two types of interneurons, the granule and periglomerular cells (or internal and external granule cells), which interact with the relay cells via reciprocal or dendro-dendritic synapses. These synapses have been studied extensively by many investigators, working in different laboratories, and their morphological characteristics are very well established[4].

In the case of the granule cells, which lack axons, the reciprocal synapses occur between large, spine-like appendages or 'gemmules', on the peripheral processes of the granule cells, and the smooth dendrites and somata of the mitral and tufted cells. The mitral (tufted) to granule portion of the synapse is characterized by a discrete cluster of synaptic vesicles in close association with an 'asymmetrical' (type I) synaptic membrane thickening, whereas the granule to mitral (tufted) portion is characterized by a large cluster of synaptic vesicles (which often fill the gemmule) associated with a 'symmetrical' (type II) membrane thickening[5-8]. With appropriate buffer concentration in the fixative or washing solutions, the vesicles in the mitral cells are observed to be spherical, while those in the granule cells are flattened or pleomorphic[6-8]. Although the reciprocity of these synapses has recently been questioned[9] it should be emphasized that several previous studies, using serial sections, indicate that a very high proportion (possibly greater than 75%) of the mitral to granule synapses are reciprocated by a granule to mitral synapse from the same gemmule[5,7,8,10].

In agreement with the morphological characteristics of the two halves of the reciprocal synapses, physiological evidence indicates that the mitral to granule synapses are excitatory while the granule to mitral synapses are inhibitory[5,11,12]. Pharmacological experiments using small electrophoretic injections also suggest that the transmittor released by granule cells is 'GABA'[13,14] and this is supported by a recent immunocytochemical study which showed that the enzyme which synthesizes GABA, glutamate decarboxylase, is present in the somata and processes of granule and periglomerular cells[15].

The synapses between the periglomerular cells and the dendritic tufts of the mitral and tufted cells occur in the glomeruli of the olfactory bulb, and are similar to those related to the granule cells. However, the periglomerular cells are relatively free of gemmules, and the reciprocating synapses are only rarely situated in close proximity to each other[16-18]. Unlike the granule cells, the periglomerular cells have axons, which form non-reciprocal synapses with the dendrites of mitral and tufted cells[19].

Apart from the olfactory nerves themselves, no other axon terminals have been found on the mitral and tufted cells, and it is likely that all other modulating influences act through the granule and periglomerular cells. These include short axon cells within the olfactory bulb[2,3] and bulbopetal fibers from the nucleus of the horizontal limb of the diagonal band, and from areas of the olfactory cortex[20-24].

OLFACTORY CORTEX

The axons of the mitral and tufted cells pass caudally in the lateral olfactory tract, and give off collaterals to each of the olfactory cortical areas: anterior olfactory nucleus, olfactory tubercle, ventral part of the tenia tecta, piriform cortex, nucleus of the lateral olfactory tract, anterior cortical amygdaloid nucleus, periamygdaloid cortex, and lateral entorhinal cortex[28-31]. This diverse array of cortical structures will collectively be referred to as the olfactory cortex. Throughout this cortex, the fibers from the olfactory bulb are sharply restricted to the superficial part of the

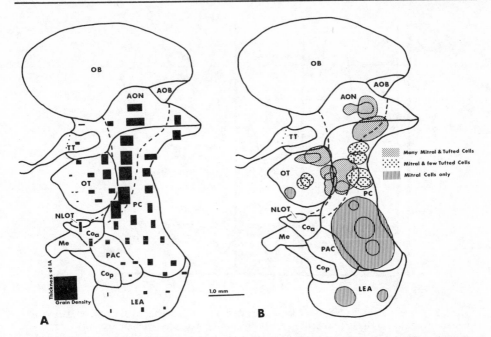

Figure 1. Unfolded, homolographic projection of the olfactory bulb and cortex of the rat. A. The distribution of anterogradely transported label in layer IA, following an injection of ^{3}H-leucine into the olfactory bulb; 7 days survival[25]. B. HRP injection sites from which mitral and tufted cells in the olfactory bulb were retrogradely labeled[26,27].

molecular layer (IA). Although no topographic organization has been found in this projection, there is a systematic variation in the density of the projection across the cortex[28,31]. Following injections of ^{3}H-leucine into the olfactory bulb, transported axonal label is heaviest deep to the lateral olfactory tract, and decreases lateral, caudal and medial to the tract (fig. 1a). Interestingly, the thickness of layer IA and the density of termination within that layer vary in parallel, so that the total projection (thickness X density) varies by two orders of magnitude between the most heavily labeled and most lightly labeled areas[25].

Although Cajal[1] believed that the axons of the tufted cells cross to the opposite olfactory bulb through the anterior commissure, this has been disproved by several investigations[32-34]. Recent experiments with the horseradish peroxidase (HRP) method of retrograde axonal tracing indicate that most, at least, of the tufted cells project through the lateral olfactory tract, although their termination is largely restricted to the rostral olfactory areas near the lateral olfactory tract (anterior olfactory nucleus,

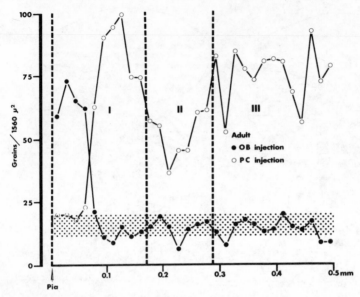

Figure 2. Grain counts made from autoradiographs of the piriform cortex in two experiments with injections of ^{3}H-leucine into the olfactory bulb or piriform cortex, to demonstrate the laminar distribution of the sensory and association fibers[27].

medial part of the piriform cortex, and lateral part of the olfactory tubercle; fig. 1b)[26]; the tufted cell projection to the lateral part of the olfactory tubercle is particularly heavy. Injections of HRP into more caudal parts of the olfactory cortex produce retrograde labeling of very few tufted cells, although mitral cells are labeled from all parts of the olfactory cortex.

The axons of mitral cells in the accessory olfactory bulb also project through the lateral olfactory tract, but terminate exclusively in layer I of the medial and posterior cortical amygdaloid nuclei; these nuclei do not receive fibers from the main olfactory bulb[29,30].

Association fibers from the olfactory cortex itself also project to all of the cortical structures which receive fibers from the olfactory bulb; the laminar termination of these fibers in layers IB and III of the cortex is precisely complementary to that of the olfactory bulb fibers in layer IA (fig.2)[28]. The association fibers also extend into neocortical areas adjoining the olfactory cortex: the infralimbic area on the medial side of the hemisphere, and the ventral and posterior agranular insular areas in the dorsal bank of the rhinal sulcus[24,25].

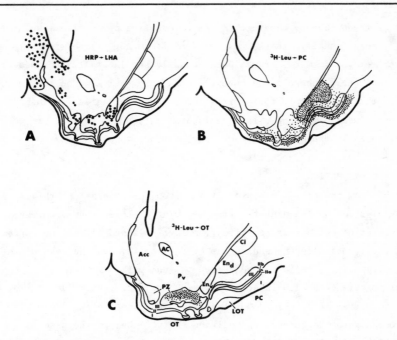

Figure 3. Cross-sectional diagrams of the anterior piriform cortex and olfactory tubercle showing: A. Retrogradely labeled cells following an injection of HRP into the lateral hypothalamus; B. Anterograde axonal label following an injection into layers I-III of the anterior piriform cortex; C. Anterograde axonal label following an injection into layers I-III of the olfactory tubercle[27,36].

The greatest number of association fibers appear to arise in the piriform cortex, although association projections have been identified from all of the olfactory cortical areas except the olfactory tubercle[24]. Experiments using the HRP method have also shown that different cellular layers in the piriform cortex give rise to different components of the association system[24]. Axons from cells in layer IIB (the deeper, more compact part of layer II) are predominantly distributed caudal to their cells of origin, whereas axons from cells in layer III are distributed rostral to their origin. Cells in layer IIA project in both directions, particularly to areas outside the piriform cortex (the anterior olfactory nucleus, olfactory tubercle, and lateral entorhinal cortex).

In the rostral part of the olfactory cortex, there is also some degree of topographic organization in the termination of the association projections[24]. Fibers from rostral areas (the anterior olfactory nucleus and the anterior piriform cortex) terminate in the cortex deep and adjacent to the lateral olfactory tract (medial part of the anterior piriform cortex, and lateral parts of the olfactory tubercle and anterior olfactory nucleus) while fibers arising more caudally (in the posterior piriform cortex) terminate in areas further removed from the tract, both medially and laterally (the medial parts of the olfactory tubercle and anterior olfactory nucleus, and the lateral part of the anterior piriform cortex and the ventral agranular insular area). The most caudal olfactory area, the lateral entorhinal cortex, projects to a small area in the medial part of the olfactory tubercle, and to the medial side of the olfactory peduncle.

EXTRINSIC PROJECTIONS

Apart from the well-known projections from the lateral entorhinal cortex to the hippocampus and dentate gyrus, extrinsic projections from the olfactory cortex do not appear to arise from layers II and III of the cortex itself, but from a heterogeneous group of deep cells. In the case of the piriform cortex, these cells may be termed the endopiriform nucleus[37]. Autoradiographic experiments with injections restricted to layers II and III of the piriform cortex invariably demonstrate labeled axons in the endopiriform nucleus deep to the cortex, in addition to the label in the association fibers in layers IB and III (fig. 3b), but do not demonstrate projections outside the cortex. However, if the injections also involve the endopiriform nucleus or other deep cells, labeled axons are found in the mediodorsal thalamic nucleus, the ventral putamen, and the lateral hypothalamus, as well as in the ventral subiculum and the medial and posterior cortical amygdaloid nuclei[35,38,39]. The last three structures, in turn, project directly to the medial hypothalamus[39].

The endopiriform nucleus is not homogeneous, and several subdivisions may be recognized within it. For example, injections of HRP into the lateral hypothalamus label cells in the ventral part of the endopiriform nucleus and in the polymorph zone deep to the olfactory tubercle, but not in the dorsal endopiriform nucleus (fig. 3a)[36]. The cells in the ventral endopiriform nucleus appear to receive fibers from the piriform cortex, while those in the polymorph zone receive fibers from the olfactory tubercle (fig. 3b,c). Because of this complexity, further experiments are required to fully define the position of the deep cells in the olfactory system. However, in view of their close relation to the overlying olfactory cortex, it may be well to consider the deep cells as the deepest layer of the olfactory cortical areas, comparable to layers V and VI of the neocortex.

(Supported by Research Grant # NS09518 USPHS)

REFERENCES

1. Cajal, S.R.   (1911)   Histologie du Système Nerveux de l'Homme et des
    Vertébrés.
    Vol. II, Maloine, Paris

2. Price, J.L. and Powell, T.P.S. (1970)
    J. Cell Sci. 7, 631-651.

3. Pinching, A.J. and Powell, T.P.S.   (1970)
    J. Cell Sci. 9, 305-345.

4. Shepherd, G.M.   (1972)
    Physiol. Rev. 52, 864-917.

5. Rall, W., Shepherd, G.M., Reese, T.S. and Brightman, M.W. (1966)
    Expl. Neurol. 14, 44-56.

6. Price, J.L. (1968)
    Brain Res. 11, 697-700.

7. Price, J.L. and Powell, T.P.S. (1970)
    J. Cell Sci. 7, 125-155.

8. Willey, T.J.   (1973)
    J. Comp. Neur. 152, 211-232.

9. Ramon-Moliner, E.   (1977)
    Brain Res. 128, 1-20

10. Landis, D.M.D., Reese, T.S. and Raviola, E.   (1974)
    J. Comp. Neur. 155, 67-92

11. Rall, W. and Shepherd, G.M.   (1968)
    J. Neurophysiol. 31, 884-915.

12. Nicoll, R.A. (1969)
    Brain Res. 14, 157-172

13. McLennan, H.   (1971)
    Brain Res. 29, 177-184

14. Nicoll, R.A. (1971)
    Brain Res. 35, 137-149

15. Ribak, C.E., Vaughn, J.E., Saito, K., Barber, R. and Roberts, E. (1977)
    Brain Res. 126, 1-18.

16. Reese, T.S. and Brightman, M.W. (1970) in Ciba Foundation Symposium
    on Taste and Smell in Vertebrates
    pp. 115-149, Churchill, London

17. Pinching, A.J. and Powell, T.P.S. (1971)
    J. Cell Sci. 9, 347-377.

18. White, E.L. (1973)
    Brain Res. 60, 299-313.

19. Pinching, A.J. and Powell, T.P.S. (1971)
    J. Cell Sci. 9, 379-409.

20. Price, J.L. and Powell, T.P.S. (1970)
    J. Anat. (Lond.) 107, 215-237

21. Price, J.L. and Powell, T.P.S. (1970)
    J. Cell Sci. 7, 157-180

22. Dennis, B.J. and D.J.B. Kerr (1976)
    Brain Res. 110, 593-600

23. Broadwell, R.D. and Jacobowitz, D.M. (1976)
    J. Comp. Neur. 170, 321-346

24. Haberly, L.B. and Price, J.L. (1977)
    J. Comp. Neur. (in press)

25. Schwob, J.E. and Price, J.L. (in preparation)

26. Haberly, L.B. and Price, J.L. (1977)
    Brain Res. (in press)

27. Abbreviations for figs. 1-3:   Acc: Nu. Accumbens; AC: Anterior Commis-
    sure; AOB: Accessory Olfactory Bulb; AON: Anterior Olfactory Nu.; Cl:
    Claustrum; Co_a: Anterior Cortical Amygdaloid Nu.; Co_p: Posterior Cortical
    Amygdaloid Nu.; En_d: Dorsal Endopiriform Nu.; En_v: Ventral Endopiriform
    Nu.; LEA: Lateral Entorhinal Cortex; LOT: Lateral Olfactory Tract; Me:
    Medial Amygdaloid Nu.; NLOT: Nu. of the LOT; OB: Olfactory Bulb; OT:
    Olfactory Tubercle; P_v: Ventral Putamen; PAC: Periamygdaloid Cortex;
    PC: Piriform Cortex; PZ: Polymorph Zone of OT; TT: Tenia Tecta

28. Price, J.L. (1973)
    J. Comp. Neur. 150, 87-108

29. Scalia, F. and Winans, S.S. (1975)
    J. Comp. Neur. 161, 31-56

30. Broadwell, R.D. (1975)
    J. Comp. Neur. 163, 329-346.

31. Skeen, L.C. and Hall, W.C. (1977)
    J. Comp. Neur. 172, 1-36

32. Lohman, A.H.M. (1963)
    Acta Anat. 53, Suppl. 49, 1-109

33. Powell, T.P.S., Cowan, W.M., and Raisman, G. (1965)
    J. Anat. (Lond.) 99, 791-813

34. Lohman, A.H.M. and Mentinck, G.M. (1969)
    Brain Res. 12, 396-413.

35. Krettek, J.E. and Price, J.L. (1977)
    J. Comp. Neur. 172, 687-722

36. Haberly, L.B., Luskin, M. and Price, J.L. (unpublished observations)

37. Loo, Y.T. (1931)
    J. Comp. Neur. 52, 1-148

38. Krettek, J.E. and Price, J.L. (1977)
    J. Comp. Neur. 172, 723-752

39. Krettek, J.E. and Price,J.L. (submitted for publication)

Olfactory centrifugal pathways

David I. B. Kerr

Department of Human Physiology and Pharmacology, University of Adelaide, Adelaide 5001, South Australia

ABSTRACT

Using the retrograde HRP method it has been confirmed that the olfactory peduncle (anterior olfactory nucleus, AON) and the horizontal nucleus of the diagonal band (HNDB) project to the olfactory bulb. In addition, regions deep to the tubercle, and much of the prepyriform cortex, also project directly to the olfactory bulb. From evoked potentials the entire basal cortex, save only the angular cortex (angular "ganglion" of Cajal), has been found to project to the olfactory bulb, partly by relay in AON. Pyriform cortex and AON contribute a low frequency component to induced waves elicited in the bulb by olfactory stimuli. Surprisingly, little or no bulbar response could be evoked by HNDB stimulation which has so far shown only marginal effects on induced waves, generally an increase in amplitude. The functional significance of the HNDB centrifugal system, which has only secondary olfactory afferent relations, remains obscure.

INTRODUCTION

Centrifugal fibers entering the mammalian olfactory bulb were originally described by Cajal in his study of the olfactory cortex[4], but their possible functional significance attracted little attention until first investigated by Hagbarth and myself some quarter century ago[21]. Disappointingly little concerning their functions has been added during the ensuing years, although it would be fair to say that there is a similar lack of general understanding concerning the functions of other centrifugal systems in the brain. The relevant anatomy, in which considerable advances have been made, has been well reviewed recently[1,2,3,15,16,24,33], and the following summary serves only as a basis for discussion of our more recent investigations of the centrifugal systems concerned in olfaction[36].

OLFACTORY AFFERENT PROJECTIONS

Axons derived from mitral and tufted cells form the afferent projection from the bulb through the lateral olfactory tract (LOT). The major LOT projections embrace the retrobulbar anterior olfactory nucleus (AON), a considerable proportion of the olfactory tubercle (OT), the anterior and posterolateral aspects of the cortical amygdaloid nucleus (CO), and the entire pyriform cortex with the exception of the angular cortex (spheno-occipital or angular ganglion of Cajal[4]). The prepyriform cortex (area 51 of Brodmann) receives a projection of larger fibers over the LOT, whilst the posterior region, which lies within the entorhinal cortex (Brodmann area 28), receives fine fibers derived as collaterals from the main LOT[19,29].

CENTRIFUGAL PROJECTIONS TO THE OLFACTORY BULB

The AON provides the major crossed projection through the anterior com-missure directed to the opposite bulb and opposite AON. Collaterals of these fibers arise at the peduncle level of the ipsilateral AON to run back into the ipsilateral bulb[34]. The commissure projection arises from the pars ext-erna, pars lateralis and pars dorsalis of AON[2,10,15]. The AON and adjacent peduncle project to the horizontal nucleus of the diagonal band (HNDB), poss-ibly the bed nucleus of the stria terminalis, and at the cortical level, tae-nia tecta, the mediolateral olfactory tubercle and the rostrocaudal extent of the pyriform cortex[2,15]. These regions in turn project back upon the AON e.g. cells in the entire olfactory cortex, including the posterior division, label with horseradish peroxidase (HRP) after injections involving AON[15,20].

A most significant advance has been the identification by Price and Powell[27] of the HNDB as a major source of the thick-fiber centrifugal system described by Cajal. This has been confirmed by HRP studies in rat, cat and rabbit[3,10,15,20], which also implicate the adjacent hypothalamus. Many of the cells in this region stain for choline esterase, and the system was hin-ted at by Schute and Lewis in their studies of cholinergic systems in the brain[31]. The results of injecting ^{3}H-leucine into the HNDB of rats show wide-spread projections to tubercle and peduncle, including AON, as well as the bulb[33]; the fibers entering the bulb are seen to run in close proximity to the LOT in confirmation of degeneration studies[27]. Divac[11] has identified neo-cortical and brain-stem projections also from HNDB, but it is not clear if the same neurones project to all three regions.

The tubercle contains islands of labelled cells after injections of HRP confined to the main bulb[10,20]. Some of these cells may well represent a caudal extension of AON. The prepyriform cortex adjacent to the peduncle blends imperceptibly with the AON and contains many labelled cells particu-larly immediately adjacent to the main LOT (PP2 of Rose) in layer II. This explains in part some of the earlier controversy[14,27] concerning the tubercle and prepyriform cortex as sources of centrifugal fibers to the bulb. Inevit-ably, a lesion encroaching on this PP2 region will affect not only the centri-fugal system running near the tract itself, but also the projection arising from the immediately adjacent cortex.

Aminergic projections involving 5HT from the raphe, and noradrenaline from the locus coeruleus have been described entering the bulb[3,7]. These projections are confirmed by labelling of cells in the locus coeruleus and raphe after deposition of HRP into the bulb[3,15,20] but their functions remain unknown.

POSSIBLE FUNCTIONS OF THE OLFACTORY CENTRIFUGAL SYSTEMS

Centrifugal input to the bulb could have an overall depressive action[5,21] on induced or resting activity, or could enhance and excite such activity by direct excitation or by disinhibition, as has been suggested by Pager et al[26]. It is also possible that the analytical and selective actions of the bulb might be influenced, e.g. by way of sharpening inhibitory surrounds or by causing a redistribution of excitability over the mitral and tufted cell receptive fields (in a manner analogous to that suggested for the centrifugal fibers to the retina in the turtle[6]), or it might be, as Granit has proposed[15], that centrifugal activity could be concerned in some way with "clearing" the system so that new messages can be written out in a "clean state". At any event, the olfactory bulb receives at least two centrifugal systems, the one derived from HNDB, the other from AON and cortex, and it seems unlikely that both these would be concerned with similar actions in the bulb particularly since HNDB has only secondary olfactory afferent relations.

From the summary in Price and Powell[28] (Fig.10), the bulbar relays of their two categories of centrifugal fibers, commissural (AC) and HNDB, are quite different. The commissural centrifugals are directed to the dendritic shafts and basal dendrites of the granule cells. These synapses are responsible for the large graded negativities recorded from the internal granule cell layer when stimulating the commissural system[12,18], and presumably would assist dendro-dendritic inhibition of mitral cells. By contrast, HNDB fibers are shown relaying with asymmetric synapses at the gemmule level on the granule cell dendrites immediately adjacent to the dendro-dendritic synapse, in which event the response to HNDB stimulation would be a positivity virtually identical to that of retrograde activation of the dendro-dendritic system by LOT stimulation, or the HNDB fibers could apply "presynaptic" inhibition to the gemmules. The interpretation of potentials evoked in the bulb by retrograde LOT stimulation is rather difficult despite the excellent work of Rall and Shepherd[30], particularly when LOT stimulation is interacted inadvertently or deliberately with the centrifugal systems originating from the cortex and AON. In the absence of barbiturate anaesthesia, "dendro-dendritic" inhibition is often absent after the first few milliseconds. Responses to paired LOT shocks do not necessarily interact in an inhibitory fashion, although, as Stewart and Scott[32] have also shown, in the presence of barbiturate this does occur. It is an old observation that the bulbar systems are peculiarly sensitive to barbiturate which reinforces inhibitory actions in the bulb[21].

ELECTROPHYSIOLOGY OF THE CENTRIFUGAL SYSTEMS

Electrical stimulation of AON, provided it does not engage the peripherally placed LOT fibers, evokes purely negative potentials of high amplitude in the olfactory bulbs, as does stimulation of the anterior commissure fibers. These potentials are most prominent in the granule cell layer, and are presumably synaptic potentials in that they summate with a sustained negativity following stimulus trains applied to the commissure[18]. Similar negative potentials are generated in the bulb by stimulation of widespread areas in the pyriform cortex and tubercle. These potentials are partly bilateral and partly ipsilateral[8,9]. The pathways involved in these effects are not well understood; some relay in the AON, and our impression is that several systems are activated in such experiments. Our anatomical studies indicate that some areas, particularly the cortex overlying the tract (PP2 cortex), project directly to the bulb without relay[2,10,15,20], but we have not been able to identify responses due unequivocally to activation of these particular cells in the anterior olfactory cortex.

Surprisingly, no significant potentials definitely assignable to the HNDB system can be identified in the bulb following electrical stimulation of HNDB under the recording conditions we employ, with bipolar recording electrodes straddling the mitral cell layer, in any of the species so far studied (cat, ferret, rat, rabbit, guinea pig and phalanger). There is indeed a remarkable paucity of bulbar evoked potentials resulting from stimulation of HNDB region, in sharp contrast to the surrounding areas which on stimulation are very effective in causing evoked potentials in the bulb[8], (Fig.5)[9], (Fig. 2), which in itself may be highly significant.

Using induced waves as an index of bulbar activity resulting from odorant stimulation, we have explored the effects of stimulating the centrifugal systems in rabbits prepared, as in all our induced wave experiments, with full local anaesthetic ritual and destruction of the mesio-diencephalic junction in the region of the central grey and central tegmental fasciculus (known to be involved in pain transmission[22]) prior to immobilization and lightening of the anaesthesia. Bulbar induced waves are readily modified by anterior commissure activation, either through olfactory stimulation of

the opposite bulb, or by electrical stimulation of the commissure[18,21].
Contra-lateral olfactory stimulation depresses induced waves if the timing is
correct[18]. The effects of electrical stimulation depend on the frequency of
stimuli applied. Low frequency stimulation drives the bulb, and the induced
waves entrain at the applied frequency, whilst high frequency stimulation
abolishes or occludes the induced waves[21]. At least part of the centrifugal
influences from pyriform cortex and tubercle are mediated through the AON,
and the results of stimulating these regions closely resemble those of stimulating the commissure itself.

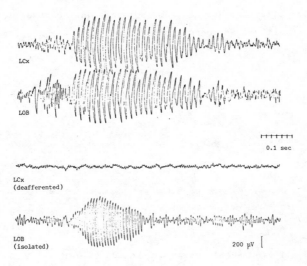

Figure 1. Removal of cortical centrifugal influences on induced waves by
bulb isolation in the phalanger.

The influence of the olfactory cortex upon bulbar activity can also be
seen (Fig. 1) where the later, lower frequency component of the induced waves
(upper records), which is closely related to parallel activity in the pyriform cortex, is eliminated by isolating the bulb with a section passing
through the rostral peduncle ahead of AON (lower records). Such an "isolated" bulb produces remarkably regular and reproducible patterns of induced
waves[36]. Since all influences, including the AON, have been eliminated this
indicates that induced waves, whatever the mechanism of their generation,
arise from intrinsic systems within the bulb, and that the later irregular
components of slower frequency are due to centrifugal influences arising from

the cortex which itself becomes inactive following isolation. The significance of this feedback is not immediately clear since this later, slower frequency component of induced waves is generally obscured in records taken from
the free moving animal.

Concomitant electrical activation of HNDB (100 Hz) during olfactory
stimulation has only marginal effects on induced waves, most often an increased amplitude (Fig.2). Here there is little effect of HNDB stimulation (S)
in the resting bulb, beyond a brief transient at the onset of stimulation.
In this experiment olfactory stimulation (O) produced only a small burst of
induced waves with little sign of the later component of cortical origin.
Combined HNDB and olfactory stimulation (SO) gave an increased amplitude of
the induced waves without any conspicuous action on their frequency or the
duration of the burst.

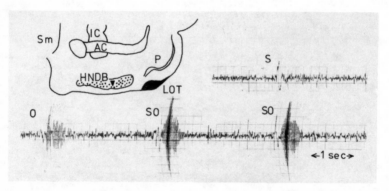

Figure 2. HNDB elicited augmentation of induced waves.

Despite the supposed major connections of the HNDB system in relation to
the dendro-dendritic synapses between mitral and granule cell, from these results one is tempted to look for removal of inhibition in some as yet unidentified synaptic region concerned in controlling the mechanism for generating
induced waves. Yamamoto and Iwama[35] saw an increased amplitude of induced
waves upon stimulating "hypothalamic" sites, probably HNDB. Also, in the
original paper[21] we saw a similar increase upon surface stimulation of the
ipsilateral basal cortex, generally delivered at HNDB levels. Many of the
interactions between olfaction and the psychological set of the animal[17,23,25,26]
are likely to be quite subtle, and it may well be that recordings of
induced waves are not at all suited to such studies. However, the present
results confirm the role of the pyriform cortex in centrifugal control of olfactory activity, and raise important questions concerning the nature and
action of the HNDB system as presently understood.

REFERENCES
1. Broadwell, R.D. (1975) J.Comp.Neurol. 164, 329-346.
2. Broadwell, R.D. (1975) J.Comp.Neurol. 164, 389-410.
3. Broadwell, R.D. and Jacobowitz, D.M. (1976) J.Comp.Neurol. 170, 321-346.
4. Cajal, S. Ramon y. (1901) Trab.lab.invest.biol. Madrid 1, 1-140,189-206.
5. Callens, M. (1965) Peripheral and Central Regulatory Mechanism of the Excitability in the Olfactory System. Thesis. Arscia Uitgaven, Brussels.
6. Cervetto, L., Marchiafava, P.L. and Pasino, E. (1976) Nature (Lond.) 260,56-57.
7. Dahlström, A., Fuxe, K., Olsson, L. and Ungerstedt, U. (1965) Life Sci. 4, 2071-2074.
8. Dennis, B.J. and Kerr, D.I.B. (1968) Brain Res. 11, 373-396.
9. Dennis, B.J. and Kerr, D.I.B. (1975) J.Comp.Neurol. 159, 129-148.
10. Dennis, B.J. and Kerr, D.I.B. (1976) Brain Res. 110, 593-600.
11. Divac, I. (1975) Brain Res. 93, 385-398
12. Duval, G. and Leveteau, J. (1974) Brain Res. 78, 395-410.
13. Granit, R. (1976) Aggressologie 17(A), 5-9.
14. Heimer, L. (1968) J.Anat.(Lond.) 103, 413-432.
15. Heimer, L. (1977) in The Continuing Evolution of the Limbic Concept, in Press, Plenum Press, New York.
16. Heimer, L. and Wilson, R.D. (1975) in Golgi Centennial Symposium Proceedings, Santini, M., Edit. pp 177-193, Raven Press, New York.
17. Hernandez-Peon, R., Lavin, A., Alcocer-Cuaron, C. and Marcelin, J.P. (1960) EEG Clin.Neurophysiol. 12, 41-58.
18. Kerr, D.I.B. (1960) Austral.J.Exp.Biol.Med.Sci. 38, 29-36.
19. Kerr, D.I.B. and Dennis, B.J. (1972) Brain Res. 36, 399-403.
20. Kerr, D.I.B. and Dennis, B.J. (1976) Austral.Physiol.Pharmacol.Soc.Proc. 7, 90.
21. Kerr, D.I.B. and Hagbarth, K.-E (1955) J.Neurophysiol. 18, 362-374.
22. Kerr, D.I.B., Haugen, F.P. and Melzack, R. (1955) Amer.J.Physiol. 183, 253-258.
23. Le Magnen, J. (1975) in Olfaction and Taste V.Proc. of the Fifth International Symposium, pp 381-388. Academic Press, New York.
24. Moliner, E., Ramon, - (1975) Advances in Neurology 12, 135-147.
25. Pager, J. (1974) Physiol.Behav. 12, 189-195.
26. Pager, J., Giachetti, I., Holley, A. and Le Magnen, J. (1972) Physiol. Behav. 9, 573-579.
27. Price, J.L. and Powell, T.P.S. (1970) J.Anat. 107, 215-237.
28. Price, J.L. and Powell, T.P.S. (1970) J.Anat. 107, 239-256.
29. Price, J.L. and Powell, T.P.S. (1971) J.Anat. 110, 105-126.
30. Rall, W. and Shepherd, G.M. (1968) J.Neurophysiol. 31, 884-915.
31. Schute, C.C.D. and Lewis, P.R. (1967) Brain, 90, 497-522.
32. Stewart, W.B. and Scott, J.W. (1976) Brain Res. 103, 487-499.
33. Swanson, L.W. (1976) J.Comp.Neurol. 167, 227-256.
34. Valverde, F. (1965) Studies on the Piriform Lobe, Harvard Univ.Press, Cambridge, Mass.
35. Yamamoto, C. and Iwama, K. (1960) Neurologia med. -chir. 2, 77-81.
36. My colleague, Dr Barbara J. Dennis has given invaluable help with all aspects of this work. Figure 1 is based on studies by Dr Peter R.Wilson in my laboratories.

Histochemical localization and identification of secretory products in salamander olfactory epithelium

Thomas V. Getchell and Marilyn L. Getchell

Department of Physiology, Yale University School of Medicine, 333 Cedar Street, New Haven, CT 06510, USA

ABSTRACT

Secretory products were identified and localized in the olfactory epithelium of the salamander. Using histochemical techniques, acidic and possibly sulfated mucopolysaccharides were found in the supranuclear region of sustentacular cells. Neutral mucopolysaccharides were found in the acinar cells of Bowman's gland. The secretory material in the sustentacular cell appeared vesicular and that in Bowman's gland appeared granular. Various mechanisms by which secretion may be initiated and the role which secretory products may play in the integrated physiological activity of the olfactory epithelium are discussed.

Initial results of an electrophysiological study investigating intracellularly recorded responses in the salamander olfactory epithelium suggested that sustentacular cells may release secretory products in response to odour stimulation[10,11]. Evidence obtained using electronmicroscopy[3,13,21,25] and extracellular recording techniques[9,21] also suggested secretory activity in other species. Histological and histochemical investigations of the salamander olfactory epithelium were performed to determine further details of the cellular organization and to locate, identify and characterize the secretory products of the sustentacular cells and Bowman's gland. This study is an extension of our research leading to an understanding of the integrated physiological activity of the olfactory epithelium.

Land-phase salamanders, Ambystoma tigrinum, were anesthetized by chilling and further immobilized with D-tubocurarine (0.05-0.1 ml, 3 mg/ml). The nasal cavities were surgically exposed by removal of the overlying skin, cartilage and dorsal epithelium. For the Golgi study, the ventral epithelium was fixed in situ with 2.5% glutaraldehyde and 0.75% OsO$_4$ in 0.1 M phosphate (pH 5.9) or acetate (pH 4) buffer. Blocks of tissue were removed, further fixed, embedded in epon and sectioned at 50 μm. Cellular impregnation was achieved by use of a combination of previously reported methods[19,30]. For the histochemical study, the ventral epithelium was fixed in situ with a few drops of

10% formalin. The animals were then decapitated and exsanguinated. Blocks
of tissue were removed and further fixed in formalin, paraffin-embedded and
sectioned at 3-5 μm. Histochemical reagents employed were toluidine blue[16],
cresyl violet[18], alcian green[24], alcian blue[16] and alcian blue-periodic-
acid-Schiff (AB-PAS)[16].

The cellular organization of the salamander olfactory epithelium resembled that described for land vertebrates in general[13]. It ranges in thickness
from 200 to 300 μm. Three cell types were present in the pseudostratified
neurepithelium (Fig. 1A): olfactory receptor, sustentacular and basal cells.
The nuclei of these cell types were generally stratified. The densely staining, elongated sustentacular cell nuclei (SC) lay distally about 20-35 μm from
the epithelial surface which was covered with mucus (MU). It was difficult to
realistically estimate the thickness of the mucus layer in fixed material, but
it appeared to be about 10-15 μm. Ovoid receptor cell nuclei (ORC) lay primarily in the intermediate zone, and the irregularly shaped basal cell nuclei
(BC) lay in close proximity to the basement membrane. Bowman's glands are
large simple tubulo-alveolar exocrine glands (Fig. 1A,D) which may consist of
more than one acinus. They usually lay at different depths within the submucosa (SM) and opened to the mucosal surface via secretory ducts which tra-
versed the neurepithelium (Fig. 1D; Fig. 2). Occasionally a complete acinus
lay within the epithelium proper. Acinar lengths ranged from approximately
100 μm for those lying intraepithelially to several hundred microns for those
lying in the submucosa. Nerve bundles, blood vessels and loosely organized
connective tissue were also present in the submucosa.

Figure 1B shows the morphology of an olfactory receptor as revealed by
the Golgi technique. The slender dendrite of the primary bipolar neuron was
approximately 80 μm long and about 2 μm in diameter. Dendritic lengths were
variable, ranging from about 50 μm to 180 μm. The soma was approximately 10
μm wide and 20 μm long. Much of the soma volume was occupied by the nucleus.
A small diameter unmyelinated axon formed at the base of the soma. The axons
have been classified as "C" fibers in other species[13]. Occasionally, the
secretory duct of the Bowman's gland became impregnated during Golgi staining.
As seen in Fig. 1D right, the distal intraepithelial portion of the duct was
relatively straight and was 8-10 μm wide. The cells lining the secretory duct
appeared distinctly different from the other cell types in the epithelium as
discussed above (see Fig. 1A,D).

Histochemical techniques showed that the supranuclear region of sustentacular cells contained vesicle-associated material which showed metachromasia

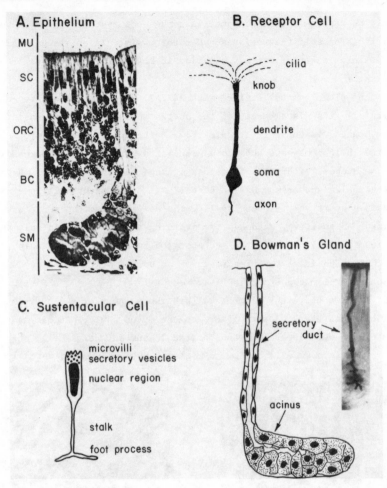

A. Epithelium

MU
SC
ORC
BC
SM

B. Receptor Cell

cilia
knob
dendrite
soma
axon

C. Sustentacular Cell

microvilli
secretory vesicles
nuclear region
stalk
foot process

D. Bowman's Gland

secretory duct
acinus

Fig. 1. Cellular organization of the salamander olfactory epithelium shown by a Heidenhain-stained section (A). Schematic drawings of olfactory receptor (B) and sustentacular (C) cells, and Bowman's gland (D) derived from Golgi and histochemical studies, and electronmicroscopy.

when stained with toluidine blue (Fig. 2A; arrows) and cresyl violet. In addition, the presumed secretory material stained positively with alcian green and alcian blue. These staining reactions indicated the presence of acidic and possibly sulfated mucopolysaccharides (MPS) as a component of sustentacular cell secretory products. In some cells, only the most apical part of the supranuclear region stained intensely with alcian blue. Between this and the nucleus was a region that was moderately PAS positive. This staining pattern was also reported for goblet cells of the tracheal mucosa where it was interpreted to represent mucosubstance in a phase of synthesis not yet bearing sialic acid or sulfated residues. Metachromasia, alcian green or blue positive staining material was not observed in Bowman's glands or other cells in the epithelium.

When the epithelium was stained with AB-PAS, the supranuclear region, and particularly its distal zone, of the sustentacular cells stained intensely blue and appeared vesicular (Fig. 2B, arrow). The acinar cells of Bowman's gland stained bright magenta and had a granular appearance. The Bowman's glands lying deepest within the submucosa stained a deeper shade of magenta, and their granular appearance was enhanced. All cells observable in a single acinus stained positively. Occasionally, the cells lining the secretory duct also stained PAS positive, although the staining appeared less intense and somewhat less granular than in the secretory cells comprising the acinus proper. The PAS positive staining reaction of Bowman's gland indicated the presence of neutral mucopolysaccharides.

Thus, the two secretory elements within the salamander olfactory mucosa may contribute different classes of MPS to the mucus sheet. Acidic and possibly sulfated MPS were identified and located in sustentacular cells and neutral MPS in the acinar cells of Bowman's glands. These results were also

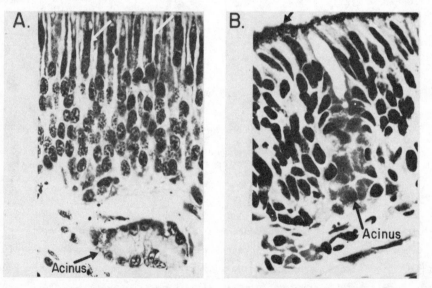

Fig. 2. Sections from the salamander olfactory epithelium stained with toluidine blue (A) and AB-PAS (B). The arrows in the upper region of each section show the location of MPS in the supranuclear region of the sustentacular cell. The acinus of Bowman's gland lies in the submucosa (A) or intraepithelially (B).

observed in the frog, mudpuppy and turtle olfactory epithelia in our studies. In contrast, in the mouse and rat olfactory epithelia, sustentacular cells showed staining reactions indicating the presence of neutral MPS, while Bowman's gland cells stained positively for both neutral and acidic MPS.

Detailed experimental results describing the ionic and organic composition of olfactory mucus have not been reported, nor have its rheological properties been thoroughly investigated. The mucus layer serves several important functions. It protects the epithelial cells from particulate, bacterial and viral contamination and dehydration. The mucus sheet appears to separate odours spatially analogous to a chromatographic-like function[14]. It also dissolves and disseminates odours. It provides a semi-rigid matrix for olfactory cilia and is the ionic environment in which the postulated binding of the stimulus to receptor molecules occurs.

The functions of specific classes of MPS, i.e., acidic and neutral MPS, are presently not well defined[2]. Acidic MPS have been implicated in a variety of activities related to their negative charge at physiological pH that could have bearing on their role in olfactory mucus. For example, acidic and sulfated MPS may provide ion-binding sites[6]. Intestinal goblet cell MPS bind calcium ions which can be displaced by sodium ions[7]. Thus, acidic MPS may function to regulate the ionic composition of mucus in the immediate environment of the apical region of the receptor cell where transduction is postulated to occur. In addition, the charges on the carboxyl or sulfate groups of acidic MPS may interact with odour molecules or with charged components on olfactory receptor proteins. Neutralization of these charges could affect the interaction of protein receptor molecules with odours[12]. Acidic MPS have also been shown to inhibit the activity of certain hydrolases through complex formation while enhancing the activity of others, possibly by stabilizing them against enzymatic breakdown[17]. Enzymes have been found in the olfactory mucus layer[5,27]. The ability of acidic MPS to inhibit or enhance enzymatic activity may regulate the postulated enzymatic degradation involved in removal of olfactory stimuli[23].

Okano and Takagi[21] reported histological evidence of sustentacular cell secretion in the bullfrog olfactory epithelium only when certain stimuli, e.g., chloroform or tert-butyl alcohol, elicited a positive electro-olfactogram. Odours which evoked negative electro-olfactograms, e.g., amyl acetate or n-butyl alcohol, caused no apparent release of secretory products from sustentacular cells. This implies that certain types of compounds preferentially release the secretory products from sustentacular cells. The secretory products, identified as acidic MPS in our study, may serve a specific function when certain stimuli generally regarded as anaesthetics or irritants are taken into the nasal cavity. The term anaesthetic is used in its pharmacological context, and the term irritant is used more broadly to include those compounds which cause relatively nonspecific perturbations in the cell membrane which may or may not evoke disagreeable odour sensations. Thus, the possible stimulus-initiated release of acidic MPS from the sustentacular cells into the mucus layer may provide a crucial protective factor for the salamander and frog olfactory epithelia by changing the composition of mucus in close proximity to the epithelial surface.

Secretory products of Bowman's glands have been characterized in many species. Neutral MPS have been found in secretory cells of Bowman's glands in the salamander, frog, axolotl, triton and lizard[22], rabbit[14,29], rhesus monkey[27], hogs and seals[14], mouse[6] and rats[4]. Acidic MPS have also been found in Bowman's gland cell of the grass snake and viper[22], mouse, rabbits and birds[6], toads and cats[20].

In a detailed ultrastructural study of Bowman's glands in a variety of mammals, Seifert[26] described the presence of two types of secretory cells in the glandular acinus, the dark and light cells. These different cell types have been postulated to represent different developmental stages or different functional states of secretory cells, or secretory vs. non-secretory cells. One may speculate that the dark cells, shown in previous studies to be PAS positive[26], correspond to neutral MPS-containing cells while the light cells correspond to those in this study which stained with alcian blue and presumably secrete acidic MPS. Further detailed studies in mammalian species are required to resolve this difficult point.

Mechanisms by which the acinar cells of Bowman's gland are induced to release their secretory products have not been investigated. Several mechanisms may be possible. Diffusion of stimuli through the secretory duct to the acinar cells may be one. Electrical activation would also be possible if it could be demonstrated that the cells of the secretory duct were electrically coupled by gap junctions and that the most distal duct cells were chemically sensitive. Although efferent innervation of the acinar cells has not been described, neural or hormonal regulation could modulate secretory activity. It is also not known whether or not the composition or concentration of the secretory product is changed by the duct cells as it traverses its way through the duct to the epithelial surface. Independent of these considerations, the secretory products of Bowman's glands may be involved in the determination of the rheological properties of the mucus layer and its long-term maintenance.

The results reported in this communication have described certain basic

histochemical properties of the secretory components of the sustentacular
cells and Bowman's glands in the salamander olfactory epithelium.   They form
the basis for continuing studies on the integrated physiological activity of
the vertebrate olfactory epithelium.   Further physiological, ultrastructural
and histochemical studies are required further to identify and characterize
the secretory products of sustentacular cells and Bowman's gland, the factors
which initiate secretion, and the effect of these secretions on the functioning of olfactory receptors and their effect on controlling the accessibility
of odours to the epithelial surface[1,11,12,15].

ACKNOWLEDGEMENT
     The authors thank Dr. William Miller for use of certain equipment
required for histological procedures and photomicroscopy, and Karen Beardsley
for assistance with the histology.   Supported by NSF Grant BNS 76-81404.

REFERENCES
1.   Bannister, L.H. (1974) in Transduction Mechanisms in Chemoreception,
     pp. 39-45, Information Retrieval Limited, London
2.   Barrett, A.J. (1971)
     Histochem. J. 3, 213-221
3.   Bloom, G. (1954)
     A. Zellforsch. 41, 89-100
4.   Bosjen-Moller, F. (1964)
     Anat. Rec. 150, 11-24
5.   Cuschieri, A. (1974)
     J. Anat. 118, 477-489
6.   Cuschieri, A. and Bannister, L.H. (1974)
     Histochem. J. 6, 543-558
7.   Forstner, J.F. and Forstner, G.G. (1975)
     Biochim. Biophys. Acta 386, 283-292
8.   Getchell, M.L. and Gesteland, R.C. (1972)
     Proc. Nat. Acad. Sci. 69, 1494-1498
9.   Getchell, T.V. (1974)
     J. Neurophysiol. 37, 1115-1130
10. Getchell, T.V. (1977)
     Brain Research 123, 275-286
11. Getchell, T.V. (1977) in Internat. Symp. Food Intake Chem. Sens.
     in press, Univ. of Tokyo Press, Tokyo
12. Getchell, T.V. and Getchell, M.L. (1977)
     Chem. Sens. Flav. 2, 313-326
13. Graziadei, P.P.C. (1971) in Handbook of Sensory Physiology,
     Vol. IV, pp. 27-58, Springer-Verlag, Berlin
14. Herberhold, C. (1968)
     Arch. Klin. exp. Ohr.-, Nas.- und Kehlk, Heilk. 190, 166-182
15. Hornung, D.E. and Mozell, M.M. (1977)
     J. Gen. Physiol. 69, 343-361
16. Humason, G.L. (1967) Animal Tissue Techniques,
     pp. 296-297, pp. 326-327, W.H. Freeman and Company, San Francisco
17. Kint, J.A., Dacremont, G., Carton, D., Drye, E. and Hooft, C. (1973)
     Science 181, 352-354
18. Luna, L.G. (1968) Manual of Histological Staining Methods of the Armed
     Forces Institute of Pathology,
     pp. 212-213, McGraw-Hill Book Company, New York

19. Morest, D.K. and Morest, R.R. (1966)
    Am. J. Anat. 118, 811-832
20. Moulton, D.G. and Beidler, L.M. (1967)
    Physiol. Rev. 47, 1-52
21. Okano, M. and Takagi, S.F. (1974)
    J. Physiol. 242, 353-370
22. Oledzka-Slotwinska, H. (1961)
    Compt. Rend. Assoc. Anat. (Nancy) 46, 876-889
23. Ottoson, D. (1963)
    Pharmacol. Rev. 15, 1-42
24. Putt, F.A. (1972) Manual of Histopathological Staining Methods,
    pp. 134-135, Wiley-Interscience, New York
25. Reese, T.S. (1965)
    J. Cell Biol. 22, 209-230
26. Seifert, K. (1971)
    Arch. Klin. exp. Ohr.-, Nas.- und Kehlk. Heilk. 200, 252-274
27. Shantha, T.R. and Nakajima, Y. (1970)
    Z. Zellforsch. 103, 291-319
28. Spicer, S.S., Chakrin, L.W., Wardell, J.R. and Kendrick, W. (1971)
    Lab. Invest. 25, 483-490
29. Winnin, K. (1964)
    J. Wakayama Med. Soc. 15, 213-221
30. Wong-Riley, M.T.T. (1974)
    J. Neurocytol. 3, 1-33

Receptor sensitivity, acceptor distribution, convergence and neural coding in the olfactory system

André Holley and Kjell B. Døving*

Université Claude Bernard, 69621 Villeurbanne, France
*Institute of Zoophysiology, Post Box 1051, Oslo 3, Norway

ABSTRACT

A synthetic view of the function of the first stages of the olfactory system is proposed to assemble recent experimental and conceptual advances in
the fields of receptor physiology, spatial distribution of sensibility, and
olfactory bulb organization. The importance of the convergence of the olfactory receptor cells onto the secondary neurons with respect to odour sensitivity and quality coding is evaluated in connection with the notion of receptor response probability. A model is described in which the spatially
heterogeneous distribution of sensitivity (chemotopy) in the olfactory mucosa is presented as a consequence of a variation in density for different
types of odorant acceptors. The topological projection of the peripheral
chemotopy onto the bulb accounts for the bulbar chemotopy and gives a spatial basis to the across fibre pattern which encodes each odour quality.

INTRODUCTION

The olfactory system of vertebrates is renowned for its high sensitivity to odours and its great capacity for discriminating stimulus quality.
Hitherto these sujects have been considered to be independent, we shall ad-
vocate a unified view. Work done in recent years has increased our understanding of the function of the olfactory system. Advances have been specially noteworthy in the fields of receptor physiology, the concept of spatial
sensitivity, and the organization of the olfactory bulb. We think that at
present it might be fruitful to relate the results of the recent studies
with the old and well established fact that thousands of receptor fibers
converge onto a common secondary neuron.

The first part of our discussion will consider the sensitivity of the
olfactory system where convergence plays, in our view, an essential role.
Secondly, we shall try to explain why we think it is necessary to give a
unified view of the concepts of sensitivity distribution, receptor properties, and convergence to understand the coding of odour quality.

We shall expose one possible solution to this problem. Finally, we shall discuss some properties of the transduction mechanisms in the olfactory system.

ODOUR SENSITIVITY

In studies of the olfactory receptors it can be shown that the responses of the receptor cells are dependent upon the concentration of the odour stimulus in a predictable manner[1-3]. The example of cell recordings from the frog olfactory mucosa in Fig. 1 will serve to illustrate this point. In the bottom trace, there is no evident response after presentation of the odorant. When the concentration is increased, a response appears as a greater density of spikes. Doubling the concentration of the odorant causes an additional augmentation of the frequency of firing. Slightly higher concentrations cause further increases in frequency. A fact to be noted is the small concentration range from no response to maximum firing frequency, the range usually being less than one decade. Three other features of the responses can be seen. These are the shortening of the response burst, the decrease in spike amplitude and the prolongation of the silent period after the initial response, all of which follow an increase in stimulus concentration. In a study of many receptor cells, most of them showed a steep increase in firing rate as a function of the concentration[3].

The maximum frequency of the initial burst is only one way of describing the relation between the response and the stimulus concentration. Another parameter of the response is the number of spikes in the burst, which reaches a maximum and then decreases[4]. This feature of the response can be seen in Fig. 1 and has been illustrated in the diagram in Fig. 2. Since different receptor cells might give the maximum number of spikes at different concentrations, Gesteland has suggested that receptors are tuned to a limited range of concentration.

These results have been obtained with relatively high odorant concentrations, far above the one at which animals usually react to the odours. Even though we lack experimental verification of this statement, it seems remote to consider that odorant detection is limited to concentrations at 1/100th to 1/10th of the saturated vapour pressure. Let us therefore consider what happens at threshold level.

At threshold concentration the response of the receptor cell is less conspicuous than at higher concentration levels. Repeating the stimulus at one and the same concentration will not necessarily lead to the same response : sometimes there is an obvious response, sometimes not. The random character

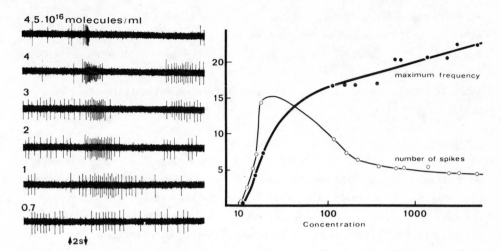

Fig. 1 : Responses of a receptor
cell to various concen-
trations of anisole.

Fig. 2 : Two ways of representing
the concentration-response
function.

of the stimulus as well as of the response comes into play. The response properties of the receptor cells and specially the statistical fluctuations of
these responses at low concentration have been studied by van Drongelen[5].
He has shown that even when there is no visible response present in the receptors, a summation of several traces demonstrates a distinct increase in number of spikes after the onset of the stimulation. In the case where the receptor cells are quiet or silent, a response can be considered as the appearance
of one or more spikes within a given period after stimulus presentation. Van
Drongelen has proposed the term response probability to describe the incerti-
tude of the response; this term indicates the fraction of odour presentations
that will lead to a response, in this case one or more spikes.

Let us consider the response characteristics in relation to convergence.
Every secondary neuron in the bulb receives input from a great number of primary fibers. The mean number of receptor axons to mitral cells has been estimated to be around 1000 : 1 in the rabbit, and seems to be of the same order
of magnitude in several other animals[6-8].The convergence will increase the
probability that a stimulus is detected at the level of the secondary neuron.
A mathematical analysis of the relation between the response probability of
the receptors cells and that of the secondary neurons shows that when 1000
receptors converge onto one secondary neuron and when these receptors have a

response probability of .001, the secondary neuron will have a response probability of .64^9. This way of considering stimulus detection in secondary neurons leads to the conclusion that, due to the convergence, odour detection in the olfactory system is liable to occur at concentrations far below the one which is commonly used to demonstrate a conspicuous response in the receptor cells.

CODING OF ODOUR QUALITY

To express the need for a unified view on odour quality coding, it might be useful to expose problems that may well be resolved by this view. As examples we can use the known properties : that the identification of any odour can take place over a wide intensity range; that for any given odour a greater part of the bulbar neurons are engaged; that odour discrimination is possible despite the mixing of sensitivities occuring in individual receptor cells, and the convergence of the receptors in the glomeruli. We shall return to these problems later but we shall first describe properties of the olfactory system that, in our view, are essential to its understanding.

As has been shown by several studies, the receptor cells respond to a great variety of odorants$^{10-12}$. Fig. 3 is an extract of the results obtained in a study^{13} of the responses of frog olfactory receptors to 20 odorants.

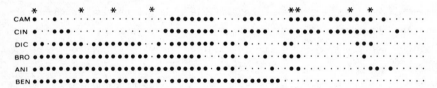

Fig. 3 : A matrix of the responses of 60 receptor cells to 6 odorants.
        (From Revial et al., 1977)

Each column represents the properties of one receptor cell; a large dot indicates a response, a small dot, no response. From this figure it is evident that benzene (BEN) and anisole (ANI) very often activate the same receptors, but also some cells will respond to one but not to the other. Thus discrimination of each will be possible. When examining another pair of odorants, camphor (CAM) and anisole (ANI), it can be seen that 25 cells respond to anisole, 14 to camphor, and 11 respond to both substances. The possibility of odour discrimination is higher than in the previous case of anisole and benzene. If the concentration used to study the receptor properties is diminished, will the cells respond in the same way? Will the odour discrimination be better at a lower concentration? In table 1 we have extracted values which concern the ability of the cells to respond to anisole and camphor from experiments made at two different concentrations.

	Concentration	
	high	low
ANI + CAM	11	2
ANI	14	8
CAM	25	18
No response	10	30
Total	60	58

Table 1   Effect of odour trials in two series of experiments at different odour concentrations.

The numbers for the responses to the high concentrations come from the study just mentioned and are extracted from Fig. 3. At the low concentration the number of cells responding to the odorants was less than in the study at high concentration and the number of cells responding to both odorants decreased from 11 to 2. The impression left by this comparison is that odour discrimination is better at lower concentration since fewer cells confuse the two stimuli. However, the statistics do not support this conclusion : the difference in distribution of the responding cells is not significant.

Again we shall consider the properties of the receptor cells in connexion with the concept of response probability. The fact that receptor cells respond in a particular fashion to an odorant indicates that they have one or several mechanisms for recognizing this stimulus. Thus an illustration of receptor cell properties, e.g. the one given in Fig. 3, is no longer only an abstract image of receptor responses but a demonstration of the physical properties of these 60 cells in relation to a particular set of odorants. The conspicuous responses will naturally decrease with diminished odour concentration, but the property of being excited will not. The response probability of the cell will follow the law given by statistics and the odour concentration. A study that uses the high concentrations will be more suitable for revealing the properties of the receptor cells than one in which the concentrations are kept at a low level, on conditions that the odour substances do not induce unspecific effects that have nothing to do with the odour recognizing mechanisms. The problem has been discussed thoroughly by Revial et al.[13].

We have discussed above the properties of the receptor cells taken as isolated elements within the system. Convergence, however, necessitates reflections in the ways in which the elements are coupled in the bulb.

Let us assume that the 60 receptor cells in the Fig. 3 have been found in one animal. What would be the consequences to discrimination in the olfactory bulb resulting from different ways of connecting these cells? One extreme case will be found when 60 cells connect to one mitral cell, when no discrimination may be possible. The other case will be when each receptor cell together with 999 others of the same type converge to one mitral cell. Thus in the bulb 60 mitral cells share the same response profiles as the 60 receptor cells shown in Fig. 3, in which case the sensitivity of the mitral cell would be greatly augmented by the effect of convergence as discussed above. The reality may lie somewhere between the two cases : neither homogeneous mixing nor complete separation of the very large number of sensitivity profiles actually represented in an olfactory mucosa.

We have first considered the receptor cells as isolated elements and then the ways in which they might be connected; now we shall examine the spatial distribution of these elements in the receptor sheet and their termination in the bulb. There are two lines of findings that will be of interest in this connection. One concerns the somatotopic projection from the mucosa to the bulb, the other is the spatial distribution of sensitivity in the mucosa and the olfactory bulb.

The somatotopic projection from the epithelium to the bulb has been demonstrated by Le Gros Clark [14] and by Land [15]. The latter study showed that cutting a small nerve bundle in the dorsal aspect of the mucosa caused a degeneration of nerve terminals in the glomeruli in the dorsal part of the bulb with an anterior posterior distribution. On the other hand, it is known that the sensitivity of the mucosa is not evenly distributed throughout the surface. This has been shown by several authors in amphibia [16-19] and in rat [20]. An example of the spatial distribution of sensitivity found in the olfactory mucosa in the rat is shown in Fig. 4. The cross-hatched areas show the region of the cribriform plate with the highest sensitivity for the odorants acetophenone, cycloundecanone, camphor and heptanal. In the bulb one should expect a certain chemotopology obtained through the somatotopic projection of the peripheral chemotopy. This has been verified experimentally, by electrophysiological means in the fish [21] and the rabbit [22-23]. With histological methods it is possible to observe morphological changes in the mitral cells after prolonged exposure of young animals to odours [24-25]. The effect named "selective degeneration" takes various spatial distributions depending upon the odorant

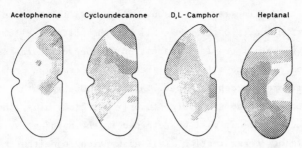

Acetophenone   Cycloundecanone   D,L-Camphor   Heptanal

Fig. 4 : The spatial distribution of the EOG responses to 4 odorants
on the cribriform plate, in the rat. (Thommesen and Døving, 1977)

and it is a clear demonstration of the non homogeneity of the olfactory bulb
in relation to odour discrimination. With the method of labeled deoxyglucose
uptake it is possible to demonstrate a spatial patterning of cell activity
resulting from a stimulation with an odour [26-28].

In view of the findings which have been briefly exposed above, we propose
a model which illustrates the concepts of spatial distribution, across fiber
pattern, odorant acceptor and convergence. The notion of "odorant acceptor"
has not been defined before but the usefulness of this concept will be evident in the last part of the discussion. This model is presented in Fig. 5.
Shown to the left of the figure are four different "acceptors" A,B,C, and D
which are unevenly distributed in the epithelium as shown to the left of the
figure. The sensitivity of the olfactory mucosa follows the spatial distribu-

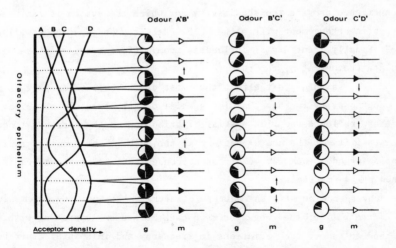

Fig. 5 : A model of the spatial distribution of the sensitivity in the
olfactory bulb.

tion of acceptor density. The receptor axons will convey information about this acceptor distribution onto the glomeruli and the mitral cells. From this point of view, the glomeruli provide a partition of the peripheral sensitivity continuum. Each glomerulus and mitral cell receives information proportional to the amount of different acceptor types. This does not imply that the receptor cells from a restricted area converge to only one glomerulus. The heterogeneity found in the epithelium will be retained in the bulb unless there is a specific principle of reorganization. This assumption is neither necessary to explain the experimental data nor useful to understanding the discriminative properties of the olfactory system. When the olfactory mucosa is exposed for example to an odorant (A'B') that fits the acceptors A and B, the mitral cells that receive the largest input from these acceptors will have the lowest threshold of firing. The mitral cells receiving a smaller input could be excited at a higher concentration but, due to lateral inhibition, it is conceivable that these cells will be inhibited by the mitral cells excited at a lower concentration. The result is an across fiber pattern of excitation and inhibition. This pattern has a spatial distribution coarsely reflecting the epithelial sensitivity. With other odorants, like the one fitting acceptors B and C and the one fitting C and D, other patterns of excited and inhibited mitral cells will emerge.

Following these lines of reasoning we can consider that both the olfactory mucosa, and the olfactory bulb code the odour quality in terms of an across fiber pattern which is spatially organized. The olfactory bulb will, by means of the convergence, provide the sensitivity for which the system is renowned. By the synaptic arrangement within the bulb [29] the response patterns will be contrasted. Finally, centrifugal influences from different areas in the brain will modulate the output of the bulb [30-31].

Our model is faithful to the fact that most of the bulb takes part in coding any odour quality in that the wide spatial distribution of the bulbar neural pattern reflects the wide spatial distribution of the peripheral acceptors. The stability of the neural pattern in the bulb, which permits stability in perception of odour quality at different concentrations of the odorants can be obtained by two mechanisms.

The convergence permits the pattern of mitral cell activity to emerge at a low concentration; the negative feed back mechanisms operating within the bulb tend to reduce the variations in frequency and in spatial distribution caused by the changes in concentration.

The sensitivity of the receptor cell is multiple. Whatever the principle

governing their connections with the mitral cells the sensitivity of the secondary neurons will also be multiple. The model explains how a set of mitral
cells with multiple and different sensitivities is able to discriminate one
odour from another. Each mitral cell can be regarded as detecting an aspect
of the properties of the odorant. A number of mitral cells can explore the
diversity of these properties, which will be sufficient to recognize the odour
as a particular quality.

The discriminative mechanisms that have been shown to operate in the olfactory system depend upon the properties of the receptor cells with respect
to the recognition of the odour molecules. Because our understanding of the
whole system will be dependent upon our understanding of the recognition mechanisms, we have introduced below a discussion of the transduction mechanisms in the receptors, focussing on the concept of acceptor.

TRANSDUCTION MECHANISMS

Apart from being important for our understanding of the neural coding of
olfactory quality, the data on the activity of primary receptors contain information relevant to studies on the odour recognizing mechanisms in the receptor cells.

Examining the responses of the 60 receptor cells in Fig. 3 shows that if
a cell responds to any one of the four odorants dichlorobenzene (DIC), bromobenzene (BRO), anisole (ANI), and benzene (BEN), it has a high probability of
responding to the other three. Thus there is a high dependency between the
stimulating properties of these substances. Since they have a benzene ring in
common one might suggest that the receptor cells carry an "acceptor" type that
recognizes the aromatic ring. In Fig. 3 one sees the responses of the 60 recep
tors to two other odorants, namely camphor (CAM) and cineole (CIN). If a receptor cell responds to one of these two, it will respond to the other also.
Thus the two odours show a high dependency. But the response of a receptor to
any one of the odorants cineole or camphor is independent of the responses to
any of the four substances with an aromatic basis. There is a distinct grouping of the odorants that we have chosen : one group has two members: cineole
and camphor; the other has four members, dichlorobenzene, bromobenzene, anisole and benzene.

In view of this partition one can imagine that there are two independently occuring recognition mechanisms representing physical entities, provisio-
naly named acceptors. This is a premature conclusion because there are some
cells that respond to a member of the group but do not respond to the other
related odorants. Such variations in receptor sensitivity could be due to

genetic variations since the results were obtained from different animals. However eight receptor cells (marked with an asterisk) have been sampled from one animal and they show different sensitivity profiles. Thus the variations in response profiles are unlikely to arise because of genetic variations between the different frogs used in the study.

At this stage we are not able to propose a unique interpretation of the findings. Several alternative explanations might be suggested. Focussing on the aromatic group, one can consider that there is a basic type of "aromatic acceptor" and that this type gives rise to a variety of more specific acceptors, all with different affinity profiles. Another way of explaining the results would be to consider that there is no specific aromatic acceptor but that several different types of acceptors share the property of recognizing the aromatic ring. It would be this common property that would determine the grouping of the aromatic substances.

Only the recent progress in olfactory physiology could allow us to begin a synthesis on our understanding of the function of the olfactory system. We hope that our essay of assembling the functional elements as a totality demonstrates the po ssibility and the necessity of a unified view of a sensory system which still carries so many riddles.

REFERENCES

1. O'Connel, R.J. and Mozell, M.M. (1969) J. Neurophysiol. 32, 51-63

2. Gesteland, R.C. (1976) in Structure-Activity Relationships in Chemoreception, pp. 161-168, Information Retrieval Ltd., London

3. Holley, A., Delaleu, J.C., Revial, M.F and Juge, A. (1976)
    2nd Congress of ECRO, Reading, U.K.

4. Gesteland, R.C. and Müller, W. (1974) Fed. Proc. 33, 1472

5. Van Drongelen, W. (1977), this volume

6. Allison, A.C. and Warwick, R.T.T. (1949) Brain 72, 186-197

7. Gemne, G. and Døving, K.B. (1969) Amer. J. Anat. 126, 457-476

8. Bhatnagar, K.P. and Kallen, F.C. (1975) Acta Anat. 91, 272

9. Van Drongelen, W., Holley, A. and Døving, K.B. (1978) in preparation

10. Gesteland, R.C., Lettvin, J.Y. and Pitts, W.H. (1965)
    J. Physiol. (London) 181, 525-559

11. Altner, H. and Boeckh, J. (1967) Z.Vergl. Physiol. 55, 299-306

12. Duchamp, A., Revial, M.F., Holley, A. and Mac Leod, P. (1974) Chemical Senses and Flavor 1, 213-233

13. Revial, M.F., Duchamp, A. and Holley, A. (1977) Chemical Senses and Flavor 2 (to be published)

14. Le Gros Clark, W.E. (1957) Proc. Roy. Soc. (London) B 146,299-319

15. Land, L.J. (1973) Brain Res. 63, 153-166

16. Mozell, M.M. (1964) Science 143, 1336-1337

17. Daval, G., Leveteau, J. and Mac Leod, P. (1970) J. Physiol. (Paris) 62, 477-488

18. Mustaparta, H. (1971) Acta Physiol. Scand. 82, 154-166

19. Kauer, J.S. and Moulton, D.G. (1974) J. Physiol. (London) 243,717-737

20. Thommesen, G. and Døving, K.B. (1977) Acta Physiol. Scand. 99,270-280

21. Thommesen, G. (1976) Acta Physiol. Scand. 96, 6A-7A

22. Adrian, E.D. (1950) Electroencephalog. Clin.Neuro-physiol. 2,377-388

23. Moulton, D.G. (1967) in Olfaction and Taste II, pp. 109-116 Pergamon, Oxford

24. Døving, K.B. and Pinching, A.J. (1973) Brain Res. 52, 115-129

25. Pinching, A.J. and Døving, K.B. (1974) Brain Res. 82, 195-204

26. Sharp, F.R., Kauer, J.S. and Shepherd, G.M. (1975) Brain Res. 98, 596-600

27. Skeen, L.C. (1977) Brain Res. 124, 147-153

28. Sharp, F.R., Kauer, J.S. and Shepherd, G.M. (1977) J. Neurophysiol. 40, 800-813

29. Shepherd, G.M. (1972) Physiol. Rev. 52, 864-917

30. Kerr, D.I.B. (1977), this volume

31. Pager, J. (1977), this volume

Odor processing mechanisms in the salamander olfactory bulb

John S. Kauer

Department of Neurosurgery, Yale University School of Medicine, New Haven, CT 06510, USA

ABSTRACT

Precise stimulus control has played a critical role in elucidating the relationship between the physiological stimulus and single unit responses in a variety of sensory modalities. We have tried to achieve similar control in the olfactory system by using step pulse and punctate odor stimulation. For these studies the salamander has been introduced as a preparation in which anatomical, physiological, and behavioral information from a single species may be obtained. By examining single unit mitral cell responses elicited by odor pulse stimulation, specific response categories consisting of suppression, excitation, and combinations of suppression and excitation have emerged. These responses are related to the concentration and duration of the applied pulses in a systematic fashion which is characteristic for each response type observed. Any one unit can give any of the response types depending on the odor presented. Any one odor elicits different responses in different units. By using punctate odor application, it has been possible to map the receptive fields of single mitral layer units. The possible relationship of the temporal and spatial characteristics of these response categories to the synaptic circuits of the olfactory bulb are discussed.

INTRODUCTION

The effective investigation of the basic neural mechanisms and odor encoding capabilities of the olfactory bulb is dependent on at least two prerequisites. One is a favorable animal preparation which is representative of the vertebrate series and which has particular advantages for studying the olfactory system. Another is the ability to control precisely the physiological stimulus such that a careful analysis of the relationship between stimulus characteristics and electrophysiological responses can be made.

In this paper the advantages of using the tiger salamander as a model system for olfactory studies are discussed and some of the single cell responses from the olfactory bulb of this animal using precise temporal and spatial control of the odor stimulus are presented.

THE SALAMANDER AS A MODEL SYSTEM FOR OLFACTORY STUDIES

The tiger salamander, Ambystoma tigrinum, has a number of characteristics which confer specific advantages on its use as a preparation in which to study olfactory function. Among the first of these is the fact that a large body of

information already exists concerning the cytoarchitecture and neural connections of the CNS of this animal. For some 25 years the brain of the tiger salamander was the focus of study by C.J.Herrick(1948). Herrick's work centered
on Golgi studies of virtually all areas of the brain. He demonstrated that to
a first approximation, the olfactory bulb of this animal shows the same cell
types in similar relationships to one another as found in mammals. Unpublished
EM and Golgi studies in our laboratory also suggest that the overall form of
both receptor and bulbar cells as well as some of their synaptic connections
(i.e. dendrodendritic reciprocal synapses,Fig.1A) are similar to the mammal.

For electrophysiological studies the salamander is an inexpensive and
easily maintained laboratory animal. Since these animals can respire through
their skin they can be immobilized with neuromuscular blocking agents or by
pithing, thus allowing intra- and extra-cellular recording to be carried out
in the absence of respiratory pulsations.

The nasal cavity of the salamander is a dorso-ventrally flattened sac
lined with olfactory receptors. The shape of the cavity allows the dorsal roof
to be removed thereby exposing the ventral receptor sheet which, in contrast
to frogs and mammals, is a flat, apparently homogeneous receptor surface.This
configuration permits odors to be delivered directly to the receptors(without
going through the external nares)via nozzles designed to present odors precisely controlled in both time and space(Kauer,1973; Kauer,1974; Kauer & Moulton,1974; Kauer & Shepherd,1975; Kauer & Shepherd,1977)(see Fig.1B).

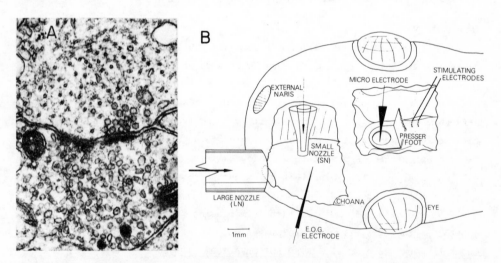

FIG.1 A.Dendrodendritic synapse in external plexiform layer of salamander olfactory bulb, probably between mitral cell and granule cell dendrites.B.Sala-
mander preparation showing odor delivery, EOG recording and olfactory bulb
recording set-up.

The olfactory bulb of the salamander shows the same sequence of laminae as seen in most other animals(Andres,1970;Shepherd,1972). However, in the salamander, these laminae are planar and are stacked in relation to one another more like a layer cake than the concentric onion-like configuration seen in frogs, reptiles, and mammals. The receptor cells and mitral/tufted bulbar output cells are larger in the salamander than in a number of other animals examined(Fink,pers.comm.;Kauer,1973;Getchell,1977). This laminar configuration of the bulb and the large size of the neural elements in both nose and bulb facilitate extra- and intra-cellular recording at several levels of this system.

An especially useful experimental organism is one in which electrophysiological and behavioral data can be obtained from the same animal. In this regard the salamander is a unique preparation in which controlled odor delivery, electrophysiological studies, and behavioral investigations can be carried out in the same species. There are a number of studies in which odor-related behavior in the tiger salamander and related species have been examined(Brodie & Gibson,1969;Nicholas,1921). In addition, preliminary experiments in our laboratory(Kauer,1973)have indicated that the salamander, unlike the frog(Mozell, pers.comm.) is amenable to odor-behavioral testing in a conventional, Y-maze, two-choice apparatus.

In conclusion, the salamander olfactory system has anatomical,physiological, and behavioral advantages which suggest that this preparation might serve as a useful model system in which significant advances in our understanding of olfactory function can be made.

SINGLE UNIT OLFACTORY BULB RESPONSES USING CONTROLLED ODOR PULSES

Single unit studies on the mitral layer cells of the salamander olfactory bulb have been carried out using an odor delivery system that controls the rise time, duration, concentration, and spatial extent of the odor pulse (Kauer,1974; Kauer & Moulton,1974; Kauer & Shepherd,1975; Kauer & Shepherd, 1977). The techniques for delivering 'square' odor pulses,'ramp' odor pulses, for monitoring the odor pulse, and for punctate odor presentation are described elsewhere, but it should be emphasized that the continued development of techniques for exerting strict control over the odor stimulus is a necessary prerequisite for making precise comparisons between various stimulus parameters and single unit responses.

These studies have shown that there are at least three major categories of activity seen in single mitral cells upon odor presentation to the ventral nasal mucosa. These categories are defined by the first response at the onset of the odor pulse and have been designated no response(N), suppression(S),and excitation(E). In the following paragraphs some of the characteristics of each of these categories will be presented.

SUPPRESSION. Suppressive responses are characterized by a cessation of spontaneous firing during an odor pulse. Examples of this activity are shown in Fig. 2. As was true for the other response types as well, all the odors tested could elicit uniform suppression in various units and any one unit could show suppression if the appropriate odor were delivered. Thus, in general, no response type was characteristic of a particular substance or unit(cf. Fig.2 with Fig.4). Suppressive responses would usually last for the duration of odor pulses up to 8 sec. long and showed no significant change in onset or duration with changes in peak concentration of the stimulus. The average onset of suppression in 127 odor applications was 300-400 msec. after the beginning of the pulse as measured by the odor monitor(Kauer & Shepherd,1977). If an odor that elicits suppression when delivered to the entire receptor sheet is presented as punctate stimulations at local regions of the mucosa, suppression is elicited at each of the sites tested as shown in Fig. 3(Kauer & Moulton,1974). Thus units showing suppression apparently show this activity as a result of odor interacting with receptors over a wide region of the nasal cavity. The units responding in this way may be termed as having wide, diffuse receptive fields when showing suppression.

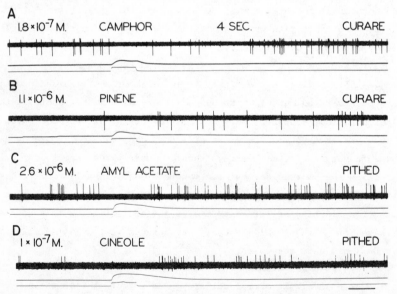

A 1.8×10^{-7} M.   CAMPHOR   4 SEC.   CURARE

B 1.1×10^{-6} M.   PINENE   CURARE

C 2.6×10^{-6} M.   AMYL ACETATE   PITHED

D 1×10^{-7} M.   CINEOLE   PITHED

FIG.2 Four different olfactory bulb units showing suppression during odor pulses of different compounds at various concentrations. Top trace is spike recording; middle trace is EOG; and bottom trace is odor monitor in this Fig. and in Fig. 4. Time mark = 4 sec.

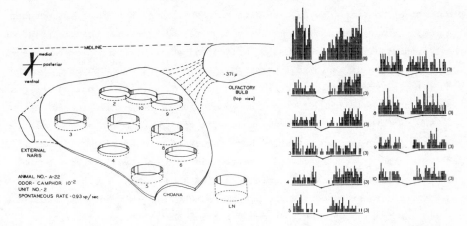

FIG. 3 Responses of a single olfactory bulb unit to stimulation of the entire receptor sheet(LN) and to stimulation of localized regions. Cylinders appearing to go down from the receptor sheet indicate suppression. PST histograms for the same responses depicted by the cylinders are shown at the right.

EXCITATION. Excitatory responses are characterized by an increase in firing at the onset of the odor pulse(Fig. 4). In contrast to suppressive responses however, excitation lasts for the duration of the pulse only near threshold. As concentration is increased the duration of the initial excitatory burst is

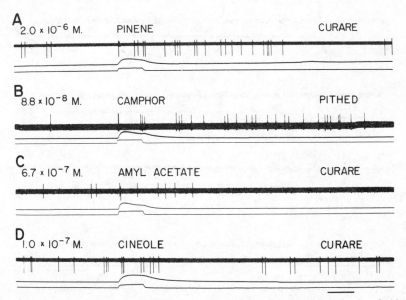

FIG. 4 Four different units showing excitation during odor pulses of different compounds at various concentrations. Note pattern of activity during the pulse consists of a brief initial burst, a period of suppression, and a return of firing during the pulse. Time mark = 4 sec.

progressively curtailed by a period of suppression, such that at high concentrations the only remnant of the excitatory response may be a single spike at the beginning of the pulse. Thus at medium concentrations the pattern of excitation consists of an initial burst followed by a period of suppression and, with relatively long pulses, of a second period of excitation during the pulse. Examples of these responses at medium concentrations are shown in Fig. 4.

The fact that excitatory responses last for the duration of the pulse only at a particular concentration near threshold, suggested that these cells had a preference for firing with a certain odor intensity. This phenomenon has been termed concentration tuning(Kauer,1973,1974). The short burst at the beginning of higher concentration pulses would thus seem to be a manifestation of this same tuning process. One could imagine that these short bursts are periods of excitation elicited as the delivered odor concentration rose from zero, through the region to which the unit was tuned and above, to where suppression was elicited. The higher the final concentration delivered, the faster the pulse would sweep through the concentration to which the unit is tuned and the shorter the initial burst would become. This interpretation was tested by delivering odor pulses of the same concentration but with different onset rise times,i.e. ramps, as shown in Fig. 5(Kauer & Shepherd,1977). One can

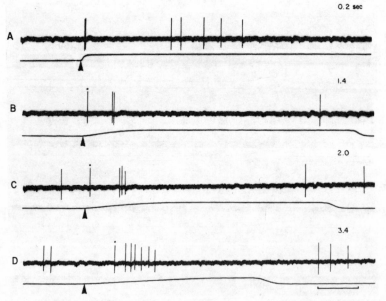

FIG. 5 Excitatory responses of an olfactory bulb unit to odor pulses of the same peak concentration with onset rise times varying from 0.2 to 3.4 sec(numbers at right). Note elongation of excitatory period with slower ramps. Dots over spikes indicate they are part of spontaneous activity. Top trace is spike recording. Bottom trace is odor monitor. Time mark = 2 sec.

see from this figure that the duration of excitation is related to the time over which the odor was at the appropriate concentration to elicit excitation, even though the peak concentration was the same in all runs. By using moderately high odor concentrations to elicit short excitatory bursts the shortest latencies of the initial excitation were in the range of 200-300 msec. after the onset of the pulse(Kauer & Shepherd,1977).

If an odor which elicits excitation by stimulating the entire receptor sheet, is delivered as a punctate stimulus, excitatory responses are seen in the unit only by stimulating particular regions of the mucosa(Kauer & Moulton, 1974). Fig. 6 shows PST histograms of activity of a bulbar unit after stimulation with camphor delivered to the sites indicated by the position of the histograms. It was found that the mucosal sites which, when stimulated locally elicited excitation from bulbar cells,were surprisingly constant in different preparations for the same odor and were in different positions for different odors in the same animal.

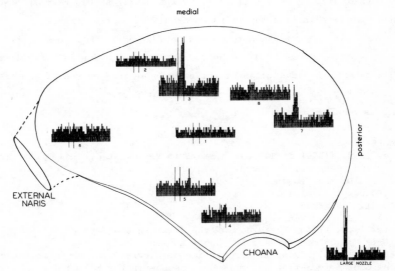

FIG. 6 PST Histograms showing excitatory activity of a bulbar unit after stimulation of the whole receptor sheet(large nozzle) and of local sites on the mucosa with camphor. Note excitation is elicited with punctate stimulation only at regions 3 and 7.

RELATIONSHIP OF ODOR RESPONSES TO BULBAR CIRCUITRY

The ability to control various parameters of the physiological stimulus for the olfactory system has begun to allow us to compare odor responses with responses obtained with electrical stimulation of the olfactory bulb. It is interesting to note that the sequence of brief excitation and following suppression seen using step pulse odor stimulation at relatively high concentrations is similar to the sequence of spike excitability in mitral cells of the rabbit using electrical stimulation(Phillips, Powell, & Shepherd,1963;Shepherd, 1963a,b;Shepherd,1972).These excitability changes have been ascribed to reciprocal dendrodendritic synapses which subserve feedback inhibition onto the mitral cells at both the glomerular and external plexiform levels. It is tempting to suggest that one is observing a manifestation of these negative feedback paths in the physiological responses to odor described above. One speculation might be that uniform suppressive mitral responses are due to lateral spread of inhibition from neighboring mitral cells which were excited. The longer onset latency of suppressive responses and the ability to elicit them over broad areas of the epithelial sheet are consistent with this interpretation. In the same way it is possible that excitatory response patterns showing a brief burst then suppression are related to initial direct excitation from the receptor axons and the subsequent self-inhibiting functions of the glomerular and external plexiform reciprocal synapses. It should be pointed out that these self-inhibiting functions apparently do not operate at the 'tuned' concentration in concentration tuned responses, for in these cases the unit continues to fire for as long as the correct concentration is maintained.

In summary, the advantages of the salamander and the use of precise stimulus control have begun to allow acquisition of data on how the olfactory system encodes odor information.

REFERENCES
1. Andres, K.H. (1970) in Taste and Smell in Vertebrates, Ciba Symposium
   pp 177-194, Churchill, London
2. Brodie, E.D. and Gibson,L.S.(1969)
   Herpetologica 25, 187-194
3. Getchell, T.V.(1977)
   Br. Res. 123, 275-286
4. Herrick, C.J. (1948) The Brain of the Tiger Salamander
   The Univ. of Chicago Press, Chicago & London
5. Kauer, J.S. (1973) Response Properties of Single Olfactory Bulb Neurons
    Using Odor Stimulation of Small Nasal Areas in the Salamander
    PhD. Thesis, Univ. of Pennsylvania
6. Kauer, J.S. (1974)
   J. Physiol. 243,695-715
7. Kauer, J.S. and Moulton, D.G.(1974)
   J. Physiol. 243,717-737
8. Kauer, J.S. and Shepherd, G.M. (1975)
   Br. Res. 85,108-113
9. Kauer, J.S. and Shepherd, G.M. (1977)
   J. Physiol. (in press)
10.Nicholas, J.S. (1921)
   Anat. Rec. 20,257-281
11.Phillips, C.G., Powell, T.P.S. and Shepherd, G.M.(1963)
   J. Physiol. 168,65-88

12. Shepherd, G.M. (1963a)
    J. Physiol. 168,89-100
13. Shepherd, G.M. (1963b)   J. Physiol. 168,101-117
14. Shepherd, G.M. (1972)   Physiol. Rev. 52,864-917

The regulatory food intake behavior: some olfactory central correlates

Jeanne Pager

Laboratoire d'Electrophysiologie, Université Claude Bernard, 43 Boulevard du 11 Novembre 1918, 69621 Lyon-Villeurbanne, France

ABSTRACT
     This paper examines how the anatomical organization of the olfacto-central pathways could subserve the achievement of regulatory behaviors. Phylogenetic and ontogenetic arguments establish that the neural tube differenciates following two gradients at least: a sensory-motor one, along the dorso-ventral axis, and a reticular-lemniscal one, from the inside to the outside. The olfactory input is related to the rest of brain by a double projection system, developed from the primitive dorso-lateral and ventro-median olfactory tracts. The mammalian lateral tract projects towards the thalamic and neocortical areas, while the median system feeds fibres into the anterior olfactory nucleus, the reticular system and the hypothalamus. There are several evidences that these tracts respectively display a mainly lemniscal/reticular structure, and could analyze the chemical/alerting dimensions of the olfactory stimulus. It is suggested that the behavior-guiding functions of odors, associated to their rewarding dimension, involves the two olfactory projection systems. The dual olfacto-central organization is illustrated by data about food intake behavior.

INTRODUCTION

     It is now generally admitted(15) that the olfactory input of Mammals is organized according to the schema previously observed in other sensory pathways. The gustatory input, for example, displays a thalamo-neocortical, as well as an extra-thalamic projection system. It was suggested that the recently discovered thalamo-neocortical olfactory pathway(9, 30) mediates adaptative and anticipatory behavioral responses. The prevailing centripetal and centrifugal olfacto-hypothalamic fibre system, on the other hand, was considered as the basis for the reflex integration of the endocrine and olfactory cues. Analysis of the olfacto-hypothalamic correlates should thus constitute a fundamental step towards understanding the mechanisms underlying the behavioral maintenance of homeostasis.

     Food intake is an example of such survival behaviors. The olfactory bulbs of hungry free-moving rats receiving food odors display an increased multiunit mitral cell activity, compared to those of the same animals when satiated. No significant difference is observed with control odors(25). The extent of the

hunger-elicited bulb activation has been correlated with the food rewarding
character of the stimulating odor(23). Cumulated data show that the percentage of positive mitral cell responses elicited by a repeated olfactory stimulus
displays a slower time-decay the more the animals are hunger-aroused and the
more palatable is the odor. The bulb response modulation thus appears as the
effect of a differential habituation. Therefore it is not sure that the nutritional modulation of mitral cell responses, a mechanism probably relevant to
the olfactory control of food intake, could be investigated merely in terms of
olfacto-hypothalamic correlates.

The anatomical organization of the olfacto-central pathways, and some
functional consequences for the olfactory regulations of behavior will be examined.

ANATOMICAL CONSIDERATIONS

It can be considered that the olfacto-central pathways are organized on-
togenetically and phylogenetically on the basis of at least two gradients. One
is a dorso-ventral gradient. A pioneer work has analyzed how the Vertebrate
neural tube differenciates along a sensory-motor gradient following its dorso-
ventral axis(11). In the sensory pole are located the highly integrative neocortical areas; the motor pole mainly controls the visceral functions. The telencephalic olfactory areas develop a double system of connection with the
rest of the brain: the dorso-lateral and the ventro-median olfactory tracts.
In adult teleost fishes (27), the two pathways correspond respectively to the
lateral and median olfactory tracts(LOT; MOT). The first tract distributes fibres to the lateral olfactory areas, which in turn project to the thalamus.
The second one sends fibres to the median olfactory areas, the hypothalamus
and the reticulate system.

An identical double frame may be recognized in Mammals(Fig. 1). The LOT
constitutes the first projecting step towards the prepiriform(PP), thalamic
(TH) and neocortical(NC) olfactory areas. The median olfactory tract reaches
the anterior olfactory nucleus(AON), itself associated with fibres of the anterior limb of the anterior commissure(AAC) and to the medial forebrain bundle
(MFB). Each pathway displays ipsilateral centrifugal fibres to the olfactory
bulb(OB), originating in the PP cortex, and the lateral hypothalamic areas(LH)
including the nucleuc of the horizontal limb of the diagonal band of Broca. In
addition, the locus coeruleus(LC) and the raphe nuclei(RN) send fibers to the
olfactory bulbs in the median projection system(5, 7). The median and lateral
olfactory pathways display interconnections at any level of projection.

Another differentiation process is a radial gradient. Studies on the pri-

Fig. 1.   <u>Simplified organization of the mammalian olfactory pathways.</u>

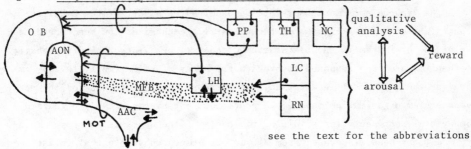

see the text for the abbreviations

mitive Fishes indicate that the whole central nervous system of Vertebrates also differentiates radially from a purely reticular tube, which gradually subdivides into concentric internal reticulate and external lemniscal structures(3, 4). A lemniscal-type sensory projection is composed of neurons with long axons, making numerous contacts with a small number of interneurons, and organized in nuclei. It also displays a topographical organization from the periphery to the cerebral cortex. Opposite characters define a reticular structure. The individualized hypothalamus corresponds to a concentration of reticular neurons basically devoted to the chemical analysis of the internal medium. It therefore displays intimate relations with the other integrating reticular structures, and with the external chemosensory receptors of the olfactory system. The reticular origin and structure of the hypothalamus have been corroborated by anatomical studies in Mammals(21).

FUNCTIONAL INVOLVEMENTS

Each gradient of differenciation leads to several physiological consequences. As a result of what has been said about the <u>radial gradient</u>, the hypothalamus is endowed with heterogeneous afferences, but not necessarily with a lack of functional specificity. Multiple inputs are likely to account for the complex overlapping behavioral effects of lesions and stimulations in hypothalamic sites. This switchboard area should then influence the probability of obtaining the various behavioral patterns by modulating the stimulus-response relations maintained elsewhere in the brain(12). In fact, the privileged correlates of the hypothalamus with the remaining reticular system indicate that other parts of the brain share functions initially attributed to the diencephalic areas alone.

Sensory neglect was first observed after lateral hypothalamic lesions(18) and was interpreted as a main feature in the LH aphagia and adypsia syndrome. But sensory, including olfactory, neglect can also result from ablations in the tectum opticum(14) and from midsagittal reticular lesions(10).

The hypothalamus must therefore be examined as a part of the behavior-controlling circuits. A review of recent data(2) emphasizes the fundamental role of the brainstem in the elaboration of adapted behaviors. The diencephalic mechanisms are then supposed to broaden the array of key-stimuli, thereby improving the behavioral integration. The corresponding hypothesis for the nervous system organization involves a continuous but hierarchically organized behavioral representation at different levels of the neuraxis. A complementary model has been elaborated from a wide set of neurophysiological investigations on food and water intake(19). It requires the joint participation of mesencephalic, diencephalic and telencephalic structures, in a complex recurrent circuit able to "modulate multimodal inputs and regulate filtering in information channels at several integrative levels in the brainstem"(20).

There is some evidence that neurons underlying food reward belong to the LH, an area regarded as being of prime importance in this respect, at least in the laboratory conditions where reward is defined(26). One may ask whether the reward-modulating sites, mainly the amygdala and the prefrontal cortex, are less fundamental than LH areas for the performance of adapted behaviors in natural conditions.

Food odor is a component of alimentary reward, and thereby a powerful guide to nutrition. It can be observed that the nutritional modulation of olfactory responses only takes place at optimal levels of general arousal and bulb excitability, when the mitral cell responses are recorded together with parameters characterizing vigilance and sleep(8). Since the modulation of olfactory responses consists of a selectively maintained bulb arousal, it is unlikely that the mesencephalic activation concomitant with LH reward is only a side effect of reinforcement.

The close relations of the olfactory bulb with the reticular system account for the high arousing ability of the olfactory stimuli, and for the bulb activation associated with mesencephalic stimulation(6). It thus seems that the median component of the olfactory input, the arousal system and the LH areas maintain privileged functional relations. As a consequence, the general arousing, sensory modulating and rewarding aspects of motivation, sometimes analyzed separately(13), can hardly be dissociated.

Some functional characteristics of the olfacto-central correlates may be regarded as the consequence of the sensory-motor gradient along the dorso-ventral axis of the differenciating neural tube. Extrapolating the interpretations of data from Fishes to Mammals leads one to consider that the lateral and the median olfactory projection systems could fulfil different functions. The LOT centripetal fibers constitute the initial steps to the neocortical olfactory areas. An improved discrimination of olfactory cues is observed along the lateral ascending pathway(30). Some topographical organization has been reported, at least in the first stages of the system(28), a feature characterizing the lemniscal-type sensory projections. Ascending fibers of the median system, on the contrary, feed the medial forebrain bundle, a reticular structure.

As the various gradients co-operate during the neural tube differenciation, a tentative synthesis can be made from the different behavioral involvements proposed up to now. The median olfacto-central system, initially devoted to the relations with the viscero-motor areas, partly through a reticulate pathway, should function more in a protopathic manner, generally called a non-specific manner. Similarly, the olfacto-central system, basically subserving the relations with sensory highly integrative neocortical areas, displays some lemniscal characters. It could mainly fulfil epicritic-like functions, generally regarded as specific functions.

Although potentials could be evoked in the OB and in the LOT during electrical stimulation of the hypothalamus, the medial forebrain bundle and the mesencephalon(1), no precise behavioral function can be ascribed to the LOT centrifugal components. Cortical associative and learning processes have been supposed to require their participation(16). The hypothesis has been tested in five food-deprived or satiated rats*. The animals bore permanent bipolar electrodes for the mitral cell multiunit recording, and had one LOT sectioned. They were trained on an aversive conditioning schedule which associated the intake of a new food with an intraperitoneal injection of Lithium chloride, on two consecutive days. During the tests, the rats were stimulated by their usual food odor, by the new aversive food odor and by isoamyl acetate or eucalyptol as control odors. The aversive food odor did not give rise to a nutritional modulation of responses, either in the control bulb or in the lesion-side bulb. These preliminary data suggest that the centrifugal LOT fibers are not concerned with the bulbar effects of an aversive learning, although further experiments are needed on this point.

The median centrifugal system might well contain a terminal effector part of circuits subserving a visceral conditioning, since the nutritional modulation disappears in one olfactory bulb after an ipsilateral lesion of centrifugal fibers passing in or near the anterior limb of the anterior commissure. The modulation is not disturbed after LOT unilateral lesions(24). It has been reported that lesions of the LOT and of the AON affected the aversive behavior of rats in opposite manners(29). Both systems are supposed to subserve the regulation of the Hamster social behavior complementarily(17). It may be pointed out that all the median olfactory projection areas give rise to self-stimulation(22). However, both the lateral and median olfacto-central pathways reach areas in the reward system: the former is mainly concerned with the MFB and LH, while the latter carries information to the dorso-median thalamus and the prefrontal cortex. Thus the olfactory projection systems both subserve the same behavioral achievements, probably not in spite of but rather, thanks to their differentiated structural and functional characteristics.

CONCLUSION

So as to propose a functional model of the olfacto-central correlates, one can suppose that different dimensions of the same odorous cue are analyzed in various parts of the olfactory circuits. In this way, they combine to elicit a determined pattern of cerebral activity at a given time. An odorous cue is probably more efficient than any other sensory cue in releasing general alertness, by activating the appropriate reticular and mesencephalic structures through the MFB neurons. An optimal general arousal level must be reached for the other operations to be performed, namely the qualitative and quantitative analysis of the stimulus, and the evaluation of its behavioral meaning by matching the memorized traces of the animal's previous experiences. Inversely, the relevance of any olfactory cue to the animal internal state is able to control the arousal level. The behavior-guiding dimension of the olfactory stimulus corresponds to its reinforcing character. The reward function has been noted previously to involve all kinds of olfacto-central pathway, either specific or non-specific. Some behavioral consequences of the olfactory bulbectomy should be appreciated by considering this functional complementarity. Finally, it must be pointed out that a dichotomic model privileges the poles of the differentiation gradients. Various amounts of "epicritic" and "protopathic" elements probably co-operate in both olfactory projection systems. The olfactory control of the Vertebrate behavior displays specific peculiarities. The relative functional preponderance, on one hand, of either type of neuronal organization in each olfactory tract, and on the other hand, of each tract among the other sensory pathways, is supposedly not irrelevant to this diversity.

REFERENCES

1. Aguilar-Baturoni, H. U., Guevara-Aguilar, R., Arechiga, H. and Alcocer-
   Cuaron, C. (1976)
   Brain Res. Bull. 1, 263-272

2. Berntson, G. G. and Micco, D. J. (1976)
   Brain Res. Bull. 1, 471-483

3. Bowsher, D. (1973)
   Brain Behav. Evol. 8, 386-396

4. Bowsher, D. (1976)
   La Recherche 7, 935-944

5. Broadwell, R. D. and Jacobowitz, D. M. (1976)
   J. Comp. Neurol. 170, 321-346

6. Cain, D. P. (1974)
   Psychol. Bull. 81, 654-671

7. Dennis, B. J. and Kerr, D. I. B. (1976)
   Brain Res. 110, 593-600

8. Gervais, R. and Pager, J. (1977) in Food and Fluid Intake,
   Proc. VIth Internat. Symp., in press

9. Giachetti, I. and Mac Leod, P. (1977)
   Brain Res. 125, 166-169

10. Greeley, H. P., Hagamen, S. J., Hagamen, W. D. and Reeves, A. G. (1975)
    Brain Behav. Evol. 12, 57-74

11. Herrick, C. J. (1910)
    J. Comp. Neurol. 20, 413-547

12. Jurgens, U. (1974) in Progress in Brain Research,
    Vol. 41, pp 445-462, Elsevier Publishing Co., Amsterdam

13. Karli, P (1973)
    Arch. Ital. Biol. 111, 668-685

14. Kirvel, R. D., Greenfield, R. A. and Meyer, D. R. (1974)
    J. Comp. Physiol. Psychol. 87, 156-162

15. Le Magnen, J. (1975) in Olfaction and Taste,
    Proc. Vth Internat. Symp., pp 301-388, Academic Press, New-York

16. Mac Leod, P. (1971) in Handbook of Sensory Physiology,
    Vol. IV, pp 182-204, Springer Verlag, Berlin

17. Macrides, F., Firl, A. C., Schneider, S. F., Bartke, A. and Stein, D. G.
    (1976)
    Brain Res. 109, 97-109

18. Marshall, J. F. and Teitelbaum, P. (1974)
    J. Comp. Physiol. Psychol. 86, 375-395

19. Morgane, P. J. (1969)
    Ann. N. Y. Acad. Sci. 157, 806-848

20. Morgane, P. J. and Stern, W. C. (1972)
    Ann. N. Y. Acad. Sci. 193, 95-111

21. Nauta, W. J. H. and Haymaker, W. (1969) in The Hypothalamus,
    Chap. IV, pp 136-209, C. C. Thomas, Springfield

22. Olds, J. A. (1956)
    J. Comp. Physiol. Psychol. 49, 281-285

23. Pager, J. (1976) in Contrôle centrifuge des réponses électriques du bulbe
    olfactif: étude chez le rat en fonction de l'état nutritionnel,
    Thèse de Doctorat d'Etat, Université Claude Bernard, Lyon

24. Pager, J. (1977)
    Brain Res., in press

25. Pager, J., Giachetti, I., Holley, A. and Le Magnen, J. (1972)
    Physiol. Behav. 9, 573-579

26. Rolls, E. T. (1975) The Brain and Reward
    Pergamon Press, Oxford

27. Sheldon, R. E. (1912)
    J. Comp. Neurol. 22, 177-339

28. Shepherd, G. M. and Haberly, L. B. (1970)
    J. Neurophysiol. 35, 643-653

29. Sieck, M. H. and Gordon, B; L. (1973)
    Physiol. Bebav. 10, 1051-1059

30. Tanabe, T., Iino, M. and Takagi, S. F. (1975)
    J. Neurophysiol. 38, 1284-1296

*   unpublished data from Royet, J. P. and Pager, J.

Interactions of olfactory stimuli and gonadal hormones in the regulation of rodent social behavior

Foteos Macrides, Andrzej Bartke and Bruce Svare

Worcester Foundation for Experimental Biology, 222 Maple Avenue, Shrewsbury, MA 01454, USA

ABSTRACT

Recent studies in mice and hamsters have demonstrated that chemosensory stimuli from females can strongly influence the hypophysiogonadal axis of males. These results, along with previous findings that male odors affect endocrine function in females, indicate that bisexual encounters are likely to produce endocrine changes in members of both sexes. In this discussion, we will examine some of the implications of these mutual interactions in the regulation of rodent social behavior.

Studies in mice and hamsters indicate that sex-related odors can affect the hypothalamo-pituitary-gonadal axis of conspecifics. It has long been known that olfactory cues from adult males can alter the estrous cycle and interrupt pregnancy in female mice[16]. Such cues can also accelerate the sexual maturation of female mice[20]. More recently, several investigators have examined the effects of stimuli emitted by females on the reproductive system of males and have observed responses analogous to those reported in females. For example, exposure to adult females causes rapid increases of plasma testosterone (T) levels in adult male mice and more prolonged exposure accelerates the growth of accessory sex organs in young males[6,10,17,19]. In the adult male hamster, exposure to vaginal odor can be as effective as pairing with females in producing rapid elevations of plasma T levels[11]. The neuroendocrine response of the adult male mouse has been attributed to female urine[14]. Physical interactions between males or exposure to the odor of another male do not produce rapid elevations of plasma T levels in these species

but male hormone levels can be altered upon establishment of a dominance relationship[2,10,15]. Plasma T levels, in turn, have been associated with the behavioral responsiveness of males toward female stimuli, their territorial behavior and aggressiveness toward other males, and the production of stimuli
which affect female endocrine function[7,9,11,12,18]. These complex interactions among sensory, hormonal and social variables can only be interpreted in
relation to the social systems in which they occur.

Although the studies in hamsters and mice clearly show that chemosensory
stimuli from females can increase circulating levels of gonadotropins and
androgen in adult males, the biological significance of these increases is not
at all obvious. Under the laboratory conditions in which these increases have
been demonstrated, the males maintain more than adequate levels of hormone to
support their sex drive and their production of sperm. One may therefore
question whether the attainment of yet higher levels yields any appreciable
increase in their eagerness or capacity to fertilize a female when they are
given the opportunity to copulate. It should be emphasized, however, that
laboratory conditions generally are "optimum" conditions and often not representative of those in the wild. Doty[4] has reviewed evidence which suggests
that the female rodent plays a more important role in the initiation and
maintenance of courtship and copulating activities than might be inferred
from laboratory experiments in which the female commonly is primed with hormones and delivered to the male by the experimenter. Although chemosensory
and social influences on gonadotropin and androgen secretion might alter the
motivational or fertilizing capacities of males, such influences may be of
greater importance for the courtship phase of sexual interactions. That is,
they might be understood as mechanisms for assessment of social relationships
during periods of competition for females, and for natural selection of mating
partners.

The production of stimuli which elicit sexual arousal in males is not critically dependent on ovarian function in either the hamster[3,13] or the mouse[10]. Maruniak and Bronson[14] have shown that urine from diestrous, proestrous, pregnant or ovariectomized female mice all produce marked elevations of LH in male mice. We had previously shown that exposure to nonreceptive females results in an elevation of plasma T levels in mice[10] and we have confirmed that non-tactile exposure to intact or ovariectomized females produces comparable elevations of plasma T. This lack of dependence of the male response on the state of fertility or the behavioral receptiveness of the female strengthens the speculation that the male response plays a role during the courtship, and not just the copulating, phase of sexual interactions. Since the estrous cycle of the female mouse can be advanced by an androgen dependent factor in the male's urine[16], the male's "response" to the female may sum with other influences on his androgen levels (e.g., his assumption of dominance in competition with other males) and contribute to his own influence on the female. We have found[10] that male mice paired with an intact female for 1 week do not have higher plasma T levels than do males that remain in all-male control groups. All of the paired males in our study mated with their females and thus by the end of the week were each residing with a pregnant (and now unreceptive) female. From the work of Maruniak and Bronson[14] we know that the urine of these pregnant females would have been capable of elevating hormone levels in other males. Moreover, we found that exposing the paired males to a new, and also unreceptive, female for 30-60 min resulted in marked elevations of the males' plasma T levels. When the males were exposed to the new females they renewed their mating attempts but were rebuffed. These findings indicate that we are not dealing with a specific endocrine response to female urine but more generally with an endocrine correlate of sexual arousal. If so, the timecourse of endocrine responses to female urine as measured in the laboratory may bear little relationship to the timecourses of such responses in the wild. The magnitude and/or duration of the male's response may depend on the character and multiplicity of the social interactions and the degree and/or duration of the male's arousal. Indeed, the female's unreceptiveness and the need for courtship may augment the male's endocrine response.

The interactions among chemosensory, hormonal and social variables which we have discussed require us to maintain a broad view of "hypothalamic functions" and to examine the regulation of pituitary output not only in relation to homeostatic mechanisms and adaptations within the organism to its environment[9] but also in relation to the interactions of organisms within a social system. Chemosensory stimuli might be conceptualized as operating in rodents on a continuum with other environmental factors such as the seasonal variations in length of daylight to coordinate the endocrine and behavioral phenomena that maintain the social system. It is interesting to note in closing that in the male hamster, prolactin appears to play a major role in mediating the recrudescence of the testes upon return to longer daylengths and the onset of the breeding season[1]. Although existing studies of chemosensory influences on gonadotropin secretion have focused on LH and FSH, it has been demonstrated in the male rat that exposure to females also elevates prolactin levels[8]. Prolactin can enhance the response of sebaceous glands, including the preputial glands, to testosterone[5]. Thus, prolactin may be involved both in sexually-relevant endocrine responses of males to the environment and in the dissemination of male odors.

ACKNOWLEDGEMENTS

Suported by NINCDS grant NS12344, NSF grant BNS75-07652, NICHD grants HD09584 and HD06867, NIH Research Career Development Award HD703699 (to A. B.) and Postdoctoral Fellowship MH05369 (to B. S.).

REFERENCES

1.   Bartke, A., Croft, B.T. and Dalterio, S. (1975) Endocrinology 97, 1601-1604.

2. Bartke, A. and Dalterio, S. (1975) Steroids 26, 749-756.

3. Darby, E.M., Devor, M. and Chorover, S.L. (1975) J. Comp. Physiol. Psychol. 88, 496-502.

4. Doty, R.L. (1974) Psychol. Bull. 81, 159-172.

5. Ebling, F.J. (1977) in Chemical Signals in Vertebrates, 1st edn, pp. 17-34, Plenum, New York.

6. Fox, K.A. (1968) J. Reprod. Fert. 17, 75-85.

7. Hoppe, P.C. (1975) J. Reprod. Fert. 45, 109-115.

8. Kamel, F., Mock, E.J., Wright, W.W. and Frankel, A.I. (1975) Horm. Behav. 6, 277-288.

9. Macrides, F. (1976) in Mammalian Olfaction, Reproductive Processes and Behavior, 1st edn, pp. 29-65, Academic Press, New York.

10. Macrides, F., Bartke, A. and Dalterio, S. (1975) Science 189, 1104-1106.

11. Macrides, F., Bartke, A., Fernandez, F. and D'Angelo, W. (1974) Neuroendocrinology 15, 355-364.

12. Macrides, F., Firl, A.C., Schneider, S.P., Bartke, A. and Stein, D.G. (1976) Brain Res. 109, 97-109.

13. Macrides, F., Johnson, P.A. and Schneider, S.P. (in press) Behav. Biol.

14. Maruniak, J.A. and Bronson, F.H. (1976) Endocrinology 99, 963-969.

15. McKinney, T.D. and Desjardins, C. (1973) Biol. Reprod. 9, 370-378.

16. Parkes, A.S. and Bruce, H.M. (1961) Science 134, 1049-1054.

17. Svare, B., Bartke, A. and Macrides, F. (unpublished).

18. Vandenbergh, J.G. (1971) Anim. Behav. 19, 589-594.

19. Vandenbergh, J.G. (1971) J. Reprod. Fert. 24, 383-390.

20. Vandenbergh, J.G. (1974) J. Sex Res. 10, 181-193.

Olfaction and Taste VI, Paris, 1977.

Neuroendocrine mediation of the effects of olfactory stimuli on estrous rhythm regulation in the rat

D. Chateau, J. Roos and Cl. Aron

Institute of Histology, Faculty of Medicine, Strasbourg, France*

ABSTRACT

5-day cyclic bulbectomized female rats failed to display reduced cycle duration on exposure to the odor of either male or female rat's urine thus indicating that the olfactory pathway was involved. However another pathway, possibly gustatory in nature, was capable of compensating for the absence of olfactory bulbs in those females which were exposed to the action of male urine. Hypothalamus ventromedial nucleus (VMN) lesions suppressed the cycle shortening action of the odor of male urine. The VMN was then supposed to constitute the pathway through which olfactory stimuli regulated estrous rhythm in the rat. Evidence was also provided that the VMN regulates estrous rhythm in bulbectomized females.

INTRODUCTION

Previous findings in our laboratory provided strong evidence that both the hypothalamic ventromedial nucleus (VMN) and olfactory stimuli were involved in estrous rhythm regulation in the rat. A change in 4-day to 5-day cyclicity resulted from VMN lesions (CARRER et al., 1973-1974 ; CHATEAU et al., 1976a). Similarly 3- to 4-month old Wistar females, when deprived of their olfactory bulbs at the age of 6 weeks, displayed a 5-day cyclicity more frequently than sham-operated or unoperated controls (ARON et al., 1971, 1972 ; ROOS et al., 1973a). Inversely, a 24-hour reduced cycle duration was shown to occur in 5-day cyclic females whose litter was sprinkled twice daily with 2 ml of either male or female urine (ARON and CHATEAU, 1971 ; CHATEAU et al., 1972).

Since females were allowed to lick their litter in the above mentioned pilot experiments it was important to determine whether the action of urine on estrous rhythm was really exerted through an olfactory pathway. A second question also arose as to whether the VMN mediated this action of urine. Thirdly we had to explore the possibility that the VMN was capable of controlling autonomously estrous rhythm in the rat.

The present paper reports on results which allow an answer to these three questions. Some of them have been published in a preliminary form in French (ROOS et al., 1973b ; CHATEAU et al., 1974).

RESULTS AND DISCUSSION

A. EVIDENCE THAT THE ACTION OF URINE ON ESTROUS RHYTHM IS
DEPENDENT ON THE OLFACTORY PATHWAY

1. Action of male urine

The data presented in table 1 show that reduced cycle duration similarly occurred in the two-thirds of the unoperated and sham operated females exposed to the action of male urine whether or not the females were prevented to lick their litter. They also indicate that cycle shortening frequency was higher in the treated females either unoperated (21/32) or sham operated (10/15) than in unoperated controls (10/32) ($\chi^2 = 9.14$; p $\langle$ 0.02 ; 2 df). Finally, they reveal that olfactory bulb deprivation only suppressed the action of male urine when the females were maintained on a grid, thus preventing them from licking the litter. By contrast reduced estrous cycle duration still occured in females placed on floor level ($\chi^2 = 5.57$; p<0.02; 1 df).

Table 1.

Modifications of oestrous cycle duration in virgin female Wistar rats (W II strain)
exposed to the action of male urine
during the 3rd, 4th and 5th cycles of a sequence of 5-day cycles

Treatment			Number of animals	Cycle shortening frequency	Shortening from 5 to 4 days of the			
					3rd cycle only	3rd, 4th and 5th cycles	4th and 5th cycles only	5th cycle only
Unoperated females	Controls	Lying on their litter	16	5/16	2	1	1	1
		Lying on a grid*	16	5/16	-	3	1	1
	Treated**	Lying on their litter	16	11/16	-	3	5	3
		Lying on a grid	16	10/16	1	6	3	-
Olfactory bulb deprived females	Treated	Lying on their litter	16	8/16	2	1	5	-
		Lying on a grid	16	1/16	-	1	-	-
Sham operated females	Treated	Lying on their litter	7	5/7	1	1	3	-
		Lying on a grid	8	5/8	1	2	2	-

* Placed at 5cm above the floor of the cage for preventing any licking
** Twice daily sprinkling of cage litter with urine

2. Action of female urine

Our data are figured in table 2. They show that cycle shortening frequency was greater in females exposed to the action of female urine than in their control counterparts ($p < 0.04$, one tailed test). They also indicate that estrous cycle duration failed to occur in olfactory bulb deprived females whether or not exposed to the action of urine (2/16 and 1/16 ; $p > 0.9$). Statistical analysis also confirmed this action of olfactory bulb removal when the effects of exposure to female urine were compared in unoperated and operated females (10/16 and 2/16, respectively ; $\chi^2 = 8.53$; p 0.01 ; 1 df).

Table 2.

Modifications of oestrous cycle duration in virgin female Wistar rats (W II strain)
exposed to the action of female urine
during the 3rd, 4th and 5th cycles of a sequence of 5-day cycles

Treatment		Number of animals	Cycle shortening frequency	Shortening from 5 to 4 days of the			
				3rd cycle only	3rd, 4th and 5th cycles	3rd and 4th cycle only	5th cycle only
Unoperated	Controls	16	5/16	-	2	1	2
	Treated[*]	16	10/16	1	2	6	1
Olfactory bulb deprived females	Controls	16	1/16	-	-	-	1
	Treated[*]	16	2/16	1	-	1	-

* Twice daily sprinkling of cage litter with urine

3. Comments

The picture which emerges from the present data is that olfactory stimuli originating from females are involved in the regulation of estrous rhythm in the rat since bulbectomized females, although allowed to lick their litter, failed to display reduced cycle duration. The situation appeared to be different when male urine was concerned. Indeed, olfactory stimuli from males were also implicated in estrous rhythm regulation. Olfactory bulb removal suppressed the effects of male urine on estrous cycle duration when the females were prevented to lick their litter. However another pathway possibly gustatory in nature, may compensate for the absence of olfactory bulbs since bulbectomized females maintained on floor level still maintained capacity to reduce cycle duration on exposure to male urine.

B. EVIDENCE THAT THE VENTROMEDIAL NUCLEUS MEDIATES THE ACTION OF OLFACTORY STIMULI ON ESTROUS RHYTHM IN THE RAT

Preliminary observations showed that female rats which had changed 4-day into 5-day cycles following VMN lesions failed to return to their initial cyclicity on exposure to male or female rat's urine whether or not they were allowed to lick their litter (CHATEAU et ARON, in press). The question then arose as to whether VMN lesions would prevent the action of olfactory stimuli in rats with a natural 5-day cycle.

A first series of experiments were designed to compare the effects of small VMN lesions, as performed by CARRER and al., (1973-74) and CHATEAU et al. (1976a), with those of sham VMN or DMN lesions in the absence of exposure to urine.

Table 3 shows that small VMN lesions did not induce any change in estrous rhythm with respect to unoperated females. By contrast, a significant increase in estrous cycle shortening was observed in sham VMN and DMN lesions taken as a whole as compared to VMN lesions (15/24 and 4/18, respectively; $\chi^2 = 8.71$; $p < 0.01$; 1 df). Therefore sham VMN and DMN lesioned females could not constitute reliable controls for studying the shortening action of urine following VMN lesions.

Table 3.

Changes in estrous cycle duration in 5-day cyclic female rats following hypothalamic ventromedial (VMN) and dorsomedial nucleus (DMN) lesions. Licking of litter not allowed.

Treatment	Number of animals	Proportion of females showing shortening from 5 to 4 days during a sequence of 3 postoperative or natural cycles.
Unoperated females	22	5/22
Small VMN lesions	18	4/18
DMN lesions	12	7/12
Sham VMN lesions	12	8/12

Table 4 summarizes results concerned with the action of male urine on estrous rhythm. A significant increase in cycle shortening was observed

152

Table 4.

Action of the odor of male urine on estrous cycle duration in 5-day
cyclic female rats following small ventromedial nucleus (VMN) lesions.
Licking of litter not allowed.

Treatment	Number of animals	Proportion of females showing shortening from 5 to 4 days during a sequence of 3 postoperative or natural cycles.
Small VMN lesioned females	14	6/14
Small VMN lesioned females exposed to the odor of urine	16	3/16
Unoperated females	16	4/16
Unoperated females exposed to the odor of urine	16	11/16

in unoperated females exposed to the action of urine as compared to the unoperated controls (11/16 and 4/16 ; $\chi^2 = 11.12$; $p < 0.001$, 1 df). By contrast small VMN lesioned females exposed to the action of urine did not differ from their lesioned counterparts (6/14 and 3/16 ; χ^2 Yates = 1.08 ; $p > 0.2$; 1 df).

We are then allowed to assume that the VMN constitutes the pathway through which olfactory stimuli regulate estrous rhythm in the rat.

C. DOES THE VENTROMEDIAL NUCLEUS CONSTITUTE AN AUTONOMOUS STRUCTURE FOR THE REGULATION OF ESTROUS RHYTHM IN THE RAT?

Table 5 shows that no cycle prolongation occurred in operated controls and bulbectomized-sham VMN lesioned females during 5 successive 4-day cycles. By contrast a 24-hour cycle prolongation or alternate 4- and 5-day cyclicity was observed in 61.1% of the bulbectomized females following small VMN lesions. Statistical analysis confirmed these data ($\chi^2 = 43.66$; $p < 0.001$; 1 df).

Table 5.

Changes in duration of two postoperative cycles following small ventromedial nucleus (VMN) lesions in 4-day cyclic female Wistar rats deprived of olfactory bulbs at the age of 6 weeks.

Treatment		Number of animals	Estrous rhythm		
			unmodified 4-day cyclicity	24-hour prolongation	Alternate 4- or 5-day cyclicity
Unoperated females [*]		42	42	0	0
Bulbectomized females	Sham VMN [**] lesions	12	12	0	0
	Small VMN [**] lesions	36	14	12	10

[*] estrous rhythm controlled during 5 successive 4-day cycles.

[**] surgery on proestrus during the third of three successive 4-day cycles.

CONCLUSIONS

The data reported here clearly demonstrate that two different pathways may be involved in estrous rhythm regulation by male urine in the rat. Previous experiments (CHATEAU et ARON, in press) using females whose cycles had changed from 4 to 5-days following small VMN lesions provided evidence that the VMN mediated the odoriferous action of urine as well as the effects related to licking of litter. Therefore the existence of two different substances capable of shortening estrous cycle by both pathways appears unlikely. However the question still arises as to whether the same urinary substance operates as a pheromone in male and female urine. Chemical information is needed to resolve this problem.

The mechanisms whereby the VMN mediates the action of olfactory stimuli on estrous rhythm have been partially elucidated. It is well known that progesterone regulates estrous rhythm in the rat. BUFFLER and ROSER (1974) showed that estrous cycle duration is dependent on blood progesterone level on the morning of diestrus II. A 5-day cyclicity appeared to be related to higher level of progesterone at this stage of the cycle than in 4-day cycles. A decrease in blood progesterone concentration was observed on the morning of diestrus II in 5-day cyclic females whose cycle duration was reduced under the influence of olfactory stimuli (CHATEAU and al., 1976b). Furthermore an increase in blood progesterone concentration occurred on the morning of diestrus II in 4-day cyclic females which displayed a 24-hour cycle prolongation following small VMN lesions (PLAS-ROSER et al., 1976). Therefore our observations suggest that the VMN mediates the action of olfactory stimuli by controlling the rate of ovarian progesterone secretion during the diestrous period of the cycle. Presumably the same mechanism is involved when the VMN autonomously regulates estrous rhythm in olfactory bulb deprived females.

Of course the nature of this hormonal control requires further investigations.

REFERENCES

1. ARON, Cl. and CHATEAU, D. (1971)
   Horm. Behav., 2, 315-323.

2. ARON, Cl., ROOS, J. and ROOS, M. (1971)
   J. Interdiscipl. Cycle Res., 2, 239-246.

3. ARON, Cl., ROOS, J., CHATEAU, D. and ROOS, M. (1972)
   Ann. Endocrinol., 33, 23-34.

4. BUFFLER, G. and ROSER, S. (1974)
   Acta Endocrinol., 75, 569-578.

5. CARRER, H., ASCH, G. and ARON, Cl. (1973-74)
   Neuroendocrinol., 13, 129-138.

6. CHATEAU, D. and ARON, Cl.
   J. Interdiscipl. Cycle Res., in press.

7. CHATEAU, D., ROOS, J. and ARON, Cl. (1972)
   C.R. Soc. Biol., 166, 1110-1113.

8. CHATEAU, D., CARRER, H., ROOS, J. and ARON, Cl. (1974)
   C.R. Soc. Biol., 167, 1973-1977.

9. CHATEAU, D., ROOS,M. and ARON Cl. (1976a)
   Neuroendocrinol., 21, 157-164.

10. CHATEAU, D., ROOS, J., PLAS-ROSER, S., ROOS, M. and ARON,Cl.(1976b)
    Acta Endocrinol., 82, 426-435.

11. PLAS-ROSER, S., CHATEAU, D. and ARON, Cl. (1976)
    J. Physiol., 72, 53A.

12. ROOS, J., CHATEAU, D. and ARON, Cl. (1973a).
    Proc. the third European Anat. Congr., Abst., 56-57.

13. ROOS, J., CHATEAU, D. and ARON, Cl. (1973b)
    C.R. Acad. Sci., 276, 2823-2826.

✳ This work has been financed by the C.N.R.S.
   (E.R.A. n° 566).

Amino acids as olfactory stimuli in fish

Toshiaki J. Hara

Freshwater Institute, Department of Fisheries and the Environment, Winnipeg,
Manitoba, Canada R3T 2N6

ABSTRACT
    Evidence is presented indicating that amino acids present in fish skin
mucus are responsible for olfactory stimulation. Electrophysiological study
of the specificity of olfactory stimulation by amino acids has established
definite structure-activity relationships. A putative amino acid receptor
site which involves two charged subsites capable of interacting with ionized
amino and carboxyl groups of amino acid molecules has been described. Chemical modification of olfactory epithelium by group specific protein reagents
suggests that the receptor for amino acids is probably a protein with a
disulfide bond in the vicinity of the active site. This disulfide can be
reduced and reoxidized with concomitant inhibition and restoration of the
response to stimulants. Sulfhydryl groups also play important roles in
olfactory transduction. Specific binding of labeled amino acids to a membrane preparation from olfactory rosettes was measured. Binding is saturable,
displaceable and stereospecific. The extent of binding of amino acids examined compares closely with their electrophysiological effectiveness.

INTRODUCTION

    Olfaction in fish, unlike in terrestrial animals, takes place entirely in

the aquatic environment. The carrier of stimulant molecules is not air but

water, therefore the spectra of chemicals detected by fish could be entirely

different from those detected by terrestrial animals. Behavioral and

electrophysiological studies indicate that amino acids, which are normally

non-odorous to terrestrial animals, are extremely effective olfactory stimuli

to fish. Odor recognition persists, however, whether water or air is the

carrier. It is not hard to imagine that the principle governing the fundamen-

tal mechanism of the olfactory process is common to all vertebrates, if one

considers evolutionary trends of olfaction in animals. An event common to

all the olfactory phenomena is the interaction of the stimulus molecule with

the receptor. Attempts have been made to study directly the binding of

stimulant amino acids to the membrane receptors of fish. My aim here is to

review recent studies on structure-activity relationships of amino acids, a putative receptor site and binding of labeled amino acids to an olfactory membrane fraction in fish, and to point out some of the advantages the study of olfaction in fish offers for understanding the primary process of olfaction.

OLFACTORY RESPONSE TO SKIN MUCUS

The skin mucus of fish, besides serving primarily as protector, plays an important role in fish behavior, influencing schooling, recognition of individuals and homing migration[1-4]. Electrophysiological studies have shown that the mucus is an effective olfactory stimulant for rainbow trout (Salmo gairdneri), and that the active components responsible for olfactory stimulation are heat stable and non-volatile, and have molecular weight less than 1000[5]. Mucus from migratory populations of Arctic char (Salvelinus alpinus) produced differential sensory responses in the olfactory bulb neurons[6,7]. Pheromone(s) have been claimed to be involved in these reactions[8]. A major component of fish skin mucus is glycoprotein similar in composition to those secreted by goblet cells of epithelial tissues in mammals[9].

Our recent chemical analyses have revealed that mucous substances collected from males and females of rainbow trout contain free amino acids totaling 36.8 ± 8.0 and 24.5 ± 8.9 μmoles/100 mg mucous substance, respectively. More than 25 different amino acids have been identified. Taurine is the most abundant amino acid, and all amino acids, except β-alanine, are present in significantly larger quantity in males than females. This is consistent with the data for whitefish (Coregonus clupeaformis), in which free amino acids total 63.0 ± 19.5 and 42.3 ± 10.2 μmoles/100 mg mucous substance in males and females, respectively. The amount of free amino acids present in the mucus seems to be fully responsible for olfactory stimulation. Artificial mucous substance, a mixture of amino aicds based on the analysis data, induces olfactory bulbar responses indistinguishable from that induced by the original mucous substance.

The role of skin mucous substance in the behavior of these species is not well understood. Whitefish can be either attracted or repelled by mucus from conspecifics. Whether this is related to the individual and/or sexual recognition is yet to be determined. An individual of schooling marine catfish eels (Plotosus anguillaris) is attracted to a "pheromone" released from the body surface of others within the school[10]. The question arises whether there still exists a single principal substance which can be identified as a pheromone, or whether the active component is merely a characteristic combination or _melange_ of free amino acids.

STRUCTURE-ACTIVITY RELATIONSHIPS OF AMINO ACIDS

Evidence has accumulated indicating that amino acids may play important roles as chemical signals in olfactory communication in fish[11]. Electrophysiological investigations of the specificity of olfactory stimulation by amino acids in trout have led to the establishment of definite structure-activity relationships[12-14]. In these studies the electrical responses from the olfactory bulb (induced response) were measured when the nares were stimulated with various stimulant chemicals. The threshold concentrations estimated for highly stimulatory amino acids range between 10^{-7} and 10^{-8}M. The requirements of amino acids for olfactory stimulation thus far determined are:

(1) Only α-amino acids, derived from proteins, are highly stimulatory. Amino acids whose amino group is located at a position other than the alpha are less effective. The stimulatory effectiveness is not directly related to the essential amino acid.

(2) Natural L-isomer of an amino acid is always more stimulatory than its D-isomer.

(3) Ionically charged α-amino and α-carboxyl groups are essential. Replacement of these groups with other functional groups or structural alterations of either or both groups result in a decreased response. Acetylation of the α-amino group or esterification of the α-carboxyl group all result in reduced activity.

(4) The α-hydrogen of amino acids must be free. Replacement of this atom by a methyl group eliminates the effectiveness. β-Hydrogens should preferably be free; replacement with other functional groups results in reduced activity.

(5) The size and polar nature of the fourth α-moiety are also important determinant factors.

The amino acids effective as olfactory stimuli are thus characterized by being simple, short and straight-chained, with only certain attached groups. Glycine is the smallest amino acid molecule that fulfills all the above requirements. Among homologous series of aliphatic amino acids, the effectiveness is maximum for alanine whose number of carbon atoms in the chain is 3, and it sharply decreases for amino acids in which overall carbon chain length is less than 3 or more than 6. The introduction of a strongly polar or bulky groups at the terminal end markedly reduces activity. All homolo-

gous oligo-peptides tested are only slightly stimulatory at 10^{-4}M. Studies
on other species, though not extensive, seem to support the above[15-17].

Under normal physiological condition, the amino acid exists in a dipolar
ion or zwitterionic form, the carboxyl group being dissociated and the amino
group associated. The degree of ionization of amino acids depends upon the
pH of the environment. The responses to amino acids are pH dependent;
responses are inhibited below pH 3 and above pH 10[18]. Although the pH-
response relationship is specific for each amino acid, highly stimulatory
amino acids display maximal activity near their isoelectric points at which
dipolar ions are at maximum and bearing no net charge.

PUTATIVE AMINO ACID RECEPTOR

It is suggested from the above that stimulatory effectiveness is
dependent upon interaction of amino acid molecules with receptor membrane
structures of definite shape, size and charge distribution. The "amino acid
receptor" in the olfactory epithelium thus can be considered to consist of an
arrangement of charged atoms or groups located within a specific region of
the molecular framework of the membrane. A putative receptor site can be
considered which involves two charged subsites, one anionic (I) and one
cationic (II), capable of interacting with ionized amino and carboxyl groups
of the stimulant amino acid molecules. These two subsites are arranged in a
specific manner around a center (III) which accommodates the α-hydrogen atom
of the amino acid molecule, thus making L-isomers more accessible to the
receptor site (Fig. 1). Three-dimensional crystal-structure analysis shows
that the conformation, bond lengths and angles about the α-carbon atom are
fairly consistent in all amino acids studied, and that the distance between
the negatively and positively charged groups is approximately 3 $\overset{\circ}{A}$[19]. Since
the size and polar nature of the fourth α-moiety of the amino acid largely
influence its stimulatory effectiveness, there must be another receptor
region which accommodates and recognizes the profile of the fourth α-moiety
(R) of the amino acid. Quality discrimination of amino acids could take
place at this region. Whitefish are able to discriminate behaviorally
between glycine and fully deuterated glycine, though both chemicals induce
bulbar responses indistinguishable from each other[20]. Also, molecular
properties other than electronic structure and force fields, such as molecular motions or dipole moments, may be involved in olfactory discrimination in
fish.

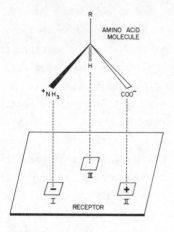

Fig. 1. A putative three-subsite amino acid receptor site. Two charged sub-sites, one anionic (I) and one cationic (II), are arranged around a center (III) which accommodates the α-hydrogen atom of an amino acid molecule. (From Hara, 1977).

The amino acid receptor site described above is similar in principle to the AH-B system proposed for human sweet taste[21]. However, the three-subsite model for fish olfactory system would seem to make the receptor more stereospecific.

CHEMICAL MODIFICATION OF OLFACTORY EPITHELIUM BY GROUP-SPECIFIC PROTEIN REAGENTS

It is generally assumed that the protein and lipid in the receptor membranes form the probable receptor molecules for chemical stimuli and that the binding of stimulant molecules is translated into permeability changes by means of conformational changes in proteins. If the receptor, and possibly other components of the stimulant-activated permeability system were protein, they might react with reagent for protein side-chain groups. Olfactory receptors of rainbow trout were treated with sulfhydryl (SH) and disulfide specific protein reagents, and the resulting modifications in activities of olfactory receptors were measured by recording the olfactory bulbar response induced by a standard stimulant. N-Ethylmaleimide (NEM), an SH-alkylating reagent, irreversibly inhibited the response. Inhibition by NEM was protected by thiol agents, but was not affected by the presence of stimulant molecules before and during treatment. This suggests that the site of NEM action is not the specific receptor site for chemical stimuli. Studies on N-substituted maleimide inactivation of the taste response in rats indicate that the site of alkylation is either intracellular or buried within the cell membrane in a region inaccessible to most extracellular fluids[22]. In fact, NEM does not significantly inhibit binding of stimulant molecules to membrane

preparations from taste epithelium of catfish[23] (see below). In contrast,
in the frog (Rana pipiens), the effect of NEM can be prevented by the presence
of an odorous substance, suggesting a competitive action on the specific receptor site[24]. It should be noted however that unlike the tight covalent interaction by NEM, the binding of stimulant molecules with receptors is
probably weak and readily displaceable nature, such as hydrophobic, electrostatic and hydrogen bonding. All mercaptide-forming reagents tested inhibited
the bulbar response. SH-oxidizing reagents alone had little effect. However,
inhibition by disulfide reagents was recovered by subsequent treatment with
oxidizing reagents. These findings suggest that the receptor for amino acids,
just as for acetylcholine, is probably a protein with a disulfide bond in the
vicinity of the active site. This disulfide can be reduced and reoxidized
with concomitant inhibition and restoration of the response to amino acids.

BINDING OF LABELED AMINO ACIDS TO A MEMBRANE PREPARATION FROM OLFACTORY EPITHELIUM

An initial event common to all the chemoreception phenomena is the interaction of the stimulus molecules - the ligand - with the receptor. We could
approach an understanding of the binding of the ligand to the receptor if we
could isolate the chemoreceptor membranes and make a direct study of the
binding of the ligand to them. The binding must show absolute specificity,
the affinity must be consistent with the biological activity of the ligand,
and the number of binding sites must be consistent with the physiological
mechanisms operative in the intact system.

Binding studies were carried out on a tissue preparation from olfactory
rosettes of brook trout (Salvelinus fontinalis) according to the method
described for catfish (Ictalurus punctatus) taste epithelium[25]. The rosettes
were dissected, homogenized, and fractionated by differential centrifugation to
obtain a tissue pellet enriched in membrane fragments and mitochondria.
(Membrane subfractions can be obtained by osmotic shock treatment of this
fraction.). After incubation of this tissue fraction with radioactively
labeled amino acids, the bound radioactivity was determined using a rapid
filtration method. Specific binding was determined by the amount of labeled
ligand that could be displaced in the presence of a large excess of non-
labeled ligand. The results obtained indicate that the specific binding
is: (1) time-dependent and saturable: half saturation occurs around
5.5×10^{-6}M for L-alanine, (2) displaceable; bound labeled amino acids
rapidly displaced by a large excess of unlabeled amino acids, (3) stereospecific as evidenced by the lack of binding by D-enatiomer, and (4) bio-

logical; preparations from brains, gills and skin exhibited minimal specific binding. The extent of binding of several amino acids tested compares closely with their electrophysiological effectiveness. Although the amount of specific binding increases linearly with protein concentration, it should be noted that acid hematein specific phospholipids are highly localized in fish olfactory neurons[26]. Phospholipids also may play a role in the transduction events either directly as part of the receptor or indirectly through their association with the membrane receptor protein.

CONCLUDING REMARKS

Both olfaction and taste in fish take place entirely in aquatic environment. Except for catfish barbels, taste receptors are usually less sensitive to amino acids compared to olfaction[27,28]. Taste receptors of catfish barbels are similar to olfactory receptors in electrical responses to amino acids[17]. Specificities of binding of labeled amino acids to a membrane preparation from catfish barbel epithelium is also comparable to those of olfactory rosettes of rainbow trout. This sensory overlap will present interesting questions as to behavioural significance for the development of two separate chemosensory systems.

If specific mixtures rather than single chemicals, such as amino acids, are responsible for the majority of intra- and interspecies behaviour responses, then one chemical may have several effects, depending on what other substances are simultaneously present. Alternatively, does single chemical mediate each specific behaviour? Two substances which induce exploratory feeding behaviour in two different species of fish have been identified in mussel and snail[29].

Most odorant molecules are amphipathic and will be adsorbed weakly to phospholipids with very weak association constants, making most binding studies unlikely to succeed[30]. Binding experiments described above satisfy the basic criteria for receptor-specific labeling, indicating that the binding is a physiologically relevant measure of an initial event of olfaction. This will offer a valid and useful system for obtaining detailed insight into the molecular interactions involved in the initial stimulant-receptor interaction.

REFERENCES

1. Wrede, W.L. (1932) Z. Vergleich. Physiol. 17, 510-519
2. Todd, J.H., Atema, J. and Bardach, J.E. (1967) Science 158, 672-673
3. Nordeng, H. (1971) Nature 233, 411-413
4. Solomon, D.J. (1973) Nature 244, 231-232
5. Hara, T.J. and Macdonald, S. (1976) Comp. Biochem. Physiol. 45A, 21-24

6. Døving, K.B. (1976) in Structure-Activity Relationships in Chemorecep-
    tion, pp. 149-160, Information Retrieval, London

7. Døving, K.B., Enger, P.S. and Nordeng, H. (1973) Comp. Biochem
    Physiol. 45A, 21-24

8. Døving, K.B., Nordeng, H. and Oakley, B. (1974) Comp. Biochem. Physiol
    47A, 1051-1063

9. Wold, J.K. and Selset, R. (1977) Comp. Biochem. Physiol. 56B, 215-218

10. Kinosita, H. (1975) in Modern Biological Science, Vol. 9, pp. 71-154,
    Iwanami, Tokyo

11. Hara, T.J. (1975) Progr. Neurobiol. 5, 271-335

12. Hara, T.J. (1973) Comp. Biochem. Physiol. 44A, 407-416

13. Hara, T.J. (1976) Comp. Biochem. Physiol. 54A, 31-36

14. Hara, T.J. (1977) Comp. Biochem. Physiol. 56A, 559-565

15. Suzuki, N. and Tucker, D. (1971) Comp. Biochem. Physiol. 40A, 399-404

16. Belghaug, R. and Døving, K.B. (1977) Comp. Biochem. Physiol. 57A,
    327-330

17. Caprio, J. (1977) Nature 266, 850-851

18. Hara, T.J. (1976) Comp. Biochem. Physiol. 54A, 37-39

19. Marsh, R.E. and Donohue, J. (1967) Adv. Protein Chem. 22, 235-257

20. Hara, T.J. (1977) Experientia 33, 618-619

21. Shallenberger, R.S. and Acree, T.E. (1967) Nature 216, 480-482

22. Mooser, G. (976) J. Neurobiol. 7, 457-468

23. Zelson, P.R. and Cagan, R.H. (1977) Fed. Proc. 36, 703

24. Getchell, M.L. and Gesteland, R.C. (1972) Proc. Natl. Acad. Sci. USA
    69, 1494-1498

25. Krueger, J.M. and Cagan, R.H. (1976) J. Biol. Chem. 251, 88-97

26. Evans, R.E. and Hara, T.J. (1977) Can. Z. Zool. 55, 776-781

27. Sutterlin, A.M. and Sutterlin, N. (1970) J. Fish. Res. Board Can. 27,
    1927-1942

28. Hidaka, I. and Kiyohara, S. (1975) in Olfaction and Taste V, pp. 147-
    151, Academic, New York

29. Sangster, A.W., Thomas, S.E. and Tingling, N.L. (1975) Tetrahedron
    31, 1135-1137

30. Dodd, G.H. (1974) in Transduction Mechanisms in Chemoreception, pp.
    103-113, Information Retrieval, London

Functional separation of smell and taste in fish and crustacea

Jelle Atema

Boston University Marine Program, Marine Biological Laboratory, Woods Hole, MA 02543, USA

ABSTRACT

In aquatic animals, the validity of a functional distinction between smell and taste is often questioned. This may be due to a lack of understanding of the role these senses play in survival. Catfish have two anatomically and functionally distinct chemical senses; taste serves a role in food localization and the consummatory phases of feeding behavior; smell is used in social behavior and in the acquisition of behavior triggered by chemical cues. A related function of the olfactory system in fish appears to be the formation of chemical search images as seen in prey odor detection in tuna and in home-stream recognition in salmon. These functions appear to have been largely preserved in adaptation to terrestrial life. There is evidence that a similar functional distinction between smell and taste exists in crustacea, and other arthropods.

INTRODUCTION

Chemical senses research has focused largely on mechanisms of chemoreception from peripheral transduction to central decoding problems. One important aspect of chemoreception has often been ignored: its evolution and biological survival function. And yet it seems obvious that an understanding of survival function could significantly contribute to elucidate the physiological mechanisms that evolved to serve that function. One question of particular relevance here is why aquatic animals evolved two or more morphologically and functionally distinct chemoreceptor organs, often analogous to the human senses of smell and taste. At the previous symposium, ISOT V, doubts were expressed as to the validity of a smell-taste distinction in aquatic animals[1]. Our recent work on chemically stimulated behavior of catfish (Ictalurus sp.), tuna (Thunnus albacares), and lobsters (Homarus americanus) provides a number of clues that may lead to a generalized concept of the biological function of smell and taste in aquatic animals.

FISH

Catfish have a well-developed nose[2,3] and an elaborate sense of taste[4-6]

which has separated into a functionally distinct external and internal sense[5] innervated by cranial nerves VII and IX/X respectively. At the cellular level[7] and in central connections through the olfactory bulb[8], fish olfactory organs are essentially similar to those of other vertebrate groups. Taste cells, taste buds[9], and central gustatory projections[6,8,10] are also essentially similar in all vertebrates.

Electrophysiological studies on catfish have shown that various amino acids can both be smelled and tasted with thresholds in the range of 10^{-8} and 10^{-11} M respectively[11]. Some alcohols, in contrast, produced olfactory but almost no taste responses in 10^{-4} M concentration[12]. Of these alcohols, morpholine has been successfully used to imprint juvenile salmon[13] and B-phenethyl alcohol was used to determine olfactory thresholds in eels[14].

Behavioral studies showed that catfish can localize a distant food source (liver juice) by taste alone[15]. The removal or occlusion of olfactory organs did not affect feeding behavior to dead bait[15,16]. However, specific deficits in the normal sequence of feeding behavior were caused by lesions in the primary taste projection areas of the brain[5]. These studies showed that facial innervated external taste is involved in guiding a catfish to the chemical food source and that it helps trigger the food pick-up reflex. Vagal and glossopharyngeal innervated internal taste appears to serve a role in final food checking, and it helps trigger the swallow reflex. Thus, catfish do not seem to need olfaction to localize and feed on dead bait. However, when their nares were blocked, they could no longer perform the previously learned task of differentiating between two individual conspecifics nor could they be trained to that task[17].

It was thus concluded that in catfish smell served a social function and taste a function in feeding behavior. However, a modified explanation for these experimental results could be that olfaction, not taste, is programmed for plasticity and learning of relatively complex tasks[2]. Preliminary results for a role of olfaction in learning are presented below.

Catfish, Ictalurus nebulosus, were kept individually in 50 l all-glass aquaria with oyster chip substrate and one shelter. The outflow of a substrate filter provided a constant flow of water to a funnel suspended over the water surface. Catfish took up a position in the shelter with their head half out. Water from the funnel was directed to flow immediately over the fish's head. Chemical stimuli could be added to the funnel and reach the fish within one second as indicated by dye tests. This procedure minimized mechanical stimulus artifacts and kept stimulus dilution within one order of magnitude.

Three stimuli were chosen: 1) the fish's own tank water (control); 2) 10^{-6} M solution of β-phenethyl alchohol; and 3) 10^{-6} M solution of glutamine, an amino acid which is both smelled and tasted at concentrations less than 10^{-8} M[11].

Fish were trained with food reward to leave their shelter and come to the surface at the far side of their tank within 10 seconds of stimulus presentation. Control tests served to avoid conditioning to other than chemical stimuli. One pair of fish (A and B) were trained to β-phenethyl alcohol and one pair (G and H) to glutamine. After a good response level was obtained and maintained for at least 2 days, one fish of each pair was made anosmic by stuffing a cotton and vaseline plug in both nasal sacs. This reversible procedure eliminates olfactory input without altering the neural circuit to the brain. The anosmic fish was tested for two days with test and control stimuli. The control fish was anesthetized but did not receive a nose plug. It was then given only control stimuli for two days to measure the effect of anesthesia and fading memory. After two days the plugs were removed and both fish tested for several days. Slight retraining was necessary in some cases. When the response level was reestablished the other fish of the pair was made anosmic while the first one served as a control. After two days of testing the nose plugs were again removed and both fish tested and retrained when necessary. In the final test one of the fish received a bilateral lesion of the facial lobes to eliminate external taste[5]. After a few days of testing the quality of the lesion was established by presenting a piece of food for them to localize and pick up. Well-lesioned fish cannot perform this task for as long as three weeks after the operation[5].

The results of these experiments are presented in Table 1. The response to phenethyl alcohol was completely abolished by nose plugging and returned after plug removal. Control fish maintained the response. In contrast, successful taste lesion did not greatly affect the trained response to phenethyl alcohol, but it abolished the ability to locate and pick up dead bait. The trained response to glutamine was also completely abolished by nose plugging, but here it was clear that the fish still sensed the stimulus as indicated by the appearance of a new behavior: they would push their heads up to the stimulus tube immediately after the glutamine solution hit them.

From these results one can conclude that the amino acid stimulus was indeed perceived both through smell and taste as predicted from electrophysiological studies. However, the trained behavioral response was mediated via the nose. In other words, to learn a new behavior in response to a chemical

TABLE 1. Results of Catfish Training Experiments: Number of correct responses/number of trials.

	B-phenethyl alcohol				Glutamine			
	Fish A		Fish B		Fish G		Fish H	
	STIM	CONT	STIM	CONT	STIM	CONT	STIM	CONT
PRE	33/36	30/30	48/50	30/30	23/26	22/28	20/24	17/23
PLUG	Control	71/74	0/41	37/37	0/46!	22/22	Control	41/41
POST	22/25	11/13	18/30*	12/12	23/36*	14/17	32/34	19/24
PRE	33/33	35/40	32/32	27/32				
PLUG	0/40	44/44	Control	51/53	Control	73/76	0/46!	45/45
POST	24/31*o	24/24	31/32o	23/24	14/15	4/5	10/16*	5/6
PRE			27/27	12/12				
LES	not successful		32/37*	14/16				

* Reminders were necessary; listed as incorrect responses.
o Some responses were slower than usual.
! New response behavior: head pushing to stimulus introduction tube.

stimulus, which can be both smelled and tasted, the olfactory system and not the taste system is utilized.

Similar conclusions on olfactory plasticity were drawn from experiments on the role of olfaction in tuna behavior[18] The general biology of these highly visual animals provides a dramatic contrast with the biology of the chemosensory catfish; this makes the similarities in the function of the olfactory system even more interesting.

Yellowfin tuna (Thunnus albacares) were maintained in 7.5 m diameter circular pools with flowing seawater (250 1/min). Their behavioral responses to prey odors were measured from videotape analysis. Odor stimuli were introduced into the tank as 20 ml slugs injected into a continuously flowing tube. Dye tests showed arrival, dilution and position of the odor cloud as it traveled around the pool during tests. By superimposing dye pictures on playback recordings of tuna responses it was possible to estimate the moment a fish encountered the odor cloud to within about 2 sec. This estimate was verified behaviorally.

Odor from natural anchovy prey caused a strong response: swimming patterns changed, swimming speed increased, head thrusts and occasional snapping were observed, and sometimes dark vertical stripes ("feeding bars") appeared on their flanks. This response declined over the two months period in which the tuna were fed on an unfamiliar California anchovy species. Odor from this latter species began to elicit very strong responses. Neither satiated nor anosmic fish (olfactory sacs filled with alginate) responded to odor introductions. It was concluded that the olfactory sense was responsible for the mediation of learned chemical cues and served to "turn-on" their search for specific prey.

When prey odor was separated into amino and non-amino fractions, either one of the fractions caused weak responses only. When the major amino acid, tryptophan, and 3 minor amino acids were presented alone in concentrations comparable to those found in whole prey odor, a very weak response was observed. Tryptophan concentration in the odor cloud when first encountered was estimated at 10^{-12} M. It was concluded that single compounds are less effective than the full mixture, as has been found elsewhere[19-22]. In other words, olfaction is programmed to recognize specific, complex chemical mixtures, and, upon recognition, to elicit specific behavior. To recognize complex mixtures fish must have a chemical search image in analogy with visual pattern recognition. These chemical search images appear to be modifiable with prey availability.

There are other examples of search images. Anadromous fish, such as salmon, that must recognize their home tributary stream are known to utilize olfaction[23]. There is little doubt that this involves recognition of a complex chemical image, or "fingerprint". Here also, imprinting to a single artificial compound, morpholine, is easily accomplished and mediated via olfaction[13]. Other chemical images that are mediated by olfaction are those involved in prey, predator, species, brood and individual recognition[24-26]. Generally in fish, social behavior seems to involve olfaction rather than taste. One example of chemically mediated sexual behavior is reflected in external morphology. Upon maturity, male <u>Cyclothone</u> <u>microdon</u>, a bathypelagic fish, develop a large olfactory apparatus, involving olfactory epithelium, olfactory bulbs and forebrain. Females remain microsmatic[27].

Fish extract chemical information from one carrier medium with smell and taste. The morphological distinction between the two chemical senses has been preserved during terrestrial adaptation. It is of some interest to see if functional distinctions found in fish have been preserved as well, since this may give us a more fundamental basis to understand their survival function than our usual criteria for smell and taste distinction: distance versus contact; low versus high threshold; air versus water medium. For the sake of brevity, I will mention one familiar example: trail following in hunting dogs. It is clear that the dog's olfactory system is capable of quick learning of complex chemical search images. Taste, on the other hand, has preserved its function as a food testing gate, adapted to the high chemical concentrations usually found in the mouth, but capable of detecting poisonous substances in low concentrations.

CRUSTACEA

Crustacea present a fundamentally different class of aquatic animals. Their main known chemoreceptor organs are antennules, maxillipeds, and dactyls. The lobster, _Homarus americanus_, is no exception, and some work on their chemoreceptive capabilities has been published. Most investigators agree that the lobster's antennules are a prominent organ for distance chemoreception whereas the dactyls are considered contact chemoreceptors. Shepheard[28] equates them with smell and taste for that reason. However, the more fundamental reasons for the existence of smell and taste, suggested above for fish and vertebrates, may be similar for crustacea and, perhaps, for other invertebrates.

Unfortunately, very little is known about the specific function of different chemoreceptor organs in crustacea. Antennules, dactyls and maxillipeds have roughly similar electrophysiological thresholds for amino acids. Antennule values range from 10^{-5} to 10^{-7} M[28-30]; dactyl thresholds range from 10^{-5} to 10^{-8} M[30,31]; maxillipeds were tested in only one instance and had thresholds of 10^{-5} M[30]. Based on threshold values either organ could serve as a distance chemoreceptor. Indeed, when both antennules were removed, lobsters still alerted to distant odor sources[32]; and antennule removal in hermit crabs was shown to result in progressively increasing dactyl sensitivity over a period of weeks[33]. Also, antennules are not always distance chemoreceptors; in some cases, they are used as contact chemoreceptors in sex recognition[34,35].

The clear morphological differences between antennular and dactyl chemoreceptors may reflect a more essential difference in biological function than one of mere distance of reception. Central connections of the antennular chemoreceptor nerve enter the medulla terminalis of the deuterocerebrum in a complex glomerular area of the brain[36], reminiscent of vertebrate olfactory bulb anatomy[37]. Antennules appear to be involved in eliciting complex behavior. Animals without antennules no longer displayed complete food searching behavior[32,38]. Localized stimulation of different chemoreceptor appendages with food juices showed that dactyls and maxillipeds responded with localized reflex actions of short duration, whereas antennule stimulation resulted in prolonged and complex search patterns[33,38,39]. Furthermore, antennules appear involved in host recognition[40,41] and in sex recognition[42,43]. A morphological reflection of the latter is found in the external morphology of enlarged male antennules of prawn[44].

From such scant information a picture nevertheless emerges, in which crustacean antennules serve a function in the recognition of odor mixtures, eliciting complex search behavior. Both their neuronanatomical connections and biological function resemble vertebrate olfaction. In contrast, the dactyl and maxilliped receptors resemble vertebrate taste in their biological function of eliciting reflex-like consummatory phases of feeding behavior. Dactyls and maxillipeds may be the functional equivalent of catfish external and internal taste respectively[5]. Insects follow the crustacean pattern; here antennae have an olfactory function, and tarsal and proboscis chemoreceptors a separate taste function. It will be interesting to follow the functional division of chemoreceptors in other taxa, particularly the rather well-studied molluscs, where multiple chemoreceptor organs are known.

APPENDIX

Several contributions to this symposium contain information relevant to the proposed concept of the functional significance of smell and taste in aquatic animals, and the preservation of these functions in terrestrial adaptation. I mention the most pertinent.
1. Zippel, H.P., et al. concluded from studies on the odor elicited activity of units in the olfactory bulb of goldfish that second order (?) neurons are mainly responsive to complex natural stimuli, and that their responses increase with prior exposure or experience (pers.comm.). They further suggest that "the pronounced and long-lasting effects mainly observed following application of natural stimuli may be due to descending influences from higher cerebral centres", or intra-bulbar circuits. Such descending influences or bulbar circuits correspond to the proposed concept of chemical search images created in the olfactory system after prior exposure or conditioning.
2. Freeman, W.J. sugggests that odor specific induced wave patterns recorded from a large surface area of the olfactory bulbs of rabbits are "related more to the expectation of an odor than to the odor per se, and that it manifests a short-term or possibly long-term memory mechanism in the bulb". Such conditioned expectations may reflect the chemical search images thought to exist in catfish, tuna, and salmon. Indeed, Freeman's method may be a (distant) measurement of the search image.
3. Little, E.E., using heart rate conditioning in channel catfish (Ictalurus punctatus), showed that olfaction mediated the conditioned response to amino acid detection. Bait shyness was induced via the gustatory system as expected.

4. Masson, C. described the complex olfactory projections of insects, corresponding in surprising detail to the olfactory morphology of crustacea and vertebrates, and the plasticity of olfactory responses.

5. Norgren, R. showed that gustatory responses in decerebrate rats are normal and highly stereotyped. This corresponds to the reflex character of the taste system proposed for fish and crustacea.

Financial support for some of the research presented in this paper was provided by grants from the U.S. Energy Research and Development Administration (E 11-1-2546) and the U.S. Environmental Protection Agency (R-803833).

I want to express my sincere appreciation to Dr. John Bardach, who created and continuously stimulated my interest in chemical senses research. I thank Nathalie Ward and Geraldine Ferris for their devoted efforts in training catfish, and all members of my research group for continued and critical support.

REFERENCES

1. Bardach, J.E. (1975) in Olfaction and Taste V, D.A. Denton and J.P. Coghlan, eds., pp. 169-171, Academic Press, New York.

2. Atema, J., Todd, J.H. and Bardach, J.E. (1969) in Olfaction and Taste III, C. Pfaffman, ed., pp. 241-251, Rockefeller University Press, New York.

3. Finger, T.E. (1976) J. Comp. Neur. 165:513-526.

4. Herrick, C.J. (1905) J. Comp. Neur. 15:375-456.

5. Atema, J. (1971) Brain Behav. Evol. 4:273-294.

6. Finger, T.E. (1975) J. Comp. Neur. 161:125-142.

7. Steinbrecht, R.A. (1969) in Olfaction and Taste III, C. Pfaffman, ed., pp. 3-21, Rockefeller University Press, New York.

8. Herrick, C.J. (1924)   Neurological Foundations of Animal Behavior, pp. 155-169, Hafner Publishing Co., New York and London, reprinted 1962.

9. Graziadei, P.P.C. (1969) in Olfaction and Taste III, C. Pfaffman, ed., pp. 315-330, Rockefeller University Press, New York.

10. Norgren, R. and Leonard, C. (1973) J. Comp. Neur. 150:217-237.

11. Caprio, J. (1977) Nature 266:850-851.

12. Caprio, J., unpublished.

13. Cooper, J.C. and Hasler, A.D. (1974) Science 183:336-338.

14. Teichmann, H. (1959) Z. Vergl. Physiol. 42:206-254.

15. Bardach, J.E., Todd, J.H. and Crickmer, R (1967) Science 155:1276-1278.

16. Atema, J. (1969) The chemical senses in feeding and social behavior of the catfish, *Ictalurus natalis*. Ph.D. thesis, University of Michigan, 134 pp.

17. Todd, J.H., Atema, J. and Bardach, J.E. (1967) Science 158:672-673.

18. Atema, J., Holland, K. and Ikehara, W. (Submitted) Chemical Search Image: Olfactory Responses of Yellowfin Tuna (*Thunnus albacares*) to Prey Odors.

19. McLeese, D.W. (1970) J. Fish. Res. Bd. Can. 27:1371-1378.

20. Mackie, A.M. (1973) Marine Biology 21:103-108.

21. Bardach, J.E. (1975) in Olfaction and Taste V, D.A. Denton and J.P. Coghlan eds., pp. 121-132, Academic Press, New York.

22. Sutterlin, A. (1975) in Olfaction and Taste V, D.A. Denton and J.P. Coghlan, eds. pp. 153-161, Academic Press, New York.

23. Wisby, W.J. and Hasler, A.D. (1954) J. Fish Res. Bd. Can. 11:472-478.

24. Teichmann, H. (1962) Ergebnisse der Biologie 25:177-205.

25. Kleerekoper, H. (1969)   Olfaction in Fishes, 222 pp., Indiana University Press, Bloomington, London.

26. Bardach, J.E. and Villars, T. (1974) in Chemoreception in Marine Organisms, P. Grant and A. Mackie, eds., pp. 49-104, Academic Press, New York.

27. Marshall, N.B. (1967) Symp. Zool. Soc. Lond. No. 19:57-70.

28. Shepeard, P. (1974) Mar. Behav. Physiol. 2:261-273.

29. Ache, B.W. (1972) Comp. Biochem. Physiol. 42A:807-811.

30. Fuzessery, Z.M. and Childress, J.J. (1975) Biol. Bull. 149:522-538.

31. Case, J. (1964) Biol. Bull. 127:428-446.

32. McLeese, D.W. (1974) Mar. Behav. Physiol. 2:237-249.

33. Hazlett, B.A. (1971) Comp. Biochem. Physiol. 39A:665-670.

34. Forster, G.R. (1951) J. Mar. Biol. Ass. U.K. 30:333-360.

35. Carlisle, D.B. (1959) J. Mar. Biol. Ass. U.K. 38:481-491.

36. Maynard, D.M. and Yager, J.G. (1968) Z. Vergl. Physiol. 59:241-249.

37. Maynard, D.M. and Sallee, A. (1970) Z. Vergl. Physiol. 66:123-140.

38. Hazlett, B.A. (1968) Crustaceana 15:305-311.

39. Atema, J., Hadlock, R. and Karnofsky, E., unpublished.

40. Ache, B.W. (1975) Mar. Behav. Physiol. 3:125-130.

41. Ache, B. and Case, J. (1969) Physiol. Zool. 42:361-371.

42. Dahl, E. Emanuelsson, H. and von Mecklenburg, C. (1970) Science 170: 739-740.

43. Ameyaw-Akumfi, C. and Hazlett, B.A. (1975) Science 190:1225-1226.

44. Kamiguchi, Y. (1972) Zoological Magazine 81:223-226.

Some properties of the fish olfactory system

Kjell B. Døving and Georg Thommesen

Institute of Zoophysiology, University of Oslo, P. O. Box 1051, Blindern, Oslo 3, Norway

ABSTRACT

A short description is given on the mechanisms employed for water sampling by the olfactory organ of fish. In one group of fishes, isosmates, the olfactory cavity is divided in two compartments, a vestibule and a gallery. The connection between the two compartments is formed by the corridors of the olfactory rosette. Water-currents are created by ciliary beats on the walls of the corridors. In another group, cyclosmates, the accessory olfactory sacs can be compressed and expanded in connection with respiratory and/or mouth movements, these volume variations force water to pass over the olfactory epithelium. Responses from the surface of the olfactory bulb elicited by natural stimuli consist of slow depolarisations upon which are superimposed regular oscillations so-called "induced waves". The responses are distributed differently for various odorants, thus amino acids elicit the greatest responses in the lateral part of the bulb surface, while the water from fish basins elicits the largest responses in the anterior/medial part of the bulb.

INTRODUCTION

Problems in the field of fish olfaction can be considered to be specific or general depending upon what questions are asked. In the presentation below we shall give some information on the specific problems that are related to the sampling of the water by the fish's nose. It will be shown that water sampling is achieved by two different mechanisms: either by a water propulsion created by ciliary activity or by the pumping action of accessory olfactory sacs. The former solution is obviously specific to the water-dwelling species, while the latter has resemblences to the air pumping in terrestrial vertebrates. Many of the general problems concerning the physiology of the vertebrate olfactory sense can be attacked at different levels in different animals, because of the consistency in the anatomical organization of the system. The comparative physiology allows a liberal choice of animals, one can use the species that is best fitted to give the information to each question asked. One such question is the spatial distribution of the responses to different odorants which can be found at different levels in the olfactory system and most probably is a general phenomenon upon which the discrimination processes are based. In the second part we shall give some of the results obtained in the fish olfactory bulb that are pertinent to the discriminatory mechanisms.

WATER SAMPLING

An understanding of how water, carrying odorous substances, passes the sensory epithelium is a prerequisite for understanding how the nervous system treats the olfactory information. Studies on the mechanisms of the water sampling has revealed that there are principally two ways by which water is made to pass the olfactory organ, either by ciliary activity or by a pumping action of accessory olfactory sacs (Burne 1909, Døving et al. 1977). The principle for water propulsion by ciliary action has been shown to be analogous to the water propulsion systems of other organs and organisms. Due to the distinct difference between the fishes which use ciliary action to force water along and those using pumping action, a specific nomenclature has been suggested: Fishes using the ciliary action for water propulsion are called isosmates, stressing the continuous sampling of water. The other group is called cyclosmates focusing on the intermittent but repeating character of water sampling in these fishes. Below is given a short description of the functional anatomy of these two types of fishes.

Isosmates. The olfactory organ of isosmates has normally two openings. The anterior nostril directs forward , and it can be tubeformed as in an eel, a funnel-shaped expansion as in the Rhinomuraena, (Holl et al. 1970), or a stout pavillon as in the carp. The posterior nostril can be found at variable distances from the anterior one, and is regularly somewhat larger, oval and bordered by a low lip.

The olfactory cavity is nearly fully occupied by the olfactory rosette which is formed by a collection of leaves situated on the bottom of the olfactory cavity at both sides of a central raphe. The anterior nostril opens to the vestibule above the olfactory rosette. Noteworthy is a valence that encloses this compartment properly named a vestibule. Outside the valence is found a peripheral compartment, the gallery. This compartment opens directly to the posterior nostril. The passage from the vestibule to the gallery can take two paths, either underneath the valence above the olfactory rosette or through the corridors that are formed by the leaves of the olfactory rosette. When a dye is used to study the water currents in the olfactory organ in a live fish one can see the dye-filament entering the anterior nostril as a continuous band. In a suitable preparation one can see the dye-filament entering one or several corridors from the vestibule, after some time the dye

appears in the gallery and later leaves the olfactory cavity via the posterior nostril. When present in the gallery the dye filament is no longer a continuous and concentrated sheet but appears dispersed and diluted. Thus a considerable stirring has occurred in the passage through the corridors. The study by Døving et al. (1977) has shown that ciliary action in the corridors is
responsible for the water propulsion.

Thus the principle behind the water flow is a division of the olfactory
cavity in to two compartments, vestibule and gallery, the water is forced
from the vestibule to the gallery by the ciliary action in the corridor walls.
The principle used in this organ is analogous to the water propulsion in fil-
terfeeding lamellibranchs (Jørgensen 1966). The inhalant and exhalant cham-
bers of these animals correspond to the vestibule and gallery of the isosmates.

As a result of the means of water propulsion the fluid is passed over
the olfactory receptors only once, this observation confirms the one made by
Bashor et al. (1974) on garfish, Lepisosteus osseus. Thus water does not re-
enter the corridors as was stated by Teichmann (1959) in a preparation of an
eel's olfactory organ in which the valence was removed.

To illustrate the construction of the olfactory organ in isosmates and
the direction of water flow a schematic diagram of a cross section of the olfactory organ of eel is shown in Fig. 1. The olfactory rosette is composed of
a variable number of olfactory leaves, which are nearly symmetrically situated on both sides of the central raphe. The outer parts of the leaves consist
of ciliated cells while the central region is composed of receptor cells
(Holl 1965, Schulte 1972). The receptor cell region is surrounded by a transient zone with a mixed cell population. The division of the olfactory cavity
in to a vestibule and gallery comes about in the eel by a valence being formed

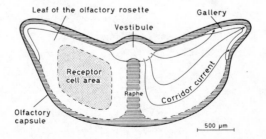

Fig. 1.   Schematic cross-section of the olfactory organ of eel, Anguilla anguilla, showing the principal water currents from the vestibule to the
gallery via the corridors. The distribution of receptor cells is taken from Holl (1965) and Schulte (1972).

by a roof of folded epithelium which fits over the leaves of the olfactory rosette. Water which can be seen to enter the central channel, the vestibule,
and distributes to the numerous corridors, enters the gallery from below, to
finally leave the olfactory cavity by the posterior naris.

Cyclosmates. The olfactory cavity has, in this type of fishes, most frequently two openings, in a few species there is only one opening (Burne 1909,
Pipping 1926). The olfactory rosette or epithelial sheet is situated just underneath the anterior opening, either stalked or on a basal epithelium. In
some fishes the basal epithelium forms a sail of connective tissue. The posterior opening is in some species equipped with a thin epithelial sheet which
serves as a valve arranged so that it may prevent water currents entering the
olfactory cavity via the posterior nostril. The volume of the characteristic
accessory sacs follows the movements of the mouth or the respiratory movements
in such a fashion that the sacs will be compressed when the mouth is closing
and expanded as the mouth opens. A characteristic form of the olfactory organ
of a cyclosmate is shown in Fig. 2. This drawing represents the olfactory organ of a Cyprinodontidae. The olfactory epithelium is situated close to the
anterior nostril and the posterior nostril is valved. In this family of fishes
one can distinguish four different types by the arrangement of the olfactory
epithelium (Zeiske 1974).

In experiments with dye-filaments the water is seen to enter the anterior
opening and leave the posterior one, in phase with the mouth movements. In
some fishes which lack the posterior valve the one-way passage may be secured
by the olfactory rosette which is situated on a sail, which may serve as a
valve, e.g. in the wrasse, Labrus bergylta. In the bar, Dicentrarchus labrax,

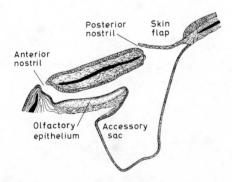

Fig. 2. The olfactory organ of a cyclosmate. Sagital section through the olfactory cavity of an oviparous Cyprinodont. Redrawn from Zeiske
(1974).

there are no valves present and water leaves and enters both openings simultaneously. But the renewal of the water will be secured as these virile fishes steadily swim around. The valves serve to secure a one-way passage of water through the olfactory cavity. The advantage of such a system is obvious in stationary fishes where the one-way passage will guarantee a renewal of the water sampled by the olfactory organ. In the fast swimming fishes as e.g. the bar, such mechanisms will be of less importance. It is however interesting to note that the macrell, Scomber scomber, and skipjack, Katsuwonus pelamis have valved posterior openings (Burne 1909, Gooding 1963).

As mentioned, there are some fishes which have only one nostril and water can be seen to flow in and out of the same opening. The mechanisms behind this particular olfactory organ have been described by Pipping (1926). As seen from her drawing reproduced in Fig. 3, the eel-pout, Zoarces viviparus, has an olfactory organ that ends in a blind cavity, the bottom of which forms a soft lining with the roof of the mouth. When water is forced into the mouth this lining expands the accessory olfactory sac, and conversely, when water is expelled from the mouth the lining bulges upwards and water leaves the olfactory cavity. A similar arrangement for water propulsion is found in the stonebiter, Anarhichas lupus.

SPATIAL DISTRIBUTION OF OLFACTORY BULB RESPONSES

Already in 1920 Holmgren suggested the existence of an "olfactory map" on the olfactory bulb of the fish. The suggestion was based on anatomical observations, and he assumed a spatial differentiation in the sensitivity of the olfactory epithelium to different odorants. The same idea emerged from an electrophysiological investigation of the olfactory bulb of some mammals by Adrian (1951). Since then the problem of spatial differentiation of specificity in the olfactory organ has been studied with a variety of techniques. On the bulbar level the principle has been confirmed by simultaneous recordings of multiunit activity (Moulton 1965), by recordings from single glomeruli (Leveteau and MacLeod 1966), by spatial mapping of the odour induced surface potential changes (Thommesen 1976, 1978), by "selective degeneration" of populations of mitral cells caused by monotonous olfactory exposure (Pinching and Døving 1974) and by autoradiographic demonstrations of spatially differentiated glucose metabolism during monotonous olfactory stimulation (Sharp et al. 1977). Electrophysiological studies on the epithelial level (Mustaparta 1971, Thommesen and Døving 1977) have confirmed the spatial differentiation of responses to different odorants. The conclusion is that receptor cells of different specificity are non-uniformly distributed in the olfactory mucosa. In the bull-

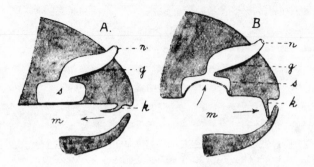

Fig. 3. Sagital sections of the nose region of the eel-pout, Zoarces viviparus during inhalation A and exhalation B. The letters indicate the
olfactory epithelium (g), the nostril (n), the accessory sac (s), the
mouth (m) and the lip (k). From Pipping (1926).

frog olfactory mucosa the problem has been investigated by a different approach, summarized by Mozell and Jagodowicz (1974). They showed that at low air
flow rates the olfactory mucosa behaves like a gas chromatograph. Differences
in the integrated response magnitude from different bundles of the olfactory
nerves correlate with response latencies and with the retention times found
across the olfactory mucosa and in a carbowax gas chromatography column. The
results support the idea that odour specific differences in the spatial distribution of receptor responses is due to the spatial distribution of the stimuli rather than to that of the receptor types.

The study of the functional organization of the fish olfactory organ is
interesting from several points of view. The stimuli are easily quantified,
water solubility being more important than volatility. Artificial respiration
is easily accomplished on paralyzed animals. The nervous structures are spatially separated so that the bulb either lies close to the epithelium, e.g.
in the Ostariophysae or close to the forebrain e.g. in the Isospondyli. These
arrangements enable the physiologist by choice of experimental animal to study
one structure at a time without electrical interference from the others. The
central connections of the olfactory system are fairly well known (Sheldon
1912, Holmgren 1920) and a spatial differentiation in nerve fiber diameter and
conduction velocity is evident in the olfactory tract (Døving and Gemne 1965).
Particularly interesting is the presence of fibers running from the bulb
through the lateral part of the medial olfactory tract to the magnocellular
part of the preoptic nucleus in the hypothalamus. This connection has been
confirmed electrophysiologically by Kandel (1964) and is likely to bring a-
bout rapid endocrine changes in the fish by olfactory cues. Cyprinidae, Silu-

ridae and Salmonidae are known to make use of their olfactory sense in social or reproductive behaviour, pheromones being strongly suspected to participate (von Frisch 1941, Todd 1971, Nordeng 1971).

The spatial differentiation of responses to different odorants has been demonstrated on the olfactory bulb of salmonids (Thommesen 1978). The experimental animal was paralyzed and the gills perfused. Monopolar DC recordings were made simultaneously from two positions on the exposed bulb surface. The ipsilateral olfactory epithelium was exposed to a continuous flow of aquarium tap water. Stimulation was performed by switching a three way stopcock to a pipette with the stimulus sample. The stimuli were L, α- amino acids and water samples from the basins where siblings of the experimental animal lived. The concentration of odorous components added to the aquarium water by the fishes was estimated by the number of fishes in the basin and the water flow through it, giving concentrations of "fish odour" up to 3.6 fish.s/ml.

The potential changes on the bulb surface consisted of two separable components as described by Ottoson (1959), a slow DC shift and regular oscillations called "induced waves" (Adrian 1950). The responses behaved as expected from synaptic events connected to the information treatment on the odorants. The relative magnitude of the responses indicated roughly the localization of these events in the bulb. Fig. 4 shows two sets of simultaneous recordings from the rostromedial and the rostro-lateral part of the olfactory bulb of a char, Salmo alpinus . The stimuli are a basin water sample with a "char odour" concentration of 1.4 fish.s/ml and 10^{-5}M of glutamine.

The responses to stimulation with the "char odour" indicate a rostral localization of information treatment, while amino acid treatment is clearly laterally located. Other amino acids, as well as mixtures of amino acids, showed the same response distribution as glutamin. In amino acid mixtures the respon-

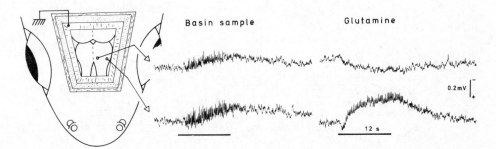

Basin sample   Glutamine

0.2 mV

12 s

Fig. 4. Simultaneous monopolar DC recordings from the left olfactory bulb of a char during ipsilateral stimulation with different odorants (see text). The relative size of the brain structure is exaggerated.

ses to each of the components were only partly additive indicating a common stimulatory feature (e.g. the L,α-amino acid group). The results indicate further that the different parts of the olfactory bulb do not act independently, but co-operate to produce one localized response even to stimulation with crude mixtures of entirely different odorants.

Results show that no substance should be judged as non-stimulatory from one part of the bulb only. The spatial variation in the response also implies that the evaluation of olfactory sensitivity of different individuals from surface response magnitude only, is unreliable unless recorded from exactly equivalent positions on the bulb.

Since the responses recorded from the surface of the bulb reflect the activity of the underlying elements, the results suggest that specific populations of mitral cells are involved by stimulation with a specific odorant. In this respect it is of interest that the location of the responses to fish odorants dominate in the region of the origin of the fibers projecting to the preoptic nucleus. Thus the "fish odour" could activate neurones which, in turn will influence the activity of neuroendocrine cells. Whether biologically significant or not, the coincidence is interesting in view of the presumed existence of fish pheromones.

The origin of the spatial arrangement of response specificity deserves attention since this may have two different origins. A non-uniform distribution of the stimulus seems unlikely in view of the mechanisms involved in water sampling which are described above. A more realistic principle in the fish olfactory organ might be a gradient of specific sensitivity over the olfactory epithelium which by somatotopic projection will secure a spatial variation of responses in the bulb. The olfactory rosette with a distinct grouping of olfactory receptor cells by the corridor compartments offers unique experimental properties for studies of this and related questions, important in the understanding of the organization and ontogenesis of the functional anatomy of the olfactory system.

REFERENCES

Adrian, E.D. (1950) EEG. Clin. Neurophysiol. 2. 377-388
Adrian, E.D. (1951) Ann. psychol. 50. 107-113.
Bashor, D.P., R.W. Beuerman and D.M. Easton(1974) Experientia 30. 777-779
Burne, R.H. (1909) Proc. Zool. Soc. London 2. 610-662.
Døving, K.B., M. Dubois-Dauphin, A. Holley and F. Jourdan (1977) Acta zool. (Stockh.) 58. 245-255.
Døving, K.B. and G. Gemne (1965) J. Neurophysiol. 28. 139-153.
Frisch, K. von (1941) Z. vergl. Physiol. 29, 46-145.
Gooding, R.M. (1963) F.A.O. Fish. Rep. 6 (3). 1621-1631.

Holl, A. (1965) Z. Morph. Ökol. Tiere 54. 707-782.
Holl, A., E. Schulte and W. Meinel (1970) Helgoländer wiss. Meeresunters. 21. 103-123.
Holmgren, N. (1920) Acta zool. (Stockh.) 1. 137-315.
Jørgensen, C.B. (1966) Biology of suspension feeding Pergamon Press, Oxford. 357 pp.
Kandel, E.R. (1964) J. Gen. Physiol. 47. 691-717.
Leveteau, J. and P. MacLeod (1966) J. Physiol. (Paris) 58. 717-729.
Moulton, D.G. (1965) Cold Spring Harbor Symposia on Quantitative Biology 30. 201-206.
Mozell, M.M. and M. Jagodowicz (1974) Ann. N.Y. Acad. Sci. 234. 76-90.
Mustaparta, H. (1971) Acta physiol. scand. 82. 154-166.
Nordeng, H. (1971) Nature. 233. 411-413.
Ottoson, D. (1959) Acta physiol. scand. 47. 149-159.
Pinching, A.J. and K.B. Døving (1974) Brain Res. 82. 195-204.
Pipping, M. (1926) Societas Scientiarum Fennica. Comm. Biol. 2. 1-27.
Schulte, E. (1972) Z. Zellforsch. 125. 210-228.
Sharp, F.R., J.S. Kauer and G.M. Shepherd (1977) J. Neurophysiol. 40. 800-813.
Sheldon, R.E. (1912) J. Comp. Neurol. 22. 177-339.
Teichmann, H. (1959) Z. vergl. Physiol. 42. 206-254.
Thommesen, G. (1976) Acta physiol. scand. 96. 6A-7A.
Thommesen, G. (1978) Acta physiol. scand. in press.
Thommesen, G. and K.B. Døving (1977) Acta physiol. scand. 99. 270-280.
Todd, J.H. (1971) Sci. Am. 224 (5). 98-108.
Zeiske, E. (1974) Z. Morph. Tiere 77. 19-50.

Abstracts of Poster Presentations

Properties of single olfactory receptors revealed by cross-adaptation
to odorants in the tiger salamander F. Baylin and D. G. Moulton,
(Monell Chemical Senses Center, University of Pennsylvania and
Veterans Administration Hospital, Philadelphia, Pa. 19104, USA.)

Since cross-adaptation to odor modifies receptor sites selectively it
offers a tool for investigating the number of types of receptor sites
for a given odorant and on a given receptor. Using this approach, we
tested four pairs of odorants: ethyl n-butyrate, methyl-n-butyrate;
butanol (BUT), propanol (PROP); benzaldehyde (BZA), nitrobenzene (NB)
and BZA, acetophenone. (Odors of members of a pair are similar). An
olfactometer delivered the paired odorants sequentially, with or without a variable interpulse interval. Of 100 units isolated, 56 responded to at least one of the test odorants. Of these 56, 30 responded to both odorants from at least one pair. All 30 showed both self-
and non-reciprocal cross-adaptation. In general, the effects were concentration-dependent and there was no correlation between the spike-
generating capacity of an odorant and the magnitude of self- and cross-
adaptation. Some receptors showed no adaptation effects even at high
concentrations suggesting that different types of receptor sites, responsive to a given odorant can coexist on a single cell. We estimated
the minimal number of site types responsive to each member of an odorant pair (such as A and B) as follows: (1) For each test odorant
(except, possibly, NB) there is a site type which responds only to it.
(e.g. there are sites responsive to each of BUT and PROP but not to
both.) (2) When odorant A cross-adapts response to B, A presumably
interacts with those sites that generate response to B. Thus a third
site type probably exists. (3) Since cross-adaptation between A and
B is non-reciprocal, a fourth site probably exists which responds to
both A and B. Thus we conclude that a minimum of two and probably
three or more site types exist which respond to each of the test
odorants. (Supported partly by NIH Grant 1-RO1 NS 10617-01).

Olfactory receptor-glomerular ratio versus olfactory acuity in mammals Kunwar
P. Bhatnagar, (Department of Anatomy, University of Louisville Health Sciences
Center, Louisville, Kentucky 40201 U.S.A.)

Despite similarities in the olfactory system throughout the vertebrate
series, a wide diversity exists in the acuity of the sense of smell in
different animals. Since macrosmatic animals tend to have more extensive
olfactory epithelial areas than microsmatic animals, it might be suspected
that these differences could be expressed in terms of ratio of receptors to
glomeruli (R:G). To test this hypothesis the present investigation has
dealt with the quantitative estimation of the number of olfactory receptors
projecting upon each glomerulus in three species of bats with differential
olfactory acuity. Measurements of olfactory epithelial surface areas (SA),
in mm^2, were made from heads serially sectioned at 10 μm and stained with
trichrome, Protargol S or cresyl violet. Every fifth section was examined.
Mean height (h) of the receptor nuclear compartment within the olfactory
epithelium, and the mean diameter (d) of a receptor nucleus, in millimeters,
were carefully determined. Total number (N) of receptors per nasal cavity
was estimated from the formula $N = SA \times h \div \pi d^3/6$, where the expression $\pi d^3/6$
represents the volume of one receptor nucleus, in mm^3. Glomeruli were counted
under the microscope and the counts adjusted using Abercrombie's formula. The
following results were obtained:

	receptors per nasal cavity	glomeruli per bulb	glomerular diameter, μm	R-G ratio
Eptesicus fuscus	1.561×10^7 (5)	970 (6)	60	16,095 : 1
Artibeus jamaicensis	8.938×10^7 (2)	1,188 (1)	130	75,240 : 1
Desmodus rotundus	9.431×10^7 (1)	1,336 (1)	80	70,595 : 1

( ) = number of animals examined

Artibeus and *Desmodus*, the Jamaican fruit-bat and the vampire bat
respectively, recognized for their far keener sense of smell and a well-
developed olfactory system when compared with the less-well endowed
insectivorous *Eptesicus*, do exhibit a much higher receptor-glomerular ratio.
These data when compared with the only other available, for rabbit (5.0×10^7;
1,900; 185; 26,000 : 1), suggest that the receptor-glomerular ratio is
directly proportional to the animal's olfactory acuity; the glomeruli are not
numerically constant amongst species. Data are currently being gathered from
many other species for a broader analysis.

Qualitative and quantitative odour discrimination by mitral cells and anterior olfactory nucleus cells.M.BOULET,G.DAVALandJ.LEVETEAU. (Université
Paris VI, U.E.R.6I,4 Place Jussieu, /5230 PARIS, FRANCE)

Chemical olfactory discrimination have been studied in the olfactory bulb
(O.B.) and the anterior olfactory nucleus (A.O.N.). The responses to odour
stimulation of 6I single mitral cells and of 64 A.O.N. units were simultaneously recorded from rabbits. The test battery consisted of 6 chemical stimuli
(benzaldehyde, butanol, isoamyl acetate, nitrobenzene, propanol, pyridine)
delivered at two intensity levels corresponding to a hundredfold difference
in concentration; they were the same as selected in previous experiments on
receptors and mitral cells by MAC LEOD et al.(I973) and HOLLEY et al. (I974)
in order to make possible a comparison between them. The between-odour paired
correlation have been calculated (Pearson's r) in the 4 cases. The ranking of
the mean r values are as follows :mitral cells, weak odours :mean r = 0.095
± 0.144〈 mitral cells, strong odours: mean r = 0.399 + 0.054 . A.O.N. cells,
weak odours mean r =0.480 + 0.I06〈 A.O.N. cells; strong odours ÷ mean r =
0.6I6 + 0.032. The odour discrimination reaches its best for the mitral cells
stimulated weakly; it decreases somewhat when the same cells cells are stimulated strongly. At A.O.N. level the odour discrimination already limited in
the case of weak stimuli, almost disappears for strong stimuli. Multidimensional analysis of the odour similarities, respectively in the O.B. and in
the A.O.N. ,reveals an unexpectedly high loading of the first axis with an
intensity factor. These results indicate that the discriminatory ability of
the mitral cells is better than the chemoreceptors one and that it is poorer in
the A.O.N.

<u>Odour preference scales in rats</u>. Richard E. Brown, (Department
of Zoology, South Parks Road, Oxford OX1 3PS, England)

An adaptation of Thurstone's law of comparative judgement
was used to formalize preference scales for social odours in
rats. Investigation time scores were recorded in pairwise odour
presentations and difference scores calculated for each pair.
Scale values were computed through the matrix of difference scores. Each scale was subjected to analysis of variance which
partitioned the total between cells variance into scale and re-
sidual variance. Post-hoc tests were used to calculate implied
scale means. Sixteen groups of adult rats (male x female ; intact x gonadectomized ; sexually experienced x naive ; mixed x
same sex housing rooms) were presented with all pairwise combinations of urine odours from estrous females (F) ; ovariectomized
females (Fo) ; intact males (M) ; castrated males (Mc) ; own
group cagemates (G) ; and a no odour control (N). Intact sexually
experienced males showed a scale with the highest values for female odours (N < G = M < Mc < Fo = F) but did not prefer estrous
to nonestrous female odours. Sexually naive intact males showed
lower scale values for female odours than experienced males
(N < G = M < Mc = Fo = F). Housing differences did not affect
male preference scales. Castrated males showed preferences of a
low magnitude in the sexually experienced group housed in a mixed sex room. The other three groups showed no scalable preferences. Intact females all showed the same scale values irrespective of sexual experiences or housing conditions (N < G = Fo =
F < Mc < M). Ovariectomized females showed no scalable odour
preferences. These results are compared· with those from ten other
studies on rat odour preferences (1).

Pre-weanling infant rats were reared with their mother alone
(Mfam) or with both their mother and their father (M+F fam). At
16-20 days of age they were given all pairwise comparisons of
soiled bedding from both types of litter (Mfam and M+Ffam) ; a-
dult males (M) ; nulliparous adult females (F) ; and clean saw-
dust (N). Those rats reared with their mother alone showed a preference scale ordered N = F < M+Ffam = M < Mfam. Those reared
with both parents showed the scale N = F < Mfam = M < M+Ffam.
Infants rats were therefore able to scale their odour preferences
and showed the highest scale values for their own family odour.

This scaling procedure provides a powerful method for the
study of odour preferences using the approach paradigm preference test. (Supported by National Research Council of Canada Pre
and PostDoctoral Fellowships, and a grant in aid of research from
Sigma Xi).

(1) Brown, R.E. Odour preference and urine-making scales in male
and female rats : effects of gonadectomy and sexual experience
on responses to conspecific odors. J.C.P.P. 1977, 91 (5).

Electrophysiological responses to odors in hamster receptor neurons Richard
M. Costanzo and Robert J. O'Connell, (The Rockefeller University, New York,
New York, USA)

Critical to an understanding of the encoding of quality information is the
selection of appropriate test odorants. Although it is usually assumed that
most mammals discriminate between, and respond to a range of different odor
qualities, the selection of a particular test odorant is often arbitrary and
unrelated to those compounds normally discriminated by the experimental animal. Recent work in this laboratory has led to the isolation and identification of several biological odorants from estrous hamster vaginal discharge.
This material contains compounds which normally elicit strong behavioral responses in the male. Since the olfactory input for these behaviors must be
initially processed by the receptors, it seemed likely that at least some receptor neurons might be more selective in their responses to these particular
compounds. Seven compounds (chemical purity > 99%) were selected for study.
Three of these compounds (n-amyl acetate, ethyl acetate, and ethyl iso-
butyrate) are traditional odors not found in vaginal discharge. The remaining compounds (dimethyl disulfide, n-butanol, n-hexanol, and ethyl n-butyrate)
are found in vaginal discharge; and one, dimethyl disulfide, is a powerful behavioral attractant for the male. The waveform and concentration of these
stimuli, as delivered by a continuous flow dilution olfactometer, were determined with a flame ionization detector. Stimuli were delivered to the exposed olfactory mucosa and extracellular responses recorded with metal microelectrodes. Most of the units studied to date were responsive to all odorants; however, the relative sensitivity to these compounds varied from neuron
to neuron. The concentration-response functions for a typical odorant usually
encompassed 1-2 log units of concentration while individual thresholds for
different compounds ranged from 3.16×10^{-8} to 1.0×10^{-4} molar. We have yet
to observe a neuron exclusively sensitive to one odor. (Supported by NIH
Grant NS 08902.)

Origins of centrifugal fibres to olfactory bulb of rat, rabbit and cat as disclosed by retrograde transport of horseradish peroxidase (HRP)

B.J. Dennis, (Department of Human Physiology and Pharmacology, The University of Adelaide, South Australia).

As a preliminary to electrophysiological investigations into the functions of olfactory centrifugal fibres, those regions giving direct input to olfactory bulb were traced by deposition of HRP into the main olfactory bulb. Adequate fixation and development of diaminobenzidine reaction product were found using 4% paraformaldehyde for fixation and making up all solutions to a final pH of 7.3 in phosphate buffer.

In the three species studied, retrobulbar regions were labelled bilaterally. On the same side as the HRP deposit, pyramidal cells of prepyriform cortex (anterior olfactory cortex), particularly in PP2 above the lateral olfactory tract, certain large cells occurring in patches throughout the peduncle (in the cat deep to tubercle proper), and the horizontal nucleus of the diagonal band (HnDB) were well labelled. The raphé nuclei and locus coeruleus also contained a few labelled cells.

When the HRP deposit involved the retrobulbar area and peduncle, labelling extended more caudally in olfactory cortex and occurred in restricted parts of the cortical amygdaloid nucleus and in "hypothalamic areas" adjacent to HnDB. Confirming its connections with retrobulbar structures, HnDB itself was particularly impressively labelled.

There is thus direct feedback to the bulb from areas such as AON and olfactory cortex which receive lateral olfactory tract fibres, and also indirect centrifugal influence from HnDB and brain stem.

The neurodynamics of the olfactory bulb. W.J. Freeman, Dept. Physiol.-Anat., Univ. California, Berkeley 94720 USA

The olfactory bulb and cortex each contain many millions of excitatory and inhibitory neurons with dense local interactions. During each inspiration the olfactory receptors deliver a volley of action potentials to the bulb that increases the firing rates of many bulbar neurons and subsequently of cortical neurons. If the animal is alert and motivated the EEG shows a sinusoidal burst at 40 to 80 Hz. It is postulated that olfactory information is transmitted from the bulb to the cortex by modulation of the firing rates of bulbar neurons at the burst frequency.

A model of the bulbar mechanism has been developed in a set of nonlinear integrodifferential equations, to simulate closely the performance of the bulb in response to electrical stimulation of its afferent and efferent nerves. With sufficiently high internal feedback gains the model enters a stable limit cycle state at frequencies characteristic of the EEG bursts.

The limit cycle can be modulated if the strengths of one or more of the connection types in the model are spatially matched as a template to the input pattern. From studies of the spatial distribution of the EEG of the bulb it is suggested that such matching may occur in the bulb during the orienting process, learning, and habituation, so that if a particular input recurs, the bulb may enter limit cycle activity more or less readily.

It is proposed that the model may be useful for pinpointing the type and manner of synaptic changes during learning and habituation, and their centrifugal controls. Supported by MHO6686.

Aggression by groups of castrated male mice against lactating or
non-lactating strangers: a urine dependent phenomenon.
M. Haug, Laboratoire de Psychophysiologie, 7 rue de l'Université ,
67000 Strasbourg.

In our previous work, we have demonstrated that urine of mice in a period
of lactation instigated an aggressive behaviour in some groups of females.
Therefore, it was logical to examine if the factor "smell" intervening in
this type of behaviour has some receptors and whether this response was
specific to females or was independent of sex. To investigate this
problem, we initially studied intact, castrated and sham-operated males in
the presence of stranger females lactating and non-lactating. The results
show that the castrated animals attack more frequently and with increased
celerity the lactating mice than the non-lactating females introduced in
their cage. Moreover, the introduction of lactating females provoked also
a rise in the frequency of fights between castrated males. In another
experiment , we have compared the aggressive behaviour of groups of
castrated, intact and sham-operated males in the presence of stranger
ovariectomized females coated with different experimental solutions:
a) physiological serum b) urine of non-lactating females c) urine of
lactating females. The results obtained show that the intact and sham-
operated males attack less frequently than do castrated males the stranger
sprayed females put in their presence. Oppositely, if the castrated males
present a very strong aggressive behaviour toward the females coated with
physiological serum or urine of lactating mice, this behaviour is quite
diminished after the coating with urine of non-lactating females. Other
experiments are in progress to specify the role of the olfactory stimuli
in the aggressive behaviour we have studied.

<u>Olfactory receptor activity</u> : Interaction between odour stimulation
and D.C. electrical polarization of the olfactory mucosa. A. Juge
and A. Holley, (Electrophysiologie, Univ. Claude Bernard, Lyon,
France).

The spike activity of frog's single olfactory receptors was found
to be a direct function of polarity and intensity of sustained D.C.
polarizations applied to the olfactory mucosa by a Ringer-agar-Ag-
AgCl electrode. The electrical influence of the surface polarizing
electrode decremented with a space constant of 150-200 μm. Interactions between chemical and electrical stimulations were investigated. When the surface electrode was positive (anodal polarization),
a current of 1-10 μA resulted in facilitation of odour responses;
conversely, cathodal polarization inhibited odour responses. Both
facilitation and inhibition were graded. The odour response threshold of some receptors was lowered during anodal polarization. Concentration / response functions were shifted according to current
polarity in a way suggesting additivity between the chemical and
electrical effects. Descriptions of interactions between odour and
electrical stimulations were simpler when neural responses were described in terms of spike frequency rather than in terms of number of
elicited spikes. When an olfactory stimulation elicited a brief response with decrementing spikes, an inhibitory electrical polarization could retard the spike decrement and increase the number of
induced spikes. The effect was the same as a stimulation at a lower
concentration. An increase in electrical excitability was sometimes
observed following odour stimulations but the more consistent effect
was a drastic reduction of current effectiveness. Following strong
stimulations with amyl acetate, cineole, anisole, and at a lesser
degree butanol, even high intensity currents failed to elicit any
spike activity. The recovery of excitability showed a time course
that depended on the nature of the odorant and its concentration.
In multiunit recordings it was observed that post-stimulus suppression of excitability was not clearly correlated with the magnitude
of the previous odour response. The effect did not seem to result
from classical inhibition of the receptors. It is suggested that the
odour stimulation caused marked changes in conductance in recorded
and / or neighbouring cells resulting in correlative changes in the
current flow pathways.

Behavioral distinctions between olfaction and taste in catfish   Edward E. Little   (Florida State University, Tallahassee, Florida   U.S.A.)

In many fish, olfaction and taste predominate as a source of information and these senses are highly developed in catfish. However, the relationship between behavior and the anatomy and physiology of the chemical senses is poorly understood. Taste has been shown to mediate feeding responses while pheromones are effective through olfaction (Atema, 1969). The stimuli of both are present in aqueous form and amino acids are a stimulator component of food and pheromones (Tucker & Suzuki, 1972). Olfactory and taste receptors are often responsive to many of the same amino acid stimuli (Caprio, 1975). In the present study olfaction and taste were distinguished using three types of behavioral experiments.

In the first experiment, cardiac deceleration was induced by amino acids which signalled electric shock. This response was mediated by olfaction since it disappeared when the olfactory tracts were sectioned or the nares temporarily blocked and reappeared when the nares blocks were removed. Of two amino acids reported to evoke strong EOG responses, cysteine was particularly potent while arginine was ineffective in conditioning. In the second experiment, fish were trained to swim from a shelter to avoid amino acid signalled shock. Arginine diluted to 10^{-10}M evoked responses and anosmic fish readily learned to avoid arginine. Thus gustation mediates this response. In the third experiment, LiCl was used to induce illness following the consumption of an amino acid. Normal and anosmic fish readily discriminated among several amino acids following illness indicating a primary role of gustation in the feeding response. Observations of the sequence of the feeding response indicate that taste receptors within the mouth are initially responsible for flavor discriminations.

<u>Relation between intramembranous particle density of frog olfactory cilia and EOG response</u> C. Masson, S. Kouprach, I. Giachetti, P. Mac Leod, (Laboratoire de Neurobiologie Sensorielle, EPHE, CNRS, (ERA 623, RCP 349) Paris. Station Centrale de Microscopie Electronique, Institut Pasteur, Paris.)

Recent freeze-etching studies of the olfactory mucosa of the mouse (KERJASCHKI and HÖRANDNER, 1976) and of calves (MENCO and al. 1976) have demonstrated numerous intramembranous particles (I.M.P.) in the cilia membranes.
By an electron microscopic investigation of freeze-cleavage carbon-platinum replicas of unfixed frog olfactory mucosa, we have measured with fair enough accuracy the size and density of I.M.P. to find significant inter-individual differences.
Two groups of frogs were food deprived for respectively 3 and 8 weeks.
I.M.P. density of frog olfactory cilia varied conspicuously : about $2,000\,\mu\,m^2$ in the short-fasting frogs vs. less than $600\,\mu\,m^2$ in the long fasting-frogs.
Corresponding EOGs were recorded in one *eminentia olfactoria* just prior to excision of the contralateral one for freeze-cleavage.
Maximum response amplitudes to stimulation by air saturated with isoamyl-acetate at 22 ° C were strikingly different : approximately 3 mV in the short-fasted frogs vs. less than 0.8 mV in the long-fasted frogs.
One could assume therefore some kind of link between I.M.P. densities and slow potentials generated by olfactory cilia. It was already demonstrated (GETCHELL and GESTELAND, 1972 ; GENNINGS and al. 1975) that chemoreception processes are somehow associated with proteinaceous receptor sites : it is not a surprise to find that a decrease of protein synthesis due to food deprivation is simultaneously followed by a loss of I.M.P. and a reduced capacity of generating electrical activity.

GENNINGS (J.N.) ; GOWER (D.B.) ; BANNISTER (L.H.) J. Endocr. <u>67</u>, 47-48, (1975).
GETCHELL (L.M.) ; GESTELAND (R.C.) Proc. nat. Acad. Sci., U.S.A. <u>69</u>, 1494-1498 (1972).
KERJASCHKI (D) ; HÖRANDNER (H) J. Ultr. Res. <u>54</u>, 420-444 (1976).
MENCO (B.P.M.) ; DODD (G.H.) ; DAVEY (M) ; BANNISTER (L.H.) Nature <u>263</u>, 597-599 (1976).

Differential response of olfactory epithelium to cigarette smoke.
Daniel H. Matulionis, (Anatomy Department, University of Kentucky, Lexington, Kentucky, 40506, U.S.A.)

Morphological responses of olfactory epithelium were studied after acute exposures to cigarette smoke in eight different strains of mice. A previous report (Matulionis, '74; Ann. Oto. Rhino. Laryngo. 83: 192) indicated that there may be an interstrain differential reaction to this insult. Different genetic strains of mice were chosen on the basis of their resistance or susceptibility to skin inflammation after topical application of carcinogenic compounds and inducibility of elevation of aryl hydrocarbon hydroxylase (AHH) activity after administration of similar carcinogenic agents. Generally, the morphology of olfactory epithelia appeared normal after exposure to cigarette smoke in those strains of mice (AKR/J, DBA/1J, DBA/2J, 129/J) which were resistant to integumentary inflammation and failed to have the AHH activity elevated after administration of carcinogenic agents. However, olfactory epithelia of mice from strains which were susceptible (CBA/J, C57L/J, C3H/HeJ, C3HeB/FeJ) to induction of an elevated AHH activity and skin ulceration by such compounds were notably altered by exposure to cigarette smoke. These alterations, restricted to the surface of the epithelium, were manifested as: 1) a reduction in number of olfactory vesicles and sensory cilia, 2) partial retraction of olfactory vesicles into the epithelium, 3) reduction of microvilli in the epithelial "border" zone, and 4) abnormal protrusion of supporting cells above the epithelial surface. It was also noted that olfactory epithelia of all animals in a particular strain did not respond equally to the smoke exposures. The present observations support and substantiate previous suggestions (Matulionis, '74) that normal olfaction is possibly impaired by cigarette smoke and that susceptibility to this insult might be genetically determined.

Quantification of nasal air flow patterns in dogs performing an odor detection task. D. A. Marshall & D. G. Moulton (Dept. of Animal Biology, Univ. of
Pennslyvania: Veterans Administration Hospital, Philadelphia; and Monell Chemical Senses Ctr. and Dept. of Physiology, Univ. of Penna., Philadelphia, Pa.
19104 U.S.A.)

We have established performance curves and the range of minimum α-ionone
concentrations detected by dogs (J. comp. Physiol. 110 (A), 287-306, 1976).
Presentation of fixed-flow test concentrations raised the question of how
sniffing - through changing volume, flow, and stimulus dispersion - may facilitate detection, and ultimately, aid in discrimination performance. To
assess the physical variables involved, we have trained Shepherds (using operant techniques, water as reward, and a two-choice apparatus) to find and signal odor position (interchanged randomly) by inserting the snout into one or
both of two odor sampling ports, each coupled to a pneumotachometer (Fleisch)
through which odorized or blank airflows pass. Analysis of pneumotachograph
records shows the internal structure and duration of sniffing bouts to differ
according to: individuals; odorant (eg. complex mixtures vs. single compounds)
odorant concentration at its source; and odor concentration at the sampling
point (from GLC measurements on samples generated by artificial sniffs). A
sniffing bout consists of alternating inspirations and expirations, typically
producing a net gain of 70-80 ml. Bouts at higher pentyl acetate concentrations differ from those at near threshold (about 10^{-7} of saturated vapor) in
mean number of sniffs (3 vs. 6.4), mean flows of peak sniffs (133 vs. 91
1/min) and in duration (0.77 vs. 1.30 sec). The mean duration of individual
sniffs (.12 vs. .10) remained similar for all concentrations. Longer bouts
at low concentrations show larger numbers of low amplitude sniffs. This may
effectively increase odor concentration at the sampling point (as seen in
GLC results) while creating maximum turbulance, possibly aiding dispersion of
odorant molecules into ethmoturbinate recesses. An increased number of sniffs
also appears to favor maximum contact of odorant molecules with receptors.

Postnatal structural development of the rat olfactory bulb and its functional significance. Esmail Meisami and Farhad Shafa, (Institute of Biochemistry and Biophysics, University of Tehran, P.O. Box 14-1700, Tehran, IRAN)

The rat, being a macrosmatic animal, possesses a highly developed olfactory bulb which, as in other vertebrates, shows a well-defined lamination and structural pattern. As a first step towards the establishment of a causal relationship between the appearance of functional olfactory capacities, and structural development of the bulb, we have studied the latter qualitatively and quantitatively on postnatal days 1, 5, 10, 25 and 60, using Nissl stained complete serial sections.

The results reveal that during the first two months birth the total number of mitral cells remain constant at about 70,000 per bulb, indicating the prenatal origin of these cells. Horse Radish Peroxidase staining of the mitral cells also reveals the existence of very well developed dendritic profiles of at least a few mitral cells even in the newborn.

In contrast to the precocious status of the mitral cell, the olfactory glomeruli show pronounced development after birth, increasing from a mean total of 350 per bulb at birth to about 3000 at two months; most of the increase occurs during the first two weeks. Mean diameter of the glomeruli also increase from about 35 at birth to 70 at two months. The glomeruli of the neonatal young bulb are found mostly in the anterior and dorsal-medial surfaces of the bulb, with the remaining surfaces filling gradually later.

It therefore appears that the rudimentary olfactory capacities of the neonate are processed by the existing olfactory glomeruli and/or by receptor-mitral interactions not requiring the contributions of glomerular cells. Furthermore it appears that during brain development, the buildup of new glomeruli may be partly responsible for the development of new functional olfactory capabilities.

Freeze-etch morphology of olfactory and respiratory cilia in rat, cow and frog

Bert Menco (Psychologisch Laboratorium; Rijksuniversiteit
Utrecht, Varkenmarkt 2, Utrecht, The Netherlands)

Cilia and microvilli hairlets of sensory and non sensory origin from rat and frog were compared to each other and to those of cow. As has been described before for mouse (1) and cow (2), also in rat, particle densities in inner intramembranous fracture faces are higher in olfactory cilia than in respiratory cilia. In frog, however, high densities in the respiratory cilia are equal or higher than in the olfactory cilia. Particle densities in both cilium types vary between 300 pp/μm^2 (rat respiratory cilia) and 2,000 pp/μm^2 (other cilium types). Particle densities never reach those of bovine olfactory cilia, which are about 5,000 pp/μm^2 (2). Furthermore, ciliary particle densities and distributions may, even within one replica, differ considerably. Both vesicles devoid of particles and vesicles densely occupied with particles are found on the olfactory cilia. Respiratory cilia usually contain only the former type. Ciliary necklaces, present at the base of the cilia, have usually more strands (about 7) in olfactory than in respiratory cilia (about 5). This study confirms the presence of rod-shaped particles, in addition to globular ones in supporting cell (rat, frog) and Bowman glandular cell (rat) apices (1). However, in contrast with previous studies (1), rod-shaped particles were also found in the microvilli of both cell types. Supporting cells in the bovine and respiratory cells in all species reveal only globular particles. Particle densities in all microvillous types may vary between 1,500 - 2,500 pp/μm^2. On the basis of this study it may be tentatively concluded that we can discriminate between the particle populations of the various nasal hairlet types.

Litt.: 1. KERJASCHKI, D. and HÖRANDNER, H. (1976) J.Ultrastruct.Res., 54, 420.
    2. MENCO, B.P.M., DODD, G.H., DAVEY, M. and BANNISTER, L.H. (1976)
       Nature, 263, 597.

Vomeronasal/accessory-olfactory system: stimulus access and unit response

M. Meredith, (The Rockefeller University, New York, N.Y., USA)

Vomeronasal organ (VNO) input appears to be particularly important in maintaining male mating behavior in the hamster. The VNO is a blind ending tube partially lined with sensory epithelium and is enclosed by a rigid bony capsule. Within the capsule, in the thickness of the sidewall of the organ is a region of cavernous vascular tissue innervated by the nasopalatine (NP) nerve. Low level NP nerve stimulation with a short train of pulses produced inflow of fluid at the narrow VN duct. This inflow was accompanied by collapse of the VNO sidewall overlying the cavernous tissue and was followed by re-expansion of the sidewall and outflow through the VN duct. Superior sympathetic ganglion stimulation produced effects similar to those of NP stimulation. These effects preceeded any increase of heart rate and were eliminated by NP section but contraction and inflow at the duct could be produced after VN section by intracarotid injection of small amounts of epinephrine. Sympathectomy prevented NP stimulation producing its normal effect. These experiments suggest that the VNO cavernous tissue constitutes, as speculated by Herzfield in 1888, a pumping mechanism for the delivery of stimulus substances to the VNO receptors. In addition, they show that this mechanism is under the neural control of sympathetic adrenergic fibers. NP nerve stimulation can be used to deliver odors to the VN receptors while recording from identified second-order neurones in the accessory olfactory bulb (AOB). Unit response time was short enough to account for reasonable behavioral response times. AOB units could respond with excitation or inhibition both to the naturally occurring chemicals in hamster vaginal discharge (HVD) and to artificial chemicals. Bilateral section of the NP nerves in the male reduced attraction to HVD in a testing situation where cues other than odor were not available but did not produce deficits in mating behavior when normally isolated males were removed from their home cages and placed with receptive females.

(Supported by The Monell Foundation and The Van Ameringen Foundation)

Response pattern of olfactory bulb neurons to single, paired or repetitive lateral olfactory tract stimulation K. Mori and S. F. Takagi,
(Dept. of Physiol. Sch. of Med. Gunma Univ. Maebashi, Gunma, Japan)

Responses of olfactory bulb neurons were studied to single, paired or
repetitive lateral olfactory tract (LOT) stimulation as an extension of
our research dealing with the synaptic mechanisms controlling mitral cell
excitability in the rabbit. Mitral cells showed an antidromic spike and
a subsequent IPSP following a single LOT stimulation, while granule layer
cells were activated synaptically by the LOT stimulation. The conduction
velocity of mitral cell axons was 10.1 m/sec (±2.4 m/sec SD, N=129).

As reported in the previous communication (K. Mori and S. F. Takagi in
Food Intake and Chemical Senses, 1976), the LOT-evoked test antidromic
spike of mitral cells failed to invade the somato-dendritic region and
the test IPSP was markedly suppressed by the conditioning LOT stimulation.
Paired LOT stimulation revealed two types of granule layer cell responses.
Following conditioning LOT stimulation, most granule layer cells showed
the depression of the test LOT-evoked EPSPs and spikes (Type I granule
layer cells). In contrast to this, some other granule layer cells did not
show the depression of their test LOT-evoked responses following conditioning LOT stimulation (Type II granule layer cells).

During repetitive LOT stimulation, type I granule layer cells showed
alternation of the amplitude of the EPSPs, while mitral cells showed that
of their IPSPs. These response patterns of mitral cells and type I
granule layer cells support the hypothesis of the dendrodendritic synaptic
interactions between mitral cell dendrites and granule cell peripheral
processes.

Olfactory receiving areas in the cerebral cortex of the cat   F. Motokizawa,
Y. Ino, Y. Tsujimoto and T. Yasuda,(Dept. Physiol., Nara Med.Coll.,Kashihara,
Nara 634, Japan)

This work was undertaken with the object of examining whether the cat cerebral
cortex outside the olfactory lobe is in receipt of olfactory afferents. Evoked
potentials were recorded in the entire cortex upon stimulation of the olfactory bulb(OB) in chloralose anesthetized cats. Three kinds of potentials
were observed; (1) a biphasic negative-positive potential in the prepyriform
cortex(PPF), (2) a triphasic positive-negative-positive potential in the orbital gyrus(ORB), (3) a biphasic positive-negative potential in the rest of the
cortex. Latencies of these responses were nearly fixed at 4 msec in all recording sites. From analysis of origin of each potential component by topical
application of KCl on the cortical surface and recording a reversal of polarity of the potential in the cortical layers it was concluded that all components in PPF and the negative and second positive components in ORB originate
from the cortex under the electrode, while the initial positive in ORB and
both components in all cortical regions except PPF and ORB represent activity
originating at PPF and conveyed to the electrode by electric spread. In the
olfactory pathway to ORB a thalamic relay is not likely involved, because
evoked responses to OB shocks in the mediodorsal nucleus, known for its connection with the fronto-orbital cortex, had a latency of 10 to 30 msec, which
is far longer than that for the response in ORB. It has been reported that the
orbital gyrus receives vagal, somatosensory and splanchnic afferents. Also in
our study such polysensory projections to ORB were confirmed and, furthermore,
mutual interactions were observed for all pairs of inputs optionally selected
from olfactory, trigeminal and vagal afferents.

Olfactory evoked brainpotentials and electro-olfactogram in man

K.H. Plattig, G. Kobal (Inst. f. Physiol u. Biokybernetik, Universitätsstr. 17, D-8520 Erlangen, FRG)

Monomodal olfactory stimulation is difficult in regard to timing and intensity of stimulation, but also in regard to the fact that disturbing auditory, thermic and pressure sensations are easily elicited by the olfactometers. To avoid extra-olfactory artifacts we improved our stimulating device which has been in use for the "pulse method" of olfactory stimulation in man within the past years by developing the "flow-method", in which the interference with disturbing somatosensory concomitants are reduced by using a constant flow of prewarmed air which is replaced by odorous air without any turbulence. Rise and fall of the stimulating odorous concentration at the nostrils occur within 20 ms (pulse method) and 40 ms (flow method) respectively. Human olfactory evoked responses from different sites of the skull are shown, elicited via the flow method by various stimuli (eucalyptol, eugenol, linalool). Disadvantages of the pulse method are demonstrated especially in the alteration of the somatosensory and olfactory responses caused by interference with additional tactile potential components. There are two clearly recognizable components, which occur at different latencies: 1) one which is probably of mainly somatosensory origin,200-280 ms after stimulus onset, often double-peaked, and 2) an olfactory one, 450-680 ms after stimulus onset. The somatosensory part is more distinct in case of the flow-method, if the odorous substances directly stimulate trigeminal nerve endings in the nose. The olfactory peak is higher in the precentral middle area of the skull; the somatosensory peak is more pronounced on the contralateral skull areas. These two components have different time courses during averaging,which indicate different courses of adaptation and habituation: Component 1 grows steadily, while the growth of component 2 is more and more decreasing so that component 2 of the averaged potential gets smaller. Sometimes component 1 is split into two peaks, which are not distributed equally over the various recording sites on the skull. To get more detailed information on the differences in time courses quoted above, we started to measure in addition the electro-olfactogram (EOG) adapting the recording and stimulating method of P. Bekiaroglou (1971).

Reference:

B e k i a r o g l o u, P., G i s d a k i s, S. (1971): Registierung elektrischer Aktivität auf der Riechschleimhaut des Menschen. S.Ber.Bay.Akad.Wiss.(math.-nat.Kl.),pp.145-157. München: Verlag der Bayerischen Akademie der Wissenschaften.

Primary odors in mice: inferences from specific anosmias Steven Price,
(Dept. of Physiology, Medical College of Virginia, Virginia Commonwealth
Univ., Richmond, Va. 23298, USA)

An active avoidance paradigm was used to test the ability of individual Swiss
mice to detect odorous compounds. Geraniol, menthol, benzaldehyde, and
salicylaldehyde, corresponding to the odors described as floral, minty,
almond, and cinnamon, respectively, were used in the primary screening.
Animals which appeared to be anosmic to one or more of these were then tested
for their ability to detect phenylethyl alcohol, a floral odorant, and menthone and carvone, both of which smell minty to humans. Anosmia to phenylethyl alcohol was found in 7 out of 14 animals anosmic to geraniol. All of
38 animals with other anosmias were able to detect phenylethyl alcohol. The
association of the anosmia to phenylethyl alcohol with that to geraniol is
highly significant (P = 0.001). Anosmia to menthone was significantly
correlated with anosmia to menthol (P = 0.0025) and to carvone (P = 0.0025),
while the correlation between anosmia to carvone and to menthol did not
quite reach the usually accepted 5% level of confidence (P = 0.10). The
results suggest that mice have receptors which correspond to those responding
to odorants described by humans as floral and other receptors which respond
to minty odorants. Therefore, primary odor categories in mice probably
resemble those in humans.
(Supported by a research grant and a Research Career Development Award from
the National Institute of Dental Research, National Institutes of Health,
and by a research grant from the National Science Foundation)

Anesthetic effect on olfactory bulb responses to olfactory tract stimulation

John W. Scott, (Department of Anatomy, Emory University School of Medicine, Atlanta, Georgia 30322, U.S.A.)

Single unit and field potential responses to paired pulse electrical stimuli of the lateral olfactory tract were analyzed in the rat. This paradigm has been used in the literature to demonstrate that the granule cells are activated by dendrodendritic synapses rather than by axon collaterals. The time course of response recovery depends upon type and depth of anesthetic. With surgical levels of barbiturates, the field potential response to the test pulse is depressed for up to 100 msec. With urethane or ether, the test response is greater than control (augmented) for similar periods. The present experiments show that: (1) Moderate levels of barbiturates prolong single unit suppression as well as field potential suppression, (2) very deep barbiturate levels block the suppression of single unit responses to the test pulse and produce an augmented field potential response to the test pulse, and (3) conditions producing an augmented response to the test pulse cause a reduction in the size of the primary response. These observations appear to reflect two processes: (1) Inhibition of mitral cells by granule cells and (2) facilitation of synaptic output of mitral cells. A similar facilitation is well known at other synapses. The field potential is generated by synaptic currents in granule cells and is related to the synaptic output of mitral cells. A reduction in the output of mitral cells can reduce inhibition and unmask the facilitation. Barbiturates prolong inhibition so that the effects of facilitation are not seen except with very large doses. These observations are important for studies of olfactory bulb responses to odors in anesthetized preparations and also suggest that the synaptic facilitation must be considered in models of the normal function of the olfactory bulb.

Odorant Responses in Gustatory NTS Neurons. R.L. Van Buskirk & R.P. Erickson
(Dept. Psychology, Univ. Wyoming, Laramie, WY 82071 USA and Dept. Psychology,
Duke University, Durham, N.C. 27706 USA)

Ingestive functions are normally accompanied by a perceptual and functional
fusion of the sensory inputs of taste, smell, and oral somatosensation
(Mozell et al, Arch.Otolaryng.,1969). A potential physiological substrate of
such a fusion is suggested by the contiguity and convergence of known odorant
sensitive intranasal trigeminal afferents (Cain, Chem.Senses & Flavor,1976;
Tucker, Handbook of Sensory Physiology, 1971) with oral afferents in dorsal
spinal trigeminal n. oralis and gustatory NTS (Van Buskirk & Erickson, Brain
Res.,1977; Neurosci.Letters,1977). In 14 female Sprague-Dawley rats, 33
taste-responsive neurons in the gustatory NTS were investigated for responses
to the odorants acetone, amyl acetate, methyl alcohol, vinegar, and the odor
of a saturated solution of sucrose. These odorants include some known to
cause nasal trigeminal responses (Tucker, 1971) and some related to food.
Twenty of the 33 taste-responsive neurons responded with a well defined
change from spontaneous firing rate to at least one of the odorants. In one
case the odorant response was stronger than the maximum taste response, but
most were 50% of the maximum taste response or less. In all but two cases
the odorant responses were statistically significant; for those two cases
not statistically significant the response was strongly biphasic, consisting
of an initial decrease from spontaneous rate followed by a well defined
increase above spontaneous rate. Most odorants elicited firing rate increases
in some neurons and decreases in others and no odorant elicited responses in
all odorant- and taste-responsive (OT) neurons. Responses were found to
acetone in 7 neurons, to amyl acetate in 5 neurons, to methyl alcohol in 11
neurons, to vinegar in 6 neurons, and to odor of sucrose in 2 neurons.
Odorant responses were paired in 10 neurons, with acetone and methyl alcohol
occuring as the most common pair (3 neurons). Eleven neurons responded to
odorants with only increases from spontaneous rate, 5 with only decreases,
and two with increases to one odorant and decreases to another. Examination
of OT neurons versus those responding only to taste stimuli (T-only) showed
no significant differences in mean breadth of response (number of stimuli
responded to) to the taste stimuli (.1M NaCl, .5M sucrose, .01M citric acid,
.01M quinine HCl), whether based on a minimum response criterion of 2 times
spontaneous rate, on 50% of the maximum response (Pfaffmann et al, Progress
in Psychobiology and Physiological Psychology, 1976), or on entropy (a
measure specifying the uncertainty of responses to different stimuli within
the same neuron (Beckman, Probability in Communication Engineering, 1967;
Travers & Smith, submitted for publication, 1977)). On the other hand, the
mean response rates of the OT neurons to the four taste stimuli were found to
be significantly lower than those for the T-only neurons (χ^2=20.29, df=3,
$p < .01$). More OT neurons showed maximum taste responses to sucrose and less
to citric acid than in T-only neurons, and many more OT neurons showed
sucrose-NaCl-citric acid (SNH) response profiles and many fewer that responded to all four stimuli (SNHQ) than occured in T-only neurons. No correlation
was found between responses to any odorants and the maximum taste responses.
In three animals the ethmoid nerve, an intranasal trigeminal afferent, was
found to have contributed at least one of the odorant responses in the OT
neurons. Although neither the function of the OT neurons nor the functional
significance (if any) of their differences from T-only neurons in NTS is
known, the OT neurons may well have a significant relationship to those
functions requiring interaction of odorant and taste information in ingestion.
Supported by NSF Grant BNS75 22692.

RESPONSES OF FROG OLFACTORY RECEPTORS TO STIMULI AT THRESHOLD CONCENTRATIONS

W. van Drongelen, Electrophysiologie, Univ. Claude-Bernard, Lyon, France

Receptor cell activity in the frog eminentia olfactoria was recorded
using metal-filled microelectrodes. Several units discharged spontaneously
with a mean frequency lower than 0.2 spikes per second, or were silent in
periods up to 5 min. in absence of stimulation. Some units had a higher
spontaneous activity, their activity could be modeled with a Poisson process.
Responses to stimuli at threshold concentrations were investigated
repeating a number of stimulations within a small concentration range.
Stimulations at threshold concentrations were sometimes followed by a
conspicuous increase   in spike frequency, sometimes not. From this
observation one might ask for the significance of weak fluctuations in
post-stimulus spike discharge. Do these modifications represent activity
caused by olfactory stimulation? If so, how can post-stimulus activity
be described quantitatively? To visualize the responses to sub-threshold
stimulations of the same unit, the neural activity obtained in a number of
individual odour trials has been superimposed.
The distribution of the number of spikes in responses to odour trials at
threshold showed a reasonable agreement with two types of Poisson
distributions. A Chi-square test indicated significance levels from 10% to
90% for a normal Poisson distribution, and from 5% to 75% for a modified
Poisson distribution. In receptor cells displaying no spontaneous discharge,
the Poisson models have been used to describe experimentally determined
response probability, i.e. the fraction of odour stimulations followed by a
response. The findings are discussed in connection with the receptor cell
transduction mechanism, and the excitation of second order neurons.

Mapping of functional olfactory pathways by autoradiography with
C14-2-Deoxyglucose. M. Verrier, I. Giachetti*, J. Leveteau, P.
Mac Leod*, (UER 61, Universite Paris 6, 9 quai St Bernard, 75005
Paris ; *Laboratoire de Neurobiologie Sensorielle, EPHE, CEN/FAR,
Fontenay-aux-Roses).

In order to compare the size and the relative importance of the
well known olfactory projections and to outline new projections
an autoradiographic survey of local metabolic rate with 14C-2-
Deoxyglucose (2-DG) was performed according to Sokoloff's method
50 µCi of 2-DG in 1 ml normal saline solution were injected in
the jugular vein under light Nembutal anesthesia. Electrical
stimulation of the lateral olfactory tract (L.O.T.) was immediately started and maintained for 45 mn. Rats were then decapitated
and their brains were removed in less than 2 mn and immediately
frozen in acetone chilled to-50°C with liquid nitrogen. 20 µm
thick sections were made in a cryostat at-18° C, quickly dried on
glass slides, and then exposed for 70 hours on X-Ray films at
4 C. After exposure, histological sections were stained with
thionin and compared to their autoradiographic prints. The autoradiographs were analyzed with an integrating microdensitometer.
Relative labelling of different structures was evaluated as percentage of optical density increase by respect to background
labelling.
The most labelled areas were : ipsilateral pyriform cortex :
157 % ; contralateral pyriform cortex : 81 % ; ipsilateral periamygdaloid cortex : 157 % ; contralateral periamygdaloid cortex :
80 % ; ipsilateral accumbens nucleus : 142 % ; contralateral accumbens nucleus : 71 % ; ipsilateral anterior olfactory nucleus
(A.O.N.), pars lateralis and pars ventralis : 129 % ; contralateral (A.O.N.) : 71 % ; ipsilateral olfactory bulb (mitral as
well as granule cell layers) : 105 % ; contralateral olfactory
bulb : 100 % ; ipsilateral far rostral lateral hypothalamus
(F.R.L.H.) : 100 % ; contralateral F.R.L.H. : 71 % ; ipsilateral
caudo-putamen nucleus : 80 % ; contralateral caudo-putamen
nucleus :57 % ; ipsilateral olfactory tubercule : 80 % ; ipsilateral cortical amygdaloid nucleus : 71 % ; contralateral cortical amygdaloid nucleus : 57 % ; ispilateral and contralateral
lateral amygdaloid nucleus : 71 %. Thalamic area appears unifor-
mly labelled. An asymetrical labelling appears only in rats with
anterior commissure section. Ipsilateral dorso-medial nucleus :
50 % ; contralateral dorso-medial nucleus : 45 % ; ipsilateral
ventro-postero-medial nucleus : 45 % ; contralateral ventro-postero-medial nucleus : 31 %.

Nonolfactory odor detection in pigeons J. C. Walker, D. Tucker & J. C. Smith,
(Florida State University, Tallahassee, Fl., U. S. A.)

Using the conditioned suppression procedure, absolute thresholds to amyl acetate were determined in three pigeons to be $10^{-4.11}$, $10^{-4.08}$ and $10^{-3.87}$ per
unit vapor saturation at $20°C$. Following radical bilateral olfactory nerve
resection, thresholds were $10^{-1.30}$, $10^{-1.34}$ and $10^{-.96}$ per unit vapor saturation respectively, reflecting increases of at least 2.7 log units. Seven sessions of discrimination training were conducted to determine if pigeons deprived of olfactory input could differentiate qualitatively between a range
of concentrations of amyl acetate and a similar range of concentrations of
butyl acetate, each relative to vapor saturation; no evidence of such an
ability was found. Postoperative testing of sensitivity to amyl acetate was
then resumed for fourteen sessions; absolute thresholds were shown to be
stable and as high as those seen immediately after nerve resection. These results were compared to previous data which indicated that pigeons, after being subjected to bilateral olfactory nerve resection, can discriminate between amyl acetate and butyl acetate and can detect amyl acetate at successively lower concentrations with continued postoperative testing. Those postoperative abilities were thought to be mediated by the trigeminal nerve. We
suggest, however, that at least some of the postoperative odor detection and
discrimination seen in previous work has been due to reconstituted olfactory
nerves, a problem prevented in the present study by a surgical procedure in
which virtually the entire length of olfactory nerves was removed. The basis
of nonolfactory odor detection in pigeons remains unknown although it is oft-
en hypothesized that the nasal trigeminal receptors are involved.

Olfactory pathway in the pigeon Bernice M. Wenzel, Lyle J. Rausch,
Angelica Macadar, and Larry V. Hutchison (School of Medicine, University of
California, Los Angeles, California, U.S.A.)

In extending our research on the pigeon's olfactory system we have studied
the effects of stimulating one olfactory nerve on electrical activity in both
olfactory bulbs and in the ipsi- and contralateral forebrain. Nerve conduction velocity is 0.2-0.4 m/sec. Ipsilateral bulbar evoked response latency
is 20-40 ms; amplitude reaches 4 mV; burst responses from mitral cells follow
single shocks to the nerve; and evoked response polarity reverses across the
mitral cell layer. Contralateral bulbar latency is 2-5 ms slower than ipsilateral; amplitude is halved by repetitive stimulation; polarity is often
inverted compared to the ipsilateral response; and a late response occurs
(>60 ms). Primary and secondary projection sites identified by bulbar
stimulation and degeneration after bulbar destruction were confirmed, viz.,
direct ipsilateral projections to cortex prepiriformis (CPP), lobus parol-
factorius (LPO), and hyperstriatum ventrale (HV), and indirect to neostriatum, hyperstriatum dorsale, and paleostriatum. Resting rates of discharge
from 93 of 110 spontaneously active cells in these sites either increase or
decrease by at least 20% when the olfactory nerve is stimulated. PST histograms for most cells showed peak firing rates or periods of inhibition at
latencies consistent with phases of the evoked potential recorded from that
site. The time course of post-tetanic changes varied among units from a few
seconds to several minutes. Active units (28) in sites not known to receive
olfactory input were not effectively modified by stimulation. Experiments
in progress using HRP injections into LPO and HV show input from ipsilateral
parahippocampal and septal areas, caudal neostriatum, paleostriatum, dorso-
medial thalamus, and ventral hypothalamic areas. A substantial contralateral
projection originates from dorsomedial thalamus. (Supported by USPHS grant
NS 10353 to B. M. Wenzel.)

Specific Anosmia: Mice Provide a Model C. J. Wysocki, D. Tucker and
G. Whitney, (Psychobiology Program, Florida State University, Tallahassee,
Florida, 32306, USA)

It has been suggested that "specific anosmias", sensitivity deficits to
certain odors in individuals with otherwise normal olfactory abilities, have
a genetic base (1). As an initial step in the isolation of a fatty acid
specific anosmia in nonhuman mammals, we tested commercially available mice
from nine genetically inbred strains for their relative sensitivities to
isovaleric acid (2). Utilizing a bait-shyness paradigm we found that mice
from two related strains appeared to demonstrate a deficit of sensitivity
to the compound. We tested mice from one of these strains (C57BL/6J) and
from a "normal" strain (AKR/J) with amyl acetate, pentadecalactone and
isovaleric acid (3). C57 mice were less sensitive to isovaleric acid than
were AKR mice, although in many experiments no significant differences were
observed between the strains with either amyl acetate or pentadecalactone.
The results of genetic analyses performed with segregating generations
derived from C57 X AKR hybridization suggested polygenic inheritance of
isovaleric acid anosmia (4). This mammalian model could facilitate an
understanding of the mechanisms underlying specific anosmias. Additionally,
this model might prove useful in evaluating the specific anosmia approach
to a general understanding of the olfactory process.

References
1. Whissell-Buechy, D. and Amoore, J. E. 1973. Nature, 242, 271-273.
2. Wysocki, C. J. and Tucker, D. 1976. Behav. Genet., 6, 122.
3. Wysocki, C. J., Whitney, G. and Tucker, D. 1977. Behav. Genet., 7,
    171-188.
4. Wysocki, C. J., Tucker, D. and Nyby, J. 1977. Behav. Genet., 7, 93.

Supported by U. S. Public Health Service grants MH 11218, NS 08814,
MH 05116 and an award from the Florida State University Committee on Faculty Research Support.

A neural pathway to the orbitofrontal cortex from the olfactory bulb
through the thalamus in the monkey   H. Yarita, S. Kogure, M. Iino and
S. F. Takagi, (Dept. of Physiol. Sch. of Med. Gunma Univ. Maebashi, Gunma,
Japan)

Spike activities of single cells in the medial subdivision of the
mediodorsal (MD) thalamic nucleus were intra-and extracellularly studied
in anesthetized monkeys to confirm earlier anatomical findings. Spike
potentials elicited by electrical stimulation of the ipsilateral olfactory
bulb (OB) had a mean latency of 32.0 msec. They were preceded by EPSPs
with rapid rising phases and were followed by long lasting IPSPs.

A single shock was applied to a central portion (which almost coincides
with the posterior orbital gyrus) of the orbito-frontal cortex (OFC) which
is located anterior to and medial to the olfactory area indicated previously
by Tanabe et al (1975). The shock elicited an antidromic spike potential
followed by an IPSP in the cell which also responded to the OB stimulation.
The mean latency was 2.64 msec. Some of the cells were activated synaptically by the OFC stimulation. Although the function of the medial subdivision is not yet certain, our physiological observations support an
anatomical finding that a neural projection exists from the subdivision of
the MD nucleus to the central portion of the OFC.

Thus, we proved in our laboratory the existence of two pathways from the
olfactory bulb. One goes to the latero-posterior portion of the orbito-
frontal cortex through the hypothalamus and the other to the central portion
through the thalamus.

Responses of single neurons in the olfactory bulb of the goldfish (Carassius auratus) during stimulation of the olfactory mucosa with natural and synthetic stimuli H.P. Zippel, W. Tiedemann, R. Schumann, W. Fiedler and K. Maier (Physiologisches Institut II, Humboldtallee 7, 3400 Göttingen, West Germany)

Previous work, in which recordings were made from single neurons, has shown that natural stimuli modulate the neuronal activity more frequently than synthetic stimuli and that laminary water currents, applied to the olfactory mucosa, cause pronounced - mainly inhibitory - effects at the level of the second neuron (ZIPPEL, H.P. and BREIPOHL, W., 1975. In: D.A. Denton and J.P. Coghlan, eds., Olfaction and Taste V. Academic Press, New York, London, pp. 163-167). The present study is an extension of this work, demonstrating that in comparison with synthetic odours (amyl acetate, coumarine, β-phenylethyl alcohol, phenol; 10^{-3} molar), natural stimuli (Tubifex extract, skin extract) not only cause a larger number of neurons to respond but also induce more pronounced and longer-lasting effects. The hypothesis that these findings merely reflect the action of low molecular weight compounds containing amino acids could not be confirmed. The application of synthetic amino acids (β-ala, DL-ala, L-arg, gly, α-phe, α-ser, tau; 10^{-3} molar) produced effects comparable with those of synthetic odours. Following dialysis of Tubifex extracts, the high molecular (retentate) as well as the low molecular (dialysate) components were capable of influencing neuronal activity, in both cases a superimposition of the observed synergistic and antagonistic actions corresponding to the effect of the crude extract. Similarly, after gel chromatography (Sephadex G-50) of Tubifex and skin extracts, the opposing actions of the different molecular weight fractions correspond to the effects of the non-fractionated extracts. The data indicate the importance of "noise" in the olfactory system. The pronounced and long-lasting effects mainly observed following application of natural stimuli may be due to descending influences from higher cerebral centres and/or reverberatory circuits in the olfactory bulb itself.

TASTE

New approaches to the problem of the trophic function of neurons

Daniel W. Berland, Joyce S. Chu, Mark A. Hosley, Lee B. Jones, Jon M. Kaliszewski, William C. Lawler and Bruce Oakley

Division of Biological Sciences, University of Michigan, Ann Arbor, MI 48109, USA

ABSTRACT

Neural innervation is a necessary factor for the maintenance and regeneration of mammalian taste buds. The mechanisms of such neurotrophic dependencies have remained obscure, although chemical agents have been suspected. We have developed a new physiological assay system for the neurotrophic effects of taste axons. In the Mongolian gerbil we have found that whereas taste responses can be recorded from an uncut IXth nerve for at least 12 hours without decline, after this nerve is transected the taste responses fail within 1-4 hours. There is a linear relationship between the length of the distal stump of the nerve attached to the tongue and the time required for the taste responses to decline. Efferent fibers in the IXth nerve are unnecessary for maintaining the physiological responses. These facts suggest 1) that chemical interactions, rather than impulse activity, are responsible for the trophic effects upon taste buds and 2) that the physiological function of taste buds is maintained by the continued orthograde or retrograde transport of chemical agents along sensory axons.

INTRODUCTION

Apart from impulse activity and its sequelae, neurons are presumed to have a trophic function which deals with the maintenance of normal morphological, physiological, and biochemical features of innervated cells. Receptor organs with accessory anatomical structures in addition to the nerve ending itself (touch corpuscles in the skin, taste buds, lateral line organs, muscle spindles, etc.) show varying degrees of neurotrophic dependence upon innervation, as do vertebrate skeletal muscle fibers.[1]

Do neurotrophic chemicals exist? No one has yet succeeded in isolating a trophic chemical from the nervous system and applying it to a denervated or trophically deficient assay system to mimic fully the normal trophic effects. As a first step, an important advance would be an unambiguous demonstration that mammalian peripheral nerves transport substances which have trophic effects upon their end organs. The neuromuscular junction--whose accessibility for many in vivo and in vitro experimental techniques has facilitated significant advances--appears at this time to have highly complex trophic dependencies with multiple controls. As recently as six years ago the prevailing view was that a neurotrophic agent(s) contributed importantly to the maintenance of vertebrate skeletal muscle. The demonstration by Lømo and Rosenthal[2] that e-lectrical stimulation of denervated rat muscle could restore the ACh sensitiv-ity of the muscle to its normal state has spawned a series of experiments in several laboratories[3-5] which have rekindled the debate on the relative role of muscle activity and putative trophic chemicals as agents responsible for maintaining the integrity of muscle fibers. Analysis of the neuromuscular system is confounded by impulse activity and its associated phenomena directed toward the end organ. In the taste system efferent fibers of the taste nerve are not necessary for maintenance of taste buds.[6,7] Since taste buds degener-ate when deprived of both efferent fibers and sensory fibers in the taste nerves, it has been concluded that taste axons have a neurotrophic role vis-à-vis taste buds.[8] We have long sought to investigate more directly the trophic mechanisms in taste, but have been thwarted by the fact that morpho-logical degeneration--the standard index of trophic dependence of taste buds--requires 1-2 weeks. The ideal assay system would be one which is not only independent of impulse mediated effects, but one which would allow evaluation of acute experimental treatments of the nerve and end organ by displaying al-tered function in a few hours. The gerbil IXth nerve preparation to be de-scribed appears to provide a rapid physiological assay for trophic effects in the taste system.

METHODS

Mongolian gerbils, Meriones unguiculatus, were anesthetized with sodium pentobarbital (50 mg/kg body wt. i.p., followed by supplementary injections of 30 mg/kg) or with ketamine HCl (325 mg/kg body wt. i.m.). In acute experi-ments a tracheal cannula was inserted and the trachea and esophagus were tied off. The animal was secured to a headholder[9] which immobilized the skull and facilitated orientation of the animal to permit exposure of the IXth cranial nerve (glossopharyngeal) near the carotid bifurcation.

Distilled water at 37°C was continually flowed over the posterior portion of the tongue at a rate of 0.2-0.3 ml/sec. Taste solutions at the same tem-perature (2-4 ml per trial) were alternated with the distilled water rinse without interruption of fluid flow. Owing to the excellent response, 0.3M NH_4Cl was typically used as the taste solution, although several other chemi-cals were frequently tested, e.g., 0.5M sucrose, 0.03M HCl, 0.3M NaCl, and 0.01M quinine hydrochloride.

Electrical activity was recorded by lifting either the intact or tran-sected IXth nerve onto a 100 μm nichrome wire electrode which led to a differential amplifier (Grass P-9B). The reference wire electrode was generally placed on the tissue adjacent to the nerve. The multi-unit action potential activity was displayed on an oscilloscope and could be monitored by means of a loudspeaker. All neural responses were tape recorded and the integrated responses displayed on-line on a polygraph with the integrator time constant set at 0.5 sec, full wave rectification. A response in this study was defined as the difference between spontaneous activity and the greatest integrated potential elicited by a given solution applied to the tongue.

RESULTS

Characteristically one can record taste responses of undiminished magnitude from transected mammalian taste nerves for 12 or more hours. This is not the case with the IXth nerve of the gerbil. Immediately after the IXth nerve is transected, taste responses to chemical stimulation of the posterior region of the tongue can be recorded, but they soon begin an irreversible decline in

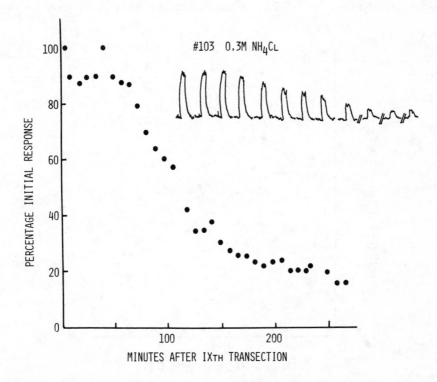

Figure 1. The decline in the summated taste response produced by cutting the IXth nerve of a gerbil. The taste stimulus (0.3M NH$_4$Cl) was applied every 4 minutes. 100%=initial response level. Inset shows the original polygraph records of summated responses beginning with the 7th response and ending with responses at 80, 100, and 120 minutes after the nerve was cut.

intensity to 0-25% of the initial response level. Figure 1 shows such a decline in response magnitude in which the taste stimulus (0.3M NH$_4$Cl) was presented every 4 minutes until, after 3.5 hours, the response was at a level less than 20% of the initial magnitude. This phenomenon occurred in most of the IXth nerves tested; less than 15% maintained the response during the recording session.

This falloff is not a consequence of drying of the nerve, since soaking it in Ringer's solution has no appreciable effect. Further, responses recorded with the nerve immersed in mineral oil also decline, and the use of a suction electrode to alter the mechanical stress and moisture conditions does not prevent the failure of the response (Fig. 2). Responses can be recorded from uncut IXth nerves for more than 12 hours.

We considered the possibility that this response failure represented a form of fatigue; that is, a loss of receptor excitability owing to repeated stimulation with taste solutions. However, the responses would often begin to

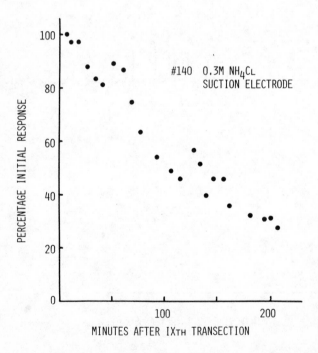

Figure 2. Decline in the response of a cut IXth nerve to 0.3M NH$_4$Cl. Impulse activity recorded with a Ringer's filled suction electrode applied to the cut end of the nerve.

decline as soon as the nerve was cut. Nor was there a detectable effect of interpolated 3 minute periods of continuous stimulation with 0.3M NH_4Cl upon the time course of the falloff in the response. Moreover, we could record for several hours from one IXth nerve and observe the response decline, and then proceed to record a normal vigorous response from the intact contralateral IXth nerve. The contralateral IXth nerve's response would also decline following nerve transection. We concluded that the cause of the response failure was not receptor fatigue.

Conceivably, the cause might lie in a failure of the axonal impulse mechanism, as might occur if a physiological concomitant of extremely rapid Wallerian degeneration spread down the nerve from the site of transection. Yet, recordings from two active electrodes on the nerve, one near the cut end and one closer to the tongue, failed to detect a spread of decay first to the proximal electrode and then to the distal electrode. The responses declined simultaneously at both electrodes. Additionally, normal compound action potentials could be electrically elicited in vitro from a IXth nerve cut 10 hours before recording (Fig. 3). The source of the response decline must lie at the level of the taste bud, and cannot be attributed to failure of the impulse mechanism in the axons themselves.

It seemed possible that transection of the IXth nerve interrupted the supply of a trophic agent(s) which was required at the level of the taste bud for maintenance of physiological excitability. Accordingly, we carried out experiments to determine whether the rate of decline of the taste response was a function of the length of the nerve stump remaining attached to the tongue

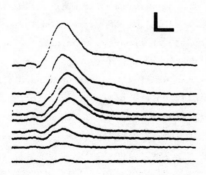

Figure 3. Oscilloscopic records of the compound action potential of the IXth nerve recorded in vitro 10 hours after nerve transection distal to the petrosal ganglion. One square wave stimulus per trace, 0.34 msec duration at (from bottom to top) 4.9, 5.0, 5.1, 5.2, 5.3, 5.4, 5.5, 5.9, and 6.4 V. Calibration lines: 0.2 mV and 0.5 msec.

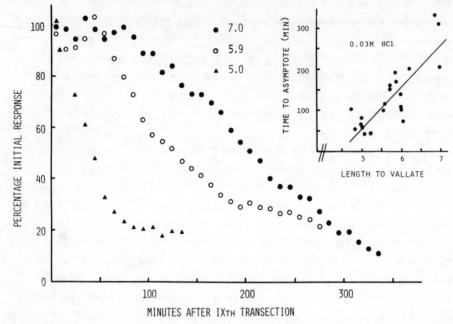

Figure 4. Decline in the taste response (0.3M NH$_4$Cl) over time for short (5.0 mm, n=11), medium (5.9 mm, n=11) and long (7.0 mm, n=5) IXth nerve stumps attached to the tongue. Records normalized with initial response set at 100%, mean length of nerves given, ± 0.3 mm. The inset shows a linear relationship between nerve length and time to reach asymptotic level (i.e. 95% down) for responses to 0.03M HCl (n=21).

after nerve transection. We found for each of the 5 chemicals tested (see Methods) that the shorter the nerve stump the more rapidly the taste response declined (Fig. 4). From the slope of the regression lines (e.g., for HCl, Fig. 4 inset) one can calculate an apparent transport velocity of 15-25 mm/day. The inference that trophic agents are transported along sensory axons is supported by experiments in which the efferent fibers in the IXth nerve were eliminated by decentralizing the petrosal ganglion. Chronic decentralization did not eliminate the taste responses. In order to determine whether the intact sensory fibers in the IXth nerve were not only sufficient but also necessary for taste responses, the chronically decentralized IXth nerve was transected distal to the petrosal ganglion. This procedure quickly resulted in the decline in the taste responses (Fig. 5, filled circles). Acute decentralization has no significant effect on taste responses recorded from the IXth nerve still attached to the petrosal ganglion. Responses continued to be elicitable for at least 6 hours (Fig. 5, open circles).

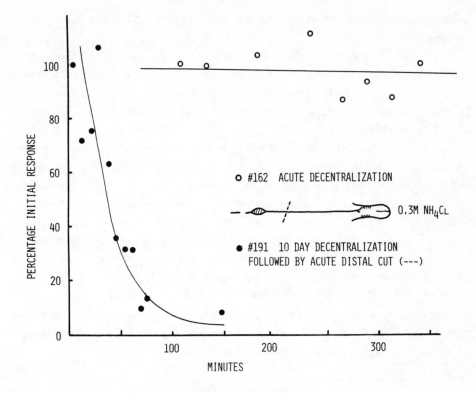

Figure 5. Effects of decentralization. Acute decentralization fails to re-duce the response of the IXth nerve to 0.3M NH$_4$Cl (open circles, gerbil #162). Gerbil #191 had the left IXth nerve cut central to the petrosal ganglion. Ten days later normal responses could be recorded from this IXth nerve. As soon as the first response was recorded, the left IXth nerve was cut distal to the petrosal ganglion (dashed line across nerve) and a decline in the taste re-sponses ensued (closed circles).

DISCUSSION

Transection of the gerbil IXth nerve causes, in 1-4 hours, an irreversi-ble 75-100 percent decline in the magnitude of the integrated taste response. This decline does not result from a failure of the axonal action potential mechanism or from excessive stimulation of the taste system. Efferent fibers in the IXth nerve are not necessary for maintaining the IXth nerve responses to taste stimulation but sensory fibers are. It is suggested that the taste responses are dependent upon a continuous supply of trophic chemical(s) trans-ported along the sensory axons. The most compelling evidence for this state-ment is that the rate of taste response decline is a linear function of the length of the nerve stump remaining attached to the tongue after nerve transection.

In other regards the IXth nerve responses to taste solutions seem quite comparable to those observed in other rodents.[10-13] Several chemicals are effective; ammonium chloride tends to be the best taste stimulus. It may well be that when sought, similar effects following nerve transection can be observed in other taste nerves. The use of shortened taste nerves might make the physiological changes more evident. Recent independent observations have shown that taste responses from the cat IXth nerve disappear more rapidly with short (22 hours) than with long nerves (28 hours).[14]

From our analysis the immediate cause of the response failure would appear to lie within the taste bud, not within the axons of the nerve. This statement does not imply that degenerative physiological changes occur within the taste receptor cells with this rapidity. The first physiological changes after interruption of neurotrophic communication might occur at the axonal terminals. The absence of a confounding role of efferent impulses and the rapidity of the response change in the gerbil IXth nerve may permit accumulation of evidence for axonal transport of a trophic chemical(s) and allow further analysis of the role and nature of such substances.

ACKNOWLEDGEMENTS

We are grateful for the assistance of Sue Igras and Linda Sorkin.

REFERENCES

1. Harris, A. J. (1974) Ann. Rev. Physiol. 36, 251-305
2. Lømo, T. and Rosenthal, J. (1972)   J. Physiol. 221, 493-513
3. Lømo, T. and Westgaard, R. H. (1975) in Symp. on Quant. Biol. The Synapse, 40, 263-274
4. Gruener, R. and Baumbach, N. (1976) J. Neurobiol. 7, 513-519
5. Cangiano, A. and Lutzemberger, L. (1977)   Science 196, 542-545
6. Donegani, G. and Gabella, G. (1967)   Soc. Ital. Biol. Sper., Boll. 47, 156-159
7. Kamrin, R. and Singer, M. (1953)   Am. J. Physiol. 207, 507-528
8. Cheal, M. L. and Oakley, B. (1977)   J. Comp. Neurol. 172, 609-626
9. Oakley, B. and Schafer, R. (1978) in Experimental Neurobiology: A Laboratory Manual, Univ. of Michigan Press, Ann Arbor
10. Oakley, B. (1967)   J. Physiol. 188, 353-371
11. Pfaffmann, C., Fisher, G. L., and Frank, M. (1967) in Olfaction and Taste II   T. Hayashi, ed. pp 361-381
12. Yamada, K. (1966)   Jap. J. Physiol. 16, 599-611
13. Frank, M. (1975) in Olfaction and Taste V, Denton, D. A. and Coghalan, J. P., eds. Academic Press, New York, pp 59-64
14. Donoso, A. and Zapata, P. (1976) Experientia 32, 591-592

A synopsis of gustatory neuroanatomy

Ralph Norgren

The Rockefeller University, 1230 York Avenue, New York, NY 10021, USA

ABSTRACT

Peripheral gustatory afferents reach the brain via the seventh, ninth, and tenth cranial nerves, and synapse in the anterior end of the nucleus of the solitary tract (NST). Cells in the caudal parabrachial area, located between the principal and mesencephalic trigeminal nuclei, receive afferents from NST and respond to gustatory stimuli applied to the tongue. From the dorsal pons, axons of these third order gustatory neurons ascend to the thalamic taste relay on the medial edge of the ventrobasal complex. Thalamic cells responding to lingual thermal and tactile stimuli are interposed between the gustatory relay medially and the remainder of the trigeminal relay laterally. On cortex, rodents maintain this proximity, but in other species at least part of the gustatory representation appears to shift to opercular cortex. In addition to synapsing in the thalamus, pontine gustatory axons pass ventrally through subthalamus and penetrate the internal capsule. Rostral to the internal capsule, the fascicles break into a maze of individual fibers which shift laterally through substantia innominata and appear to end in the central nucleus of the amygdala. Some axons, however, communicate via the stria terminalis with another terminal field in the bed nucleus of the stria terminalis.

In mammals taste buds occur within the oral cavity, pharynx and larynx. Gustatory receptors on the anterior tongue and palate are innervated by the chorda tympani and greater superficial petrosal nerves, respectively[11,20], which pass into the medulla via the intermediate nerve, the visceral afferent division of the facial nerve. On the posterior tongue, the lingual branch of the glossopharyngeal nerve (IX) innervates the circumvallate and most of the foliate papilla. The fungiform papilla near the circumvallates and a few foliates probably receive axons from the chorda tympani[6,30]. The afferents from epiglottal and other laryngeal taste buds travel in the superior laryngeal branch of the vagus (X)[1]. Other nerves distributing to the pharynx, primarily the tonsilar branch of IX and the pharyngeal of X, probably contain gustatory afferents, because taste buds occur scattered within their peripheral fields.

The gustatory afferent nerves terminate in the lateral division of the nucleus of the solitary tract (NST)[2,16,35,40]. Some axons in these nerves also descend along the dorsal border of the spinal trigeminal nuclei. Their function remains unknown, but has been equated with the somatosensory component of these cranial nerves. In some species, primary gustatory afferents may ascend through the medulla and terminate in caudal pons[7,10,22,34]. To date, however, the anterior pole of the solitary nucleus remains the only well documented first central gustatory relay[14,19,33].

Axons of secondary gustatory neurons in the solitary nucleus ascend ipsilaterally in the reticular formation just ventral to the vestibular nuclei until they reach the trigeminal motor nucleus. At this point they turn dorsally, pass through the supratrigeminal area, and terminate dorsal, ventral, and within the brachium conjunctivum[28,29] (Norgren, in preparation). Within this area, the caudal end of the parabrachial nuclei (PBN), small neurons respond to sapid stimuli (Fig. 1) in a manner not fundamentally different from gustatory neurons recorded in the solitary nucleus or peripheral nerves[30,32]. As in the solitary nucleus, the pontine taste area is circumscribed (0.6 - 0.7 mm dia.), and overlaps with neurons which respond to either tongue tactile or thermal stimuli. In fact, some cells respond to more than one of these lingual modalities, but none respond to a combination of gustatory and non-lingual (trigeminal) stimuli. As mentioned above, in several species some peripheral gustatory afferents may terminate directly in a caudal pontine gustatory relay, suggesting an analogy to the organization of trigeminal afferents which synapse on neurons in both medullary and pontine nuclei.

From the caudal parabrachial nuclei gustatory neurons project, again primarily ipsilaterally, via the central tegmental bundle into the postero-medial ventrobasal complex of the thalamus[25,29]. Within the thalamus substantial crossing occurs

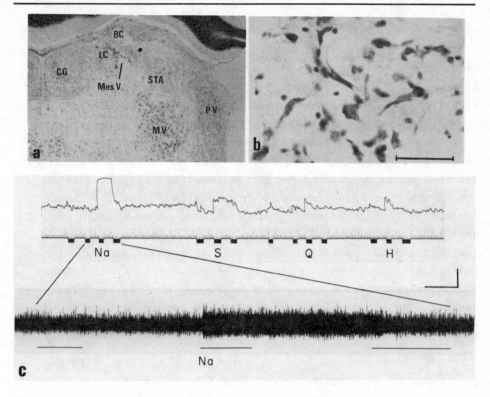

Fig. 1. Gustatory relay in the dorsal pons. (a) Low power
photomicrograph of a section through the dorsal pons (Cresyl violet). Parabrachial nuclei surround the brachium conjunctivum
(BC) dorsal to the supratrigeminal area (STA) and the mesencephalic trigeminal nucleus (Mes V). (b) Higher power photomicrograph of the section in (a) depicting neurons in the parabrachial nuclei. These cells are located on the edge of the brachium
conjunctivum just lateral to the dot (●) in (a). Neurons in the
area seldom exceed 25 μ in their greatest dimension, and are
typically bi- or tri-polar. Others appear bipolar, but in fact,
have two small dendrites on each end (cell near center of b).
Calibration equals approximately 1.0 mm in (a) and 50 μ in (b).
(c) Multiunit responses to sapid stimuli recorded from the parabrachial nuclei. The electrode tip was located at the dot in
(a). The upper trace is a continuous integrated record with
time and stimulus application marks below. The filmed oscilloscope trace in the lower record shows the multiunit activity
which generated the integrated response when NaCl was applied to
the anterior tongue. Unlabeled marks in both records represent
water rinses. Time marks in upper record are at 1.0 sec. intervals. Calibration for lower record equals 2.0 sec. and 100 μV.
Abbreviations: CG, central gray; H, 0.003 N HCl; LC, locus
coeruleus; MV, trigeminal motor nucleus; Na, 0.25 M NaCl; PV,
principal sensory trigeminal nucleus; Q, 0.003 M quinine HCl; S,
0.5 M sucrose. The lower panel (c) was taken from Norgren and
Pfaffmann, Brain Research (1975) 91: 99-117 with permission of
the publisher.

to the mirror image area contralaterally. This small celled, medial extension of the ventrobasal complex boasts a variety of names depending on the species and investigator. Nevertheless, in several of those species (rat, cat and monkey) it has been satisfactorily identified as the thalamic gustatory relay[8]. Consistent with the neuroanatomy of the system, thalamic gustatory neurons have receptive fields located ipsilaterally on the tongue[3,13]. Immediately lateral to the purely taste responsive neurons, and connecting them to the remainder of the thalamic somatosensory relay, are cells which respond to tongue thermal and tongue tactile stimuli[3,13]. Some neurons respond to both sapid and thermal stimuli. Since similar units occur in both the solitary and parabrachial nuclei, it remains unclear if the thalamic response results from convergence of separate lingual modalities, or merely reflects convergence at lower levels. Gustatory afferents also invade the more lateral tongue tactile relay, but apparently without the synaptic density necessary to drive neurons (Norgren, unpublished observation).

Despite the homology of the thalamic gustatory relay in many mammals, gustatory cortex appears to be organized differently in the lissencephalic and gyrencephalic species investigated to date. In the rat, taste cortex forms a thin band along the ventral edge of the main somatosensory projection (SS I) at the juncture of the middle cerebral artery and the rhinal sulcus (see Norgren and Wolf for references)[31]. In both rat and rabbit this area appears to be coextensive with the anterior third of Rose's granular insular cortex[17,42], and rostral to the second somatosensory area (SS II)[12,41]. In cats and monkeys two cortical gustatory areas have been distinguished, one on the lateral convexity subjacent to primary trigeminal cortex (SS I), and the other buried in the anterior operculum rostral to SS II[4,5,9]. Burton and Benjamin[8] hypothesize that pure gustatory cortex lies buried, and that the lateral area represents a convergence of lingual and gustatory modalities. Anatomical and electrophysiological data from other laboratories tend to support their conclusions[18,21,37,39].

Although the gustatory cortex of rats occupies a position analogous to the lateral area in primate, it is cytoarchitec-

tonically similar to the opercular area[38]. The efferent distribution from rodent taste cortex, however, resembles the pattern
of primary sensory cortex, i.e. it projects to each of the subcortical gustatory relays[27]. With so little electrophysiological data available from gustatory cortex, and most of that from
lissencephalic animals[42], it is not possible to determine whether primates possess a distinct cortical gustatory area, or have
physically separated functions present in the cortical gustatory
area of rodents.

Gustatory afferents also reach the forebrain more directly
than via the traditional thalamo-cortical pathway. Axons from
the same population of pontine neurons that project to the
gustatory thalamus ascend further through the subthalamus and,
after apparently giving off collaterals into lateral hypothalamus
(LTH), pierce the internal capsule (IC)[29]. Upon exiting rostral-
ly from IC, these fascicles break into small bundles and fill the
substantia innominata (SI). They extend laterally into the an-

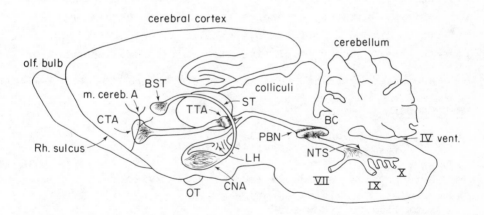

Fig. 2. Basic pathways of the central gustatory system superimposed on a parasagittal section of the rat brain. Abbreviations: BC, brachium conjunctivum; BST, bed nucleus of the stria
terminalis; CNA, central nucleus of the amygdala; CTA, cortical
taste area; IV vent., fourth ventricle; IX, glossopharyngeal
nerve; LH, lateral hypothalamus; m. cereb. A, middle cerebral
artery; NTS, nucleus of the solitary tract; olf. bulb, olfactory
bulb; OT, optic tract; PBN, parabrachial nuclei; Rh. sulcus,
rhinal sulcus; ST, stria terminalis; TTA, thalamic taste area;
VII, intermediate (facial) nerve; X, vagus nerve. The figure
was kindly supplied by Dr. Carl Pfaffmann.

terior amygdala where many apparently terminate throughout the
central nucleus of the amygdala (CNA). Another terminal zone
exists in the bed nucleus of the stria terminalis, and it connects to CNA via a component of the stria terminalis (Fig. 2)[25].
Some axons of this elaborate network convey gustatory information, because parabrachial neurons which respond to sapid stimuli can be antidromically activated by electrical stimulation in
LTH, IC, SI and CNA[24,25]. Similar evidence indicates that some
pontine gustatory neurons send collaterals to both the thalamic
taste area and the ventral forebrain.

Stimulation of the parabrachial gustatory area elicits
short latency evoked potentials (4-10 msec.) in ventral forebrain areas which closely match the axonal distribution from PBN
(Norgren et al., in preparation). Units in lateral hypothalamus
respond to gustatory stimulation, but often as not to other peripheral stimuli as well[23]. Neurons in both LTH and SI respond
during feeding behavior, but their activity can be influenced by
the sight as well as the taste of the food[15,36]. What little
evidence exists, then, suggests that, unlike the thalamo-cortical systems, gustatory afferents to ventral forebrain may be
integrated into a functional system with direct or indirect access to other sensory modalities important to feeding behavior[26].

Supported by grants from NIH (NS 10150) and NSF (BNS76-81401).

REFERENCES

1. Andrew, B.L. and Oliver, J. (1951)
    J. Physiol. (London) 114, 48-49P

2. Astrom, K.E. (1953)
    Acta Physiol. Scand. 29 (suppl. 106), 209-320.

3. Benjamin, R. (1963) in Olfaction and Taste,
    MacMillan Co., New York

4. Benjamin, R.M. and Burton, H. (1968)
    Brain Res. 7, 221-231.

5. Benjamin, R.M., Emmers, R. and Blomquist, A.J. (1968)
    Brain Res. 7, 208-220

6. Bernard, R. (1964)
    Am. J. Physiol. 206, 827-835.

7. Bernard, R.A. and Nord, S.G. (1971)
    Brain Res. 30, 349-356

8. Burton, H. and Benjamin, R.M. (1971) in Handbook of Sensory
    Physiology, Vol. IV, Chemical Senses, Part 2, Taste
    Springer-Verlag, Berlin

9. Burton, H. and Earls, F. (1969)
    Brain Res. 16, 520-523

10. Car, A., Jean, A. and Roman, C. (1975)
    Exp. Brain Res. 22, 197-210

11. Cleaton-Jones, P. (1976)
    Archs. Oral Biol. 21, 79-82

12. Donaldson, L., Hand, P.J. and Morrison, A.R. (1975)
    Exp. Neurol. 47, 448-458

13. Emmers, R. (1966)
    Proc. Soc. Exp. Biol. Med. 121, 527-531

14. Halpern, B.P. and Nelson, M. (1965)
    Am. J. Physiol. 209, 105-110

15. Hamburg, M. (1971)
    Am. J. Physiol. 220, 980-995

16. Kerr, F.W.L. (1962)
    Arch. Neurol. (Chicago) 6, 264-281

17. Krettek, J.E. and Price, J.L. (1977)
    J. Comp. Neurol. 171, 157-192

18. Landgren, S. (1957)
    Acta Phys.Scand. 40, 210-221.

19. Makous, W., Nord, S., Oakley, B. and Pfaffmann, C. (1963)
    in Proceedings of the First International Symposium on
    Olfaction and Taste, pp. 381-393, Pergamon Press, Oxford

20. Miller, I.J.,Jr. and Porcelli, L.J.,Jr. (1976)
    Anat. Rec. 184, 480.

21. Morrison, A.R. and Tarnecki, R. (1975) in Olfaction and
    Taste, V, pp. 247-249, Academic Press, New York

22. Nageotte, J. (1906)
    Rev. Neurol. Psychiat. 4, 472-488

23. Norgren, R. (1970)
    Brain Res. 21, 63-77

24. Norgren, R. (1974)
    Brain Res. 81, 285-295

25. Norgren, R. (1976)
    J. Comp. Neurol. 166, 17-30

26. Norgren, R. (1977) in Chemical Signals in Vertebrates,
    pp. 515-528, Plenum Press, New York

27. Norgren, R. and Grill, H. (1976
    Neurosci. Abstr. 2, 124

28. Norgren, R. and Leonard, C.M. (1971)
    Science 173, 1136-1139

29. Norgren, R. and Leonard, C.M. (1973)
    J. Comp. Neurol. 150, 217-238

30. Norgren, R. and Pfaffmann, C. (1975)
    Brain Res. 91, 99-117

31. Norgren, R. and Wolf, G. (1975)
    Brain Res. 92, 123-129

32. Perrotto, R. and Scott, T. (1976)
    Brain Res. 110, 283-300

33. Pfaffmann, C, Erickson, R., Frommer, G. and Halpern, B.
    (1961) in Sensory Communication, M.I.T. Press and Wiley
    & Sons, New York

34. Rhoton, A.L. (1968)
    J. Comp. Neurol. 133, 89-100

35. Rhoton, A.L.,Jr., O'Leary, J.L. and Ferguson, J.P. (1966)
    Arch. Neurol. 14, 530-540

36. Rolls, E.T., Burton, M.J. and Mora, F. (1976)
    Brain Res. 111, 53-66

37. Ruderman, M.I., Morrison, A.I. and Hand, P.J. (1972)
    Exp. Neurol. 37, 522-537

38. Sanides, F. (1968)
    Brain Res. 8, 97-124

39. Sudakov, K., MacLean, P.D., Reeves, A. and Marino, R. (1971)
    Brain Res. 28, 19-34

40. Torvik, A. (1956)
    J. Comp. Neurol. 106, 51-141

41. Welker, C. and Sinha, M.M. (1972)
    Brain Res. 37, 132-136

42. Yamamoto, T. and Kawamura, Y. (1975)
    Brain Res. 94, 447-463

Taste discrimination in the monkey

Masayasu Sato, Yasutake Hiji and Hirosumi Ito

Tokyo Metropolitan Institute for Neurosciences, Fuchu, Tokyo, Japan and Kumamoto University Medical School, Kumamoto, Japan

ABSTRACT

Analysis of single taste nerve fiber responses in the macaque indicates the presence of a coding system highly specific for taste of sucrose or quinine and its ability of tasting a variety of sweeteners. These are considered to be two of the basic properties of the taste discriminatory mechanism characteristic to the macaque monkey. In agreement with these properties the macaque responded neurally and behaviorally to both aspartame (L-aspartyl-L-phenylalanine methyl ester) and stevioside, which are 100-200 times sweeter than sucrose in humans. There is a large individual variation in the sensitivity to these sweeteners among macaques, but evidence that the sweeteners bind to the same receptor molecule as that for sucrose is presented. Studies of neural and ingestive responses to sugars indicate that taste effectiveness of varying sugars are different from that in other mammals including the squirrel monkey. Therefore, the macaque is unique in its taste sensitivity and preference for various sweeteners and sugars, and can serve as a model for the study of human taste sensation.

INTRODUCTION

Evidence presented in the past by electrophysiological studies of the taste system in a number of mammals has shown that, although there are some taste nerve fibers which respond specifically to only one of the four basic stimuli representing acid, bitter, salty and sweet tastes, a majority of fibers are responsive to two or more stimuli. Therefore, in most mammals the nature of the chemical stimuli cannot be signalled by the system of specifically labelled lines. Consequently, this led to the concept of coding by the relative activity among fibers firing simultaneously. Dr. Erickson formulated this concept into the across-fiber pattern principle[1].

On the other hand, certain behavioral experiments indicate that there are species differences in taste sensitivity among various mammals. The difference is especially marked in sensitivities to sweeteners. The existence of such species-specific taste sensitivity in mammals led us to investigate response properties of taste nerve fibers in certain species of macaque monkeys, which are phylogenetically closer to men than are rodents or squirrel monkeys. The results of our study, which were already reported in ISOT V in Melbourne[2] and elsewhere[3], indicate first that in macaque monkeys the specifically labelled line coding system for 'sweet' (sucrose) and 'bitter' (quinine) stimuli is developed. This contrasts properties of taste nerve fibers in most other mammals including the squirrel monkey, where fibers responsive best to sucrose or quinine possess sensitivities to acids and salts[4]. The second conclusion, which were derived from the correlation taste profiles constructed from responses in a large number of chorda tympani nerve fibers to a variety of taste stimuli, was that some of the non-sugar sweet-tasting compounds produce in the macaque taste quality similar to that induced by sucrose.

Such broad taste sensitivity to a variety of sweeteners in macaque monkeys, which most other mammals do not possess[5,6], has also been demonstrated by Dr. Hellekant and his collaborators. They showed that sweet-tasting proteins, monellin and thaumatin, elicited significant chorda tympani nerve responses in the green monkey (Cercopithecus aethiops) but neither in the guinea pig and rat[7] nor in the dog, hamster, pig and rabbit[8]. They further demonstrated that neither monellin nor thaumatin produced response in the Saguinus midas tamarin monkey, that belongs to the new world monkey[9]. Therefore, the macaque appears to be different from the new world monkey in its good taste sensitivity to a variety of sweeteners and its characteristic patterns of taste nerve fiber sensitivities to the four basic taste stimuli.

INGESTIVE AND NEURAL RESPONSES TO ASPARTAME AND STEVIOSIDE IN MACAQUE MONKEYS

Since an ability of tasting a variety of sweeteners, which most other mammals cannot taste, is a property specifically ascribed to the macaque monkey, we next examined ingestive and neural responses in Japanese macaques (Macaca fustaca) to some sweet-tasting compounds including aspartame (L-aspartyl-L-phenylalanine methyl ester) and stevioside (a glycoside extracted from leaves of a plant Stevia rebaudiana), both of which are about 100-200 times sweeter than sucrose in humans[10-12].

Fig.1 shows ingestive responses to 0.3 M sucrose(Su), 6 mM saccharin(Sa), 10 mM aspartame(As) and 0.5 mM stevioside(St) in four Japanese macaques, measured with 30 min-single stimuli tests[13]. Each filled block represents the mean of measurements in two consecutive days. Empty blocks show ingestion amounts of water, measured between successive two testing days, while the horizontal line indicates the mean of water intakes in each animal. The

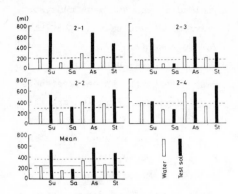

Fig.1 Ingestion of four sweeteners by four Japanese macaques

bottom figure shows the mean amounts of ingestion of the test solutions. Mean and SD of the water intake is shown by horizontal lines. Monkeys showed a preference for 10 mM aspartame as high as that for 0.3 M sucrose, and a moderate preference for 0.5 mM stevioside, but 6 mM saccharin was less preferred than water by the monkeys. Similar results were obtained in other series of experiments, although in these tests 1-3 mM stevioside was less preferred than water while 1-3 mM saccharin was often preferred by the monkeys.

In agreement with the results of the behavioral experiments, most of the macaques showed good chorda tympani nerve responses to aspartame and stevioside, while nerve responses to these sweeteners were scarcely observed in the

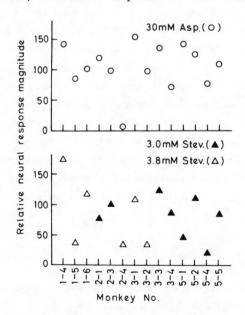

Fig.2 Relative magnitudes of integrated chorda tympani nerve responses to aspartame and stevioside in 14 macaques

rat, which is unable to discriminate 0.1-0.8 % (3.4-27.3 mM) aspartame from water[14]. In 14 monkeys consisting of 12 Japanese and two crab-eating macaques we recorded nerve responses to 0.5 M sucrose, 30 mM aspartame and 3.8 or 3 mM stevioside. The magnitudes of responses to the latter two sweeteners, expressed relative to that for 0.5 M sucrose are shown in Fig.2. Except for No. 2-4 all the monkeys responded to 30 mM aspartame with a magnitude almost similar to that for 0.5 M sucrose. Also 3 or 3.8 mM stevioside produced a response almost similar in magnitude to that for 0.5 M sucrose. However, there was a large variation in the relative magnitude of response to stevioside. Five monkeys among 14

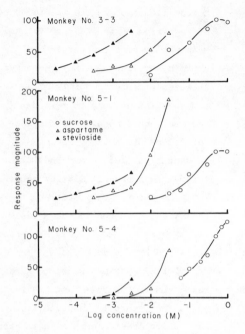

Fig.3 Concentration-neural response
relations for sucrose, aspartame and
stevioside

yielded a response magnitude for
stevioside less than half of that
for sucrose (Fig.2).

More detailed features of the
responses to the three sweeteners
and individual variation are shown
in the concentration-response relations in three monkeys, shown in
Fig.3. In monkey No. 3-3 (top
figure) 3 mM stevioside and 30 mM
aspartame produced a response almost
similar in magnitude to that for
0.3 M sucrose, and therefore, in
this monkey aspartame is about 10
times and stevioside is about 100
times more effective than is
sucrose. The thresholds for stevioside, aspartame and sucrose appear
to be less than 0.01, 0.1 and 10 mM,
respectively. In monkey No. 5-1
(middle figure) 30 mM aspartame

produced a response much greater in magnitude than that to 0.5 M sucrose while
3 mM stevioside yielded a much smaller magnitude of response. However, the
thresholds for the three sweeteners are almost of the same orders of magnitude
as those observed in the top figure. On the other hand, the monkey No. 5-4
(bottom figure) appears to possess higher thresholds for all the three sweeteners than those demonstrated in the first and second ones, although sensitivities to aspartame and stevioside, relative to that to sucrose, are more or
less similar to those shown in the top figure.

NEURAL AND INGESTIVE RESPONSES TO SUGARS IN MACAQUE MONKEYS

Although in some macaques the magnitude of neural response to stevioside
or aspartame was relatively small, these macaques showed good neural responses
to various sugars. The magnitudes of responses to nine sugars of 0.5 M in
seven macaques, expressed relative to that for 0.5 M sucrose, are presented in
Fig.4. There is a large variation in response magnitudes for sugars among
individual animals. Especially in monkeys No. 2-4 (empty triangles) and 2-3
(empty circles) the magnitude of responses to maltose and galactose is large,

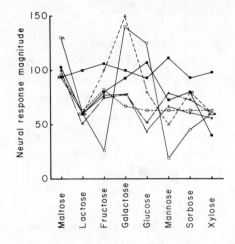

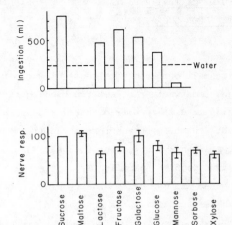

Fig.4 Neural response magnitudes for
sugars in seven Japanese macaques

Fig.5 Ingestive and neural responses
to sucrose in Japanese macaques. ±S.E.

while responses to fructose and mannose are very small in the latter.

The mean values of the magnitudes of neural responses to sugars in seven
monkeys are demonstrated in Fig.5(lower figure), which indicates the order,
maltose ≑ sucrose > lactose for disaccharides and galactose > glucose ≑ fructose >
sorbose > mannose > xylose for monosaccharides. The mean amounts of ingestion
of 0.3 M sugars during 30 min-period in two monkeys are also presented in
Fig.5(upper figure). The animals preferred sugars to water in the order,
sucrose > fructose > galactose > lactose > glucose, but rejected mannose.

The order of effectiveness of sugars determined electrophysiologically is
different from that in dog[15], rat[16,17], hamster[18] and Mongolian gerbil[19,20],
where the order of fructose > mannose > glucose > galactose was obtained for
monosaccharides and maltose is far less effective than sucrose. The order of
intake amounts is also different from the intake order for sugars in rats,
which prefer glucose to fructose[21] and possess little preference for
lactose[22]. The effectiveness of sugars in the squirrel monkey and two species
of Callithricidae was determined by Snell[23] and Glaser[24] by the chorda tympani
nerve response magnitude and the preference threshold, respectively. These
studies indicate that maltose and galactose are much less effective stimuli
than sucrose and fructose. Therefore, the macaque monkeys are also different
from the new world monkeys in possessing high taste sensitivity and preference
for maltose and galactose.

EVIDENCE THAT ASPARTAME AND STEVIOSIDE BIND TO THE SAME RECEPTOR MOLECULE AS THAT FOR SUCROSE

We mentioned earlier that a large individual variation exists in the magnitude of response to stevioside (Fig.2) and its ingestion by the monkey is small compared with those of sucrose and aspartame (Fig.1). This raises a question whether or not the binding site in the receptor molecule for stevioside is different from that for sucrose and aspartame. In order to answer this question, the effect of application of alloxan to the tongue on chorda tympani nerve responses to sweeteners were examined, because alloxan has been known to bind specifically to the sweet receptor molecules in the rat and thereby to depress chorda tympani nerve responses to sugars without affecting those to salts, acids and quinine[25]. The results of an experiment on the alloxan effect on chorda tympani nerve responses to the four sweeteners in a monkey are shown in Fig.6. In this experiment the effects of 0.5 M sucrose, 0.5 M glucose, 30 mM aspartame, 3 mM stevioside or 50 mM NaCl was tested for about 15 min immediately after 0.6 M alloxan had been applied to the tongue

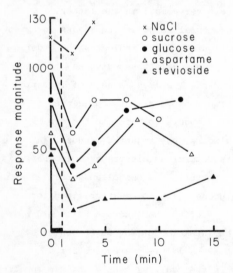

for 1 min (thick horizontal bar) and rinsed with water. As seen in the figure, there is a marked depression of the responses to all the four sweeteners immediately after the alloxan treatment, while no significant depression can be seen in NaCl response. These results would indicate that alloxan specifically affects the binding site of the receptor molecules, which is common for sucrose, glucose, aspartame and stevioside.

Fig.6 Depression of neural responses to sweeteners after alloxan

Consequently, a large individual variation in the magnitude of the neural response to stevioside in the macaque may be due to other factors. One possibility is that stevioside stimulates not only the 'sweet' taste receptors but also other kinds of receptors because it has been known to produce a saccharin-like taste[13] and in our experiment most of the macaques rejected it when its concentration was as high as 3 mM.

That aspartame and stevioside bind to the same receptor molecule as that for sucrose was substantiated by the biochemical experiment carried out by Dr. Hiji to measure absorbancy changes in the protein extracted from the tongue epithelium of the macaque on addition of the three sweeteners[26,27]. In this experiment the 60 % ammonium sulfate fraction[28,29] was prepared from the homogenate of the epithelium of the tongue of the monkey, and the difference spectral absorbancy at 278 mμ(Δ OD$_{278}$) on addition of sucrose, aspartame and

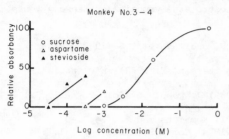

Fig.7 Absorbancy changes on addition of sweeteners to the extract of a monkey tongue epithelium

stevioside of varying concentrations was measured. Fig.7 is an example of the results of the experiments, in which relationships between the concentration of sweeteners and the Δ OD$_{278}$ value were obtained from one and the same monkey. In this figure sucrose produced an increase in Δ OD$_{278}$ above 1 mM, aspartame above 0.3 mM and stevioside above 0.03 mM. The three relationships in this figure are similar in threshold and general feature to those between the neural response magnitude and the concentration, presented above. In addition, the results shown in Fig.7 would possibly provide evidence that both stevioside and aspartame bind to the same receptor protein that forms complexes with sucrose.

CONCLUSION

In agreement with the characteristic property of tasting a variety of non-sugar sweeteners the macaque responded behaviorally and neurally to both aspartame and stevioside. The taste sensitivity to these sweeteners in the macaque is as high as in the case of men, but a large individual variation exists. A variety of sugars produced good responses in the macaque, but taste effectiveness of sugars are different from that in other mammals including the new world monkey. Neurophysiological and biochemical experiments indicate that the receptor molecule for the two sweeteners is the same as that for sucrose.

REFERENCES

1. Erickson, R.P., Doetsch, G.S. and Marshall, D.A.(1965) J. gen. Physiol. 49, 247-263
2. Sato, M.(1975) in Olfaction and Taste V, pp. 23-26, Academic Press, New York

3. Sato, M., Ogawa, H. and Yamashita, S.(1975) J. gen. Physiol. 66, 781-810
4. Frank, M.(1974) Chem. Sens. Flav. 1, 53-60
5. Carpenter, J.A.(1956) J. comp. physiol. Psychol. 49, 134-144
6. Fisher, G.L., Pfaffmann, C. and Brown, E.(1965) Science, 150, 506-507
7. Brouwer, J.N., Hellekant, G., Kasahara, Y., van del Wel, H. and Zotterman, Y.(1973) Acta physiol. Scand. 89, 550-557
8. Hellekant, G.(1976) Chem. Sens. Flav. 2, 97-105
9. Hellekant, G., Glaser, D., Brouwer, J.N. and van del Wel, H.(1976) Acta physiol. Scand. 97, 241-250
10. Cloninger, M.R. and Baldwin, R.E.(1970) Science, 170, 81-82
11. Cloninger, M.R. and Baldwin, R.E.(1974) J. Food Sci. 39, 347-349
12. Ishima, T. and Katayama, O.(1974) Abstr. 4th Symposium on Sensory Tests, 113-120 (in Japanese)
13. Maller, O.(1973) Folia primat. 20, 72-77
14. Okuizumi, K., Kuribara, H., Ogawa, H. and Tadokoro, S.(1977) Folia pharmacol. Japon. 73, 1-13
15. Andersen, H.T., Funakoshi, M. and Zotterman, Y.(1963) in Olfaction and Taste, pp. 177-192, Pergamon Press, Oxford
16. Hagstrom, E.C. and Pfaffmann, C.(1959) J. comp. physiol. Psychol. 52, 259-262
17. Noma, A., Goto, J. and Sato, M.(1971) Kumamoto med. J. 24, 1-9
18. Noms, A., Sato, M. and Tsuzuki, Y.(1974) Comp. Biochem. Physiol. 48A, 249-262
19. Jakinovich, W., Jr.(1976) Brain Res. 110, 481-490
20. Jakinovich, W. Jr. and Goldstein, I.J.(1976) Brain Res. 110, 491-504
21. Maller, O. and Kare, M.R.(1965) Proc. Soc. Exp. biol. Med. 119, 199-203
22. Richter, C.P. and Campbell, K.H.(1940) J. Nutri. 20, 31-46
23. Snell, T.C.(1965) The responses of the squirrel monkey chorda tympani to a variety of taste stimuli. Brown Univ., Rhode Island
24. Glaser, D.(1970) Folia primat. 13, 40-47
25. Zawalich, W.S.(1973) Comp. Biochem. Physiol. 44A, 903-909
26. Sato, M., Hiji, Y., Ito, M. and Imoto, T.(1977) in Chemical Senses and Nutrition, Academic Press, New York, in press
27. Sato, M., Hiji, Y., Ito, M., Imoto, T. and Saku, C.(1977) in Food Intake and Chemical Senses, Univ. Tokyo Press, Tokyo, in press
28. Dastoli, F.R. and Price, S.(1966) Science, 154, 905-907
29. Hiji, Y., Kobayashi, N. and Sato, M.(1971) Comp. Biochem. Physiol. 39B, 367-375

Qualities in hamster taste: behavioral and neural evidence

Geoffrey H. Nowlis and Marion Frank

The Rockefeller University, 1230 York Avenue, New York, NY 10021, USA

ABSTRACT

Most substances are called sweet, salty, sour, or bitter and mixtures can be analyzed into their component tastes by man. To study quality coding neurophysiologically, however, other animals must be used and it is necessary to determine how they structure their taste worlds. A taste profile is determined for any stimulus, to which an animal learns an aversion, by the extent of generalization of the aversion to sucrose, NaCl, HCl, and quinine, prototypes of man's 4 qualities. Generalization to other compounds can also be measured. Hamsters and rats sense 4 qualities and classify many compounds just as man does; yet, there are some species differences. Also, an aversion to a two component mixture generalizes less to each component alone, if both are novel, and to the novel as much as to the mixture, if one is familiar. Chorda tympani and glossopharyngeal taste neurons of these creatures can be divided into 4 classes, each with a characteristic response profile centered at one of the stimulus prototypes. Thus, it is possible there are 4 neural elements mediating 4 kinds of taste experience.

INTRODUCTION

Psychophysicists have generally found that man classifies taste stimuli into 4 categories: sweet, salty, sour, and bitter. This description of his subjective experience led to a spatial model of taste quality, Henning's taste tetrahedron. In this model, each of the 4 corners represent one taste quality, and relatively pure stimulus prototypes of these qualities are sucrose, NaCl, HCl, and quinine hydrochloride.

In order to determine the neurophysiological basis of taste quality, however, other animals must be used. These other species may not divide up their taste worlds exactly as man does, and, therefore, it is necessary to discover how they classify taste stimuli before studying sensory coding.

BEHAVIORAL TASTE PROFILES

One effective way of estimating how similar two stimuli taste to an animal is to teach a specific response to one stimulus and test for its generalization to the other stimulus[1,2]. If the hamster divides taste stimuli into 4 categories, as man does, an estimate of how similar one stimulus is to each of four prototypic stimuli should yield an adequate description of the taste quality of that stimulus.

Thirteen groups of 12 hamsters were taught an aversion[3] to one of 13 different compounds which had been shown to be effective stimuli in human psychophysical studies[4], and for activity in hamster chorda tympani single fibers[5]. After each animal had 5 minutes to drink a stimulus solution, it received an injection of apomorphine hydrochloride (30 mg/kg), which produces an aversion for a specific stimulus tasted before injection[3]. In sequential daily sessions, solutions of sucrose, NaCl, HCl, or quinine were presented to test for generalization of the learned aversion. A control group of 12 which received water to drink before its apomorphine injection, provided the standard for amount drunk of each test stimulus. Amount of generalization is expressed as a "percent suppression" score based on the ratio of the amount the experimental group drinks to the amount the control group drinks of each test stimulus. This score can be considered a quantification of the similarity between the conditioned and test stimulus: the greater the percent suppression, the greater the similarity of the stimuli.

The 4 percent suppression scores for each of the 13 conditioned stimuli are shown in Figure 1, in the form of a taste profile. If these similarity measurements are an adequate estimate of how sweet, salty, sour, or bitter these stimuli taste to the hamster, do they bear any resemblance to psychophysical measurements of how sweet, salty, sour or bitter these stimuli taste to man? Human subjects[4] judge sucrose, fructose, and saccharin to be sweet, and not salty, sour, or bitter. NaCl and $NaNO_3$ are salty, somewhat sour, and $NaNO_3$ is somewhat bitter. The three acids are primarily sour, but only citric acid is also somewhat bitter. Acetic acid and HCl are slightly salty, and not bitter. Quinine, urea, $MgSO_4$, and, to a lesser extent, KCl and NH_4Cl are all bitter, but among these stimuli only urea and $MgSO_4$ are somewhat sour. Both KCl and NH_4Cl taste salty to humans, but the conditioned aversions of hamsters to these 2 stimuli generalize not to salt, but to acid.

Thus, if our test solutions are restricted to solutions representing the 4 human taste categories, a considerable array of solutions are classified very nicely by the hamster in terms of similarity to these 4 solutions. If psychophysical judgements are restricted to the 4 classical taste categories, humans classify the same array of solutions into very similar classes, with a few notable exceptions.

Taste profiles of rats for some compounds have been determined in exactly the same way. Differences in the two rodents include a lesser response to sweet and a greater and more specific response to bitter stimuli in rat than

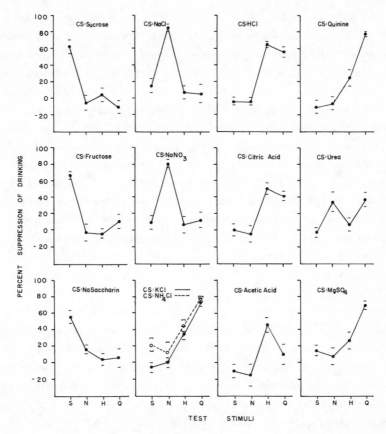

Figure 1. Hamster taste profiles: generalizations of learned aversions. Molarities of conditioned stimuli (CS's) for experimental groups (E's) were .1 sucrose, .3 fructose, .001 saccharin, .1 NaCl, .1 NaNO₃, .3 KCl, .3 NH₄Cl, .01 HCl, .01 acetic acid, .003 citric acid, .001 quinine HCl, 3.0 urea, and .1 MgSO₄. Test stimuli were sucrose (S), NaCl (N), HCl (H), and quinine (Q) at the above molarities. CS for a control group (C) was distilled water. Percent suppression of a test stimulus is 100 X (1 - amount drunk by E/amount drunk by C). Horizontal lines bracketing points show standard error of mean.

in hamster. Percent suppression of sucrose drinking after learning an aversion to sucrose or fructose is about 50% in rat and 65% in hamster. Rats generalize a quinine aversion only to quinine of the 4 stimuli, and quinine drinking is suppressed less after an aversion is taught to HCl (about 15% in rat and 60% in hamster). In fact, rats will not drink enough .001 M quinine, so 1/10 that molarity was the stimulus used for their profiles. Two of three artificial sweeteners taste different to these species than to man. Na-saccharin is similar to sucrose for both; Na-cyclamate (.025M) is similar to sucrose, but more to NaCl for hamster, and only to quinine for rat; and aspartame (.01 M), has a slight taste similar to quinine for hamster and rat.

In order to find out if hamsters can recognize pure components in mixtures, aversions were taught to each of the 6 two-component mixtures of the 4 prototypic stimuli and generalizations to the 4 stimuli presented alone measured. As a rule, drinking was suppressed to both components; an exception was the quinine-NaCl mixture for which only NaCl drinking was suppressed, but, if the quinine concentration was tripled, both were suppressed. In another experiment, an aversion to a sucrose-NaCl mixture generalized less to the parts than to the mixture itself. But, if one of the components was familiar (present in drinking water for 7 days before conditioning), the mixture aversion generalized only to the novel component and the mixture itself. In fact, generalization to the novel component was as great as to the mixture which suggests that this taste mixture is analyzed into component parts and not synthesized into a qualitatively unique sensation, as is the case for mixtures of colored lights.

MULTIDIMENSIONAL SCALING OF DISSIMILARITIES

If hamsters do not divide taste stimuli into 4 classes as man does, taste profiles based on 4 prototypic stimuli will not adequately describe the quality of a compound. In a subsequent study, 21 stimuli were used both as stimuli to which aversions were learned (CS's) and as test stimuli for generalizations. Each of 21 groups (n=6) learned an aversion to one stimulus, was tested on 4, was reconditioned with the same stimulus, tested on 4 others, etc. A control group's CS was water. The resulting 21 X 21 ratios of amount drunk by experimental and control animals were interpreted as measures of dissimilarity in a computer program (KYST-2)[6], which constructs a configuration of stimulus points in n-dimensional space whose distance represents dissimilarity. "Stress" (badness of fit) was minimized with 3 dimensions. A similar program had been used by Schiffman and Erickson[7] for analyzing taste similarities of humans.

Figure 2 is a perspective drawing of the resulting taste space. That 3 dimensions adequately describe the data strongly suggests there need only be 4 channels for taste quality. This space may be viewed as an isointensity slice through a 4-dimensional space (intensity of stimulation of each channel) which would describe all taste experience, quality and intensity. Since the stimuli used were approximately of equal intensity, the 4 intensity dimensions need not be represented. A 3-dimensional slice of a 4-dimensional space is a tetrahedron. Each corner of this taste tetrahedron may represent stimulation of one sensory channel or receptor type alone. The 3 dimensions

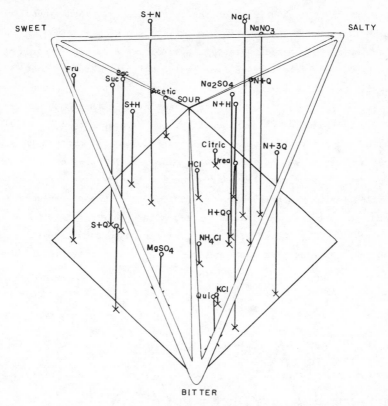

Figure 2. Taste space: multidimensional scaling of generalizations of learned aversions. The 3 dimensional space, drawn in perspective, generated by the KYST-2 program (6) with results of an experiment in which each stimulus was used as a CS and test stimulus. Ratios of amount drunk by E / amount drunk by C were used as measures of dissimilarity. A tetrahedron is drawn in the space to suggest its form. Stimuli were the 13 CS's and all 6 of the 2-component mixtures of the test stimuli described in Fig. 1, a mixture of N and 3Q (.003 M quinine), and .41 M NaSO₄. New abbreviations are Suc = sucrose, Qui = quinine, Fru = fructose, Sac = saccharin, Citric and Acetic are acids.

of the tetrahedron do not correspond to any of the 4 sensory channel dimensions. A tetrahedron with corners sweet, salty, sour, and bitter has been superimposed over points for the stimuli. Near the sweet corner, sucrose, fructose, and saccharin cluster, and there are also bitter, salty and sour clusters. Mixtures lie between appropriate clusters, as do compounds with mixed tastes such as urea.

NEURAL RESPONSE PROFILES

Studies of how 4 categories of taste experience are represented in responses of chorda tympani nerve fibers, which innervate taste receptors in

the fungiform papillae on the front of the tongue, and glossopharyngeal nerve
fibers, which innervate taste buds in the foliate and circumvallate on the
sides and center of the back of the tongue, have been numerous. Chorda tympani fibers have been typically described as being broadly tuned; that is,
not exclusively sensitive to one of the stimulus prototypes[8,9]. Because of
this observation, an across fiber pattern of activity in the whole population
of neurons was proposed as the representative of taste quality[8,10].

  But species studied varied, test stimuli varied, and the numbers of observations from a given nerve end species were often small. When stimuli are
chosen which are at about the middle of a compound's effective range, and response profiles for many single chorda tympani fibers of hamster recorded so
that experimental error is reduced, three repeating patterns of response
emerge (Figure 3)[5]. For instance, if profiles for neurons most sensitive to
NaCl in the population sampled are superimposed upon each other (A), it can

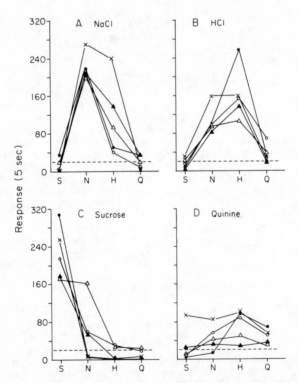

Figure 3. Hamster chorda tympani response profiles. Profiles of the 5 units
most sensitive to (A) .03 M NaCl: N, (B) .003 M HCl: H, (C) .1 M sucrose: S,
and (D) .001 M quinine hydrochloride: Q are shown of 79 sampled. From (5),
with permission of the Journal of General Physiology.

be seen that they respond best to NaCl, and second best to HCl. Neurons of hamster chorda tympani most sensitive to HCl (B), and sucrose (C) also show typical patterns; but, those most sensitive to quinine (D) do not.

When all neurons which respond best to each of the four prototypic stimuli are averaged, a response profile for a typical sucrose-best, NaCl-best, HCl-best, and quinine-best peripheral taste unit is described. Figure 4 shows mean profiles for rat units sampled from both chorda tympani[9] and glosso-pharyngeal nerves. Not only do certain response patterns occur repeatedly in one of the taste nerves of rat, but no matter whether chorda tympani or glossopharyngeal fibers are sampled, or whether they innervate fungiform, foliate, or circumvallate papillae; sucrose-best (A), NaCl-best (B), or

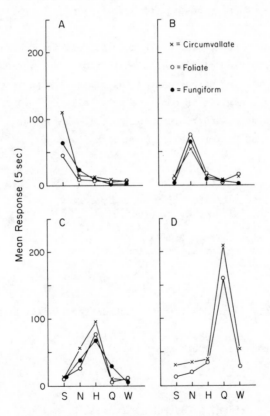

Figure 4. Rat peripheral taste nerve mean response profiles. There are 10, 11, and 12 sucrose-best (A); 11, 6, and 25 NaCl-best (B); 12, 13, and 11 HCl-best (C); and 19, 10, and 0 quinine-best (D) units innervating the circumval-late, foliate, and fungiform papillae, respectively; represented. Test molar-ities varied from .1 to .5 sucrose (S), .1 to .3 NaCl (N), .001 to .01 HCl(H), .001 to .02 quinine (Q), and W is distilled water. Fungiform data from (9).

HCl-best (C) units have similar response profiles. As there was no evidence for a quinine-best pattern in hamster chorda tympani, there is none in rat; but, this response pattern is commonly found among glossopharyngeal fibers which innervate foliate and circumvallate taste buds (D). The main difference in the fibers which innervate the three tongue areas lies in the numbers of each of the 4 patterns which are found. For instance, NaCl-best units occur most frequently in the chorda tympani and are about 50% of that population; whereas, quinine-best units occur most frequently in the glossopharyngeal branch innervating the circumvallate and are about 40% of that population. Any one of these typical profiles shows a nearly exclusive sensitivity to just one of the 4 stimulus prototypes, the notable exception being that acid-sensitive units (C) also respond to NaCl.

CONCLUSION

Thus, hamster or rat peripheral taste neurons fall into 4 classes, just as these creatures' perception of similarities in taste of a variety of compounds can be accounted for with 4 categories of taste experience. By making an analogy to taste in man, it is convenient to call the 4 behavioral categories sweet, salty, sour, and bitter, and to call the 4 neuron classes sweet, salty, sour, and bitter specific neural pathways.

REFERENCES

1. Morrison, G. R. (1967)
   Can. J. Psychol. 21, 141-152
2. Tapper, D. N., and Halpern, B. P. (1968)
   Science 161, 708-710
3. Garcia, J., and Ervin, F. R. (1968)
   Recent Advances in Biological Psychiatry 10, 284-293
4. McBurney, D. H., and Shick, T. R. (1971)
   Perception and Psychophysics 10, 249-252
5. Frank, M. (1973)
   J. Gen. Physiol. 61, 588-618
6. Kruskal, J. B. (1976) in Statistical Methods for Digital Computers,
   Wiley, New York
7. Schiffman, S. S., and Erickson, R. P. (1971)
   Physiology and Behavior 7, 617-633
8. Pfaffmann, C. (1955)
   J. Neurophysiol. 18, 429-440
9. Ogawa, H., Sato, M., and Yamashita, S. (1968)
   J. Physiol. (Lond.) 204, 223-240
10. Erickson, R. P., Doetsch, G. S., and Marshall, D. A. (1965)
    J. Gen. Physiol. 61, 588-618

Information processing in the taste system

Thomas R. Scott

Department of Psychology and Institute for Neuroscience and Behavior, University
of Delaware, Newark, DE 19711, USA

ABSTRACT

   The neural code for taste quality and intensity has been studied in
first-order (chorda tympani) and second-order (bulbar) cells. Here, the analysis is extended by single cell recordings among third-order (pontine) and
fourth-order (thalamic) neurons. A logical progression of quality coding
emerges across these four synaptic levels, with basic grouping determined at
the bulbar level and finer discriminations made by pontine and thalamic cells.
Intensity appears to be related to total neural activity through the pons,
but its thalamic representation is unclear.

   The neural code for taste quality and intensity has been analyzed in
several species at the first- and second-order levels. My intention is to describe the coding characteristics of higher-order taste neurons in the pons
and thalamus of the rat, and to speculate on their possible roles in processing gustatory information.

   The pontine taste area (PTA) has evolved during the past six years to re-
place the dotted lines anatomy books show between the solitary nucleus (NTS)
and thalamus. Its neurons are small and densely packed, yet the region is a
rather diffuse one incorporating areas around and apparently within the brachium conjunctivum. Trigeminal afferents signalling oral proprioception and
temperature to help define the taste area's ventral and anterior boundaries.
Seventy-nine single neurons were isolated by tungsten microelectrodes and recordings were taken using standard techniques. Stimuli were primarily salts
and acids plus sucrose and quinine. Pontine taste neurons can be characterized as broadly tuned, offering moderate response rates (higher than those of
all other taste levels with the exception of NTS) and rather short latencies
of 25-30 ms near the center of the region. Inhibitory responses are uncommon,
and when they occur it is typically in peripherally located neurons (3).

   Patterning theory asserts that taste quality is represented by the relative rate of discharge across a neural population (the "shape" of the activity envelope) while intensity is coded by the total area under the curve (the "height" of the envelope). It is implicit that for taste constancy to be maintained, the shape of the envelope must not be altered with concentration changes. Theoretically, each neuron should increase its discharge rate proportionally to some function of concentration. In studies of both chorda tympani (CT) and NTS neurons, Ganchrow and Erickson report just such increases with a corresponding maintenance of the integrity of the response envelope's shape (2). Among third-order cells of the PTA we find close agreement with their results (Figure 1). The total response of our pontine sample increases in an orderly fashion with a power function exponent of approximately .2 for all qualities. Across intensities, the evoked pattern for .59 M NaCl correlates with that of .24 M NaCl at the .98 level, with .13 M NaCl at the .96 level, and even with .01 M NaCl at the .88 level. Taste constancy would seem to be preserved among third-order neurons.

Neurons in the fourth-order thalamic taste relay are located

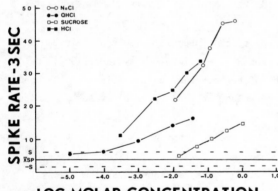

Fig 1. Mean intensity-response functions for 40 PTA neurons. From Perrotto and Scott (in preparation).

at the medial tip of the ventroposterior nucleus. Lateral to the taste area are neurons sensitive to oral somesthetic input, while cells between purely gustatory and somesthetic regions seem to receive common input from both modalities. Thalamic sensitivities and response characteristics differ in several ways from those of the first three synaptic levels of the taste system (4). First, overall evoked response rates to the standard salts and acids are sluggish, being slightly below those recorded from CT even though spontaneous activity is four times as great in the thalamus. Second, 10% of the 79 units we have isolated show a clearly specific sensitivity to one stimulus

quality. We wonder if other unresponsive units might have been selectively
tuned to stimuli we never used. Third, quinine and sucrose, both notoriously
poor at activating lower-order taste cells, achieve rough parity with the
salts and acids. Fourth, the prominent transient discharge seen at lower
levels is virtually gone in the thalamus (when inhibitory responses are included in the calculation). Fifth, response latencies are typically 60-300 ms
(range=30-3000 ms). Sixth, inhibition of neural discharge occurs in at least
8% of the stimulus applications, these tending to occur in cells where spontaneous activity is high such that prominent reduction can occur. In the interactions classified as inhibitory, the mean decrease was from 10 to 2 spikes
/sec. Finally, increased response rates are recorded to the water rinse following nearly one-third of all stimulus applications, and after almost two-
thirds of the inhibitory responses. The rat CT does not possess water fibers,
and no such responses are seen at lower levels. It seems likely that some
activity is evoked by somesthetic components which may impinge on many of the
thalamic taste neurons. But the high incidence of water responses following
inhibition suggests another factor: an "off" discharge analogous to those
seen in other sensory systems. So thalamic cells introduce several new complexities into the system, including specific sensitivities, increased responsiveness to sucrose and quinine, a decreased transient, inhibitory responses,
and occasional bursts of activity to the water rinse.

     One possible analysis of the neural code for taste quality can be deriv-
ed from patterning theory. The degree of similarity between two stimuli is
described by the correlation coefficient between the two neural patterns they
evoke. Thus a high coefficient indicates poor discriminability. Behavioral
and cross-adaptation studies support this notion. The progression of correlations among stimulus patterns indicates specialized analytical functions at
the various synaptic levels. Figure 2 shows the mean correlations among three
"salty" salts (NaCl, LiCl, Li_2SO_4), two acids (HCl, HNO_3), and three "bitter"
salts (KCl, $CaCl_2$, NH_4Cl). Also shown are mean correlations between the salty
and bitter salts, the salty salts and acids, and the bitter salts and acids,
and all are calculated for the second, third, and fourth-order neural populations. Decreased correlation implies easier discriminability. The obvious
message from NTS is that all stimuli representing the same basic quality form
a tight group, and, with the exception of bitter-sour interactions, the distance between these clusters is enormous (1). But this first-order analysis
must be refined, and the process occurs in two stages: the salty and sour
stimuli are picked apart by the pons, and the bitter stimuli by the thalamus.

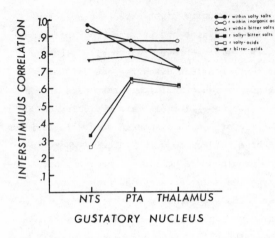

INTERSTIMULUS CORRELATION

NTS PTA THALAMUS

GUSTATORY NUCLEUS

r within salty salts
r within inorganic acids
r within bitter salts
r salty- bitter salts
r salty- acids
r bitter- acids

Fig 2. Comparison of correlations "within" and "between" stimulus groups at successive levels of the taste system. NTS data from (1), PTA from (3), thalamic from (4).

Correlations within salty salts at the three levels are .97, .81, and .81. A coherent but impenetrable block of stimuli has been exploded, possibly through neural amplification of the small differences that do exist at the NTS. Acid correlations are .94, .87, and .88, indicating a similar, though less dramatic cleavage. Concurrently, as stimuli within the salty and sour groups diverge, the groups themselves become less distinct. Salty-bitter correlations are .33, .66, and .62, and salty-sour values are .26, .64, and .61. The bitter group is not broken until the thalamic level (.86, .87, and .69) at which point it also diverges from the similar sour stimuli (.77, .79, and .69). That the distinction is never thorough can be attested to by the psychophysicists who routinely report confusion, involving more than simply linguistic labels, between these modalities. Thus there is a logical progression of sequential analysis in which the CT establishes groupings, NTS confirms, tightens, and completes the preliminary analysis, and the pons and thalamus make the finer discriminations within modalities.

Concerning intensity coding, the patterning hypothesis is a simple one: perceived concentration is proportional to the total activity evoked from a neural population. While the pontine data uphold this notion, thalamic recordings are deviant. Hydrochloric acid, KCl, and QHCl show clear increases in overall evoked activity as stimulus concentration is raised (these are the bitter-sour stimuli to which it was just proposed the thalamus may be attending). But sodium saccharin and glycine change little with intensity, and sucrose and NaCl respond non-monotonically. A comparison across synaptic levels shows that thalamic response rates are equal to or above those of CT for all weak stimuli except NaCl, but this situation is reversed at high concentrations indicating reduced sensitivity to intensity in the thalamus

(Figure 3). The general shape of the intensity-response function is similar at CT, NTS, and PTA (not shown), but, the thalamus is radically different. To insure that our sample is a random one, truly representative of the thalamic population, we took 11 multiunit recordings from cell groups, integrated the output and measured the size of the evoked response. Through this, our averaged unit data were confirmed both in terms of relative sensitivities to the various taste qualities, and in the shape of the intensity-response functions.

Among individual units, many do show direct increases with concentration. Others appear to code intensity through latency. But many show no apparent relationship in terms of spike rate or time course between their responses and stimulus concentration. With many neurons increasing with concentration, others decreasing, and some uninfluenced, there are considerable changes in the shape of the response pattern. This would indicate a lack of the taste constancy which is so evident at the lower-order levels. What role could the thalamus be playing in intensity coding? There are several possibilities. It may be coding in the same fashion as other levels, but its normal activity may be interfered with by the Flaxedil and Xylocaine administered during recording. Second, intensity may be well determined by the pontine level, and thalamic neurons may not be concerned with it. There are precedents for this suggestion in other sensory systems. Finally, the intensity code could be relayed through some reliable, but obscure transform that is not yet recognizable.

The deviation of thalamic responses from theories which adequately explain gustatory coding through three neural levels raises a larger point: why are there at least five synaptic levels of the mammalian taste system? The major theories were developed from neural data recorded from peripheral taste nerves, and take support from their ability to predict behavior. If first-order neurons predict the final outcome, we are left with the proposition that higher levels either passively transmit the code in a linear manner, alter it to a form not yet recognizable to us, or adulterate it in such a way that it no longer accurately relates to behavior. In fact our behavior data show that thalamic responses predict the time required for rats to make discriminations among simple salts and acids more poorly than NTS responses. But we may be getting incorrect answers from the thalamus because we ask the wrong questions. Discriminating between inorganic salts may be a first, second, or third-order responsibility. Complex judgments about organic foods may be reserved for thalamic and cortical processes, which may differ according to the ecological niche of the species. Also, the thalamus could be designed

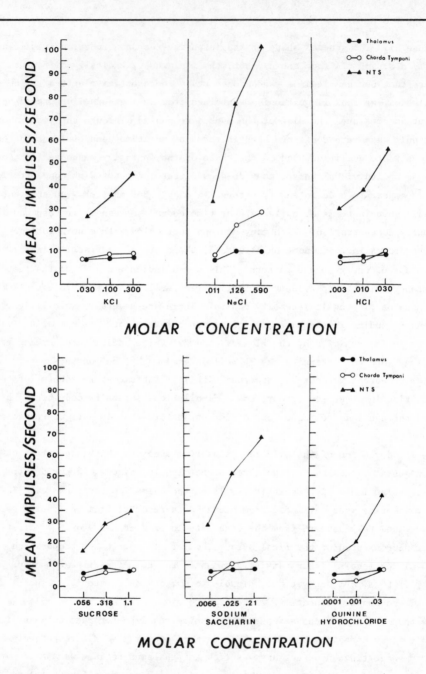

Fig 3. Mean intensity-response functions at 3 synaptic levels. CT and NTS data from (2), thalamic from Scott and Yalowitz (in preparation).

to serve more than a purely gustatory function. Olfaction and somesthesis are behaviorally allied with taste and are known to project to the ventro-basal complex, yet both are minimized by experimental procedures. Perhaps thalamic taste cells integrate information from these several senses, and so are sensitive to a greater range of input than present coding theories would suggest. In any case to better understand its code, the thalamus (and cortex) should be studied using more ethologically relevant stimuli in a wider variety of animals whose nervous systems are not debauched with paralytics and anesthetics.

This research was supported by grant NS 10405 from the National Institutes of Health.

REFERENCES

1. Doetsch, G. S. and Erickson, R. P. (1970)
   J. Neurophysiol. 33, 490-507.

2. Ganchrow, J. R. and Erickson, R. P. (1970)
   J. Neurophysiol. 33, 768-783.

3. Perrotto, R. S. and Scott, T. R. (1976)
   Brain Res. 110, 283-300.

4. Scott, T. R. and Erickson, R. P. (1971)
   J. Neurophysiol. 34, 868-884.

Physiological characteristics of cortical taste area

Takashi Yamamoto and Yojiro Kawamura

Department of Oral Physiology, Dental School, Osaka University, 32 Joancho, Kitaku, Osaka 530, Japan

ABSTRACT

The projection from both sides of chorda tympani to the cerebral cortex of the rat consists of 2 separate areas; one is the area anterior to the middle cerebral artery and the other is posterior to it. The anterior part is a band extending antero-posterior direction, while the posterior part is ovoid in its shape. Lesions of either of these anterior or posterior areas did not induce any significant effect on the conditioned taste aversions, while lesions of both areas induced a complete loss of taste aversion, and severe degeneration of thalamic taste neurons was observed. Comparison of response characteristics of the cortical units and those of chorda tympani nerve fibers revealed no obvious difference between them in the relative amounts of units responding to one, two, three or four of the conventional four tastes. Random distribution of sensitivities to four tastes was recognized in both units. Correlation coefficients of the cortical units to 14 different chemical stimuli were much higher than those of the chorda tympani fibers.

INTRODUCTION

The cortical gustatory area has been delineated in several animals[1-8]. Distribution of cortical responses evoked by electrical stimulation of the taste nerves have revealed two discrete projection areas in the squirrel monkey[1] and the cat[4]. One is confined to the appropriate part of the somatotopic pattern of Somatic Sensory Area I and the other is buried in the anterior operculum in monkeys and in the lateral bank of the presylvian sulcus in cats. Burton and Benjamin[9] suggested that the former was related to spatial localization of the gustatory stimulus and the latter was important for taste quality discrimination. On the other hand, in rat cortex[3] only one taste nerve projection area has been reported, and the taste area of the rat delineated by several investigators[3,6,10,11] has not been well matched. In the present experiment, more precise localization of the cortical projection of the tongue nerves was studied in the rat, and the effects of cortical ablation on conditioned taste aversion were examined through the behavioral experiments.

In addition to recordings of cerebral evoked potential, recordings and quantitative analyses of the cortical unit activities responding to taste stimulation are essentially important to reveal cortical processing of taste information. One approach to clarify the response characteristics of the cortical taste units is to compare them with those of the first order taste neurons. We recorded the activities of chorda tympani single fibers in the rabbit and tried to compare them with those of the cortical taste units of the rabbit which had been recorded previously[8].

SURFACE EVOKED POTENTIAL

The distribution of surface positive cortical potentials evoked by electrical stimulation of the chorda tympani and lingual nerve was mapped on the rat cerebral cortex. The animal was anesthetized by intravenous injection of pentobarbital sodium (40 mg/kg) and urethane (150 mg/kg). To stimulate the nerves, the whole chorda-lingual trunk was stimulated with bipolar electrode, and to stimulate the chorda tympani, the lingual nerve was cut central to the branching of the chorda tympani and to stimulate the lingual nerve, the chorda tympani was cut central to the branching of the lingual nerve. A 0.1 msec duration, 4-8 V square pulse was presented at 1.5 sec intervals. The nerves were stimulated supramaximally with about twice the voltage necessary for a maximal cortical response.

After exposure of the cortical surface, evoked responses were recorded with glass micropipette electrodes (1-2 μm tip diameter) filled with either 2M NaCl or 2.5% lithium carmin and depth recording was performed with the same electrode when necessary. The cortex was mapped in approximately 0.25 mm steps. The response was averaged 30 times. The location of each penetration was marked in relation to the surface blood vessels on an enlarged photograph of the rat brain under study.

Variability in the position and size of the cortical responses evoked by electrical stimulation of the chorda tympani and lingual nerve was very small. The data from 3 recordings in each nerve were mapped on the antero-ventro-lateral view of the cerebral cortex of the rat in Fig. 1. In each case, the projection was spatially discrete; one is anterior to the middle cerebral artery as shown by solid line and the other is posterior to it as shown by broken line.

Anterior area is a band extending antero-posteriorly, and lingual projection is located more dorsally than chorda projection with a slight overlap, while posterior area forms an ovoid shape slightly extending dorso-ventrally and situated more dorsally than the anterior area. The posterior area of lingual and chorda tympani projections greatly overlaps. As shown by inlet actual

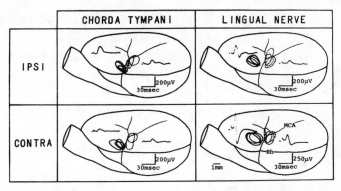

Fig. 1   Areas responsive to electrical stimulation of both sides of chorda
tympani and lingual nerves.

recordings, the latency of initial positive phase of the evoked potential recorded in the anterior area was shorter than that in the posterior area. Average values in the anterior area were 10.5 and 8.1 msec in ipsilateral and
contralateral chorda tympani, 8.0 and 7.5 msec in ipsilateral and contralateral
lingual nerves, and in the posterior area were 15.2 and 10.8 msec in ipsilateral
and contralateral chorda tympani, 12.5 and 9.5 msec in ipsilateral and contralateral lingual nerves, respectively. The ipsilateral and contralateral chorda
projections are very similar, while the lingual projection is more dominant in
contralateral side than ipsilateral one judging from magnitude of evoked potential.

According to the somatotopic organization of somatic sensory area I shown
by Welker[12] in the rat, the anterior projection of the chorda tympani corresponds to the lower limit of the tongue tactile area, and it corresponds well
with the area reported by Benjamin and Pfaffmann[3] and Norgren and Wolf[10].
Posterior area corresponds with the area reported by us[11]. Recently, Giachetti
and Mac Leod[13] suggested that olfactory input reached this posterior area.

A depth analysis both at the anterior and posterior areas revealed that
surface positive wave was reversed to negative wave and it was largest at a
point 500-600 μm beneath the surface, which was shown to be within the IVth
layer of cortex by histological survey. Evoked potentials recorded from the
anterior and posterior areas decreased their magnitudes when the electrode was
penetrated deeper, and at the depth beyond 1 mm evoked potential was negligibly
small. This fact suggests that chorda tympani inputs terminate mainly in the
IVth layer of the cortex. Together with the histological findings of the termination of the degenerated fibers after ablation of the thalamic gustatory
nucleus by Norgren and Wolf[10], it seems to be improbable that claustrum, which

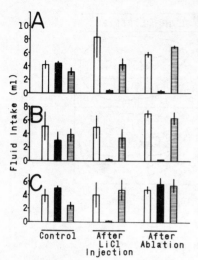

Fig. 2
Effects of cortical ablations
on learned taste aversion.
A: anterior taste area ablation, B: posterior taste area
ablation, C: both areas ablation, Open bar: 0.00002M
Quinine-HCl, Solid bar: 0.1M
NaCl, Striped bar: 0.1M Su-
corse, Ordinate: mean±S.D.
fluid intake of each solution
for 5 min.

Benjamin[14] suggested to be a candidate for a
pure taste area, is related to taste function.
In single unit analysis, we could obtain a few
units responding to chemical stimulation of
the tongue in both anterior and posterior
areas within the neocortex. Unitary discharges
to different lingual modalities are currently
under investigation in the rat.

BEHAVIORAL TEST

In order to reveal the functional significance of these anterior and posterior taste
areas, effects of separate or combined ablations of these two areas on conditioned taste
aversions were examined in the rat. The procedure is briefly described as follows, daily
5-min single bottle drinking tests with quinine-HCl, NaCl and sucrose solutions were
given in an individual box. These test solutions were presented in this sequence every
day. The fluid intake at the end of 5 min
per each solution was recorded. After about
one week of control period, rats were given
intraperitoneal injection of LiCl to produce sickness immediately after drinking NaCl[15]. Then, after another one week lesions of either anterior taste area,
posterior taste area or both areas were given to the rat. After recovery from
the operation, these 3 solutions were given, and the fluid intake was recorded.

The results are shown in Fig. 2. After injection of LiCl, rats learned
aversion to NaCl. Figure 2A shows one example of effects of anterior taste
area ablation on conditioned taste aversion. No effects of the lesion was
observed. Also, no effects of posterior area ablation on conditioned taste
aversion was recognized (Fig. 2B). Histology showed only slight degeneration
of the thalamic taste neurons in these rats. However, in some rats with ablation of the posterior area, a complete loss of aversion was observed. This may
be attributed to the destruction of gustatory thalamo-cortical fibers which
approach from a dorsal and somewhat posterior angle[10]. A further and careful
study should be done on this point. When ablation included both projection
areas, there was a complete loss of the aversion (Fig. 2C). And, once both

projection areas were ablated, the rat no longer could learn aversion to taste cues even after second injection of LiCl. In this case, histology showed severe retrograde degeneration of the thalamic taste neurons.

As already indicated by Benjamin and Burton[1] in the squirrel monkey, two cortical taste projection areas may receive inputs from the thalamic taste nucleus, and simaltaneous ablations of the two cortical areas may be necessary to cause complete degeneration of thalamic taste neurons. The present results on behavioral study indicated that both anterior and posterior areas were necessary for discriminating taste quality. Besides chorda tympani, taste informations are conveyed via the glossopharyngeal nerve which innervates the foliate and vallate taste buds, the vagus nerve innervating taste buds in the pharynx and the palatal nerves which innervate palatal taste buds. These nerves are supposed to project to spatially separate areas in the cortex other than the chorda tympani projection area. However, the present behavioral study strongly suggests that these nerves project exclusively to those same anterior and posterior areas.

SINGLE UNIT ANALYSIS

Thirty-five chorda tympani single fiber activities were recorded in the rabbit and were compared with 24 cortical taste unit activities of the rabbit which had been recorded previously[8]. Taste solutions and rinsing water were applied to the flow-chamber which covered the anterior part of the tongue. As test chemical stimuli, 0.5M sucrose, 0.25M DL-alanine, 0.3M Na-saccharin, 0.5M, 1M and 2M NaCl, 0.5M NH_4Cl, 0.5M KCl, 0.5M $MgCl_2$, 0.5M $CaCl_2$, 0.01M HCl, 0.1M tartaric acid, 0.02M quinine-HCl and distilled water were used. About 25 ml of a test solution were passed by gravity flow, followed after each stimulation by tap water. In order to avoid the effect of the preceding stimulus, the interval between successive stimulations was at least 1 min. Each chemical stimulation was applied 2 or 3 times and we applied as many stimulants as possible during the time that recordings from the unit could be maintained. The taste solutions and rinsing water were kept at 27-30°C.

We examined responsiveness of the chorda tympani fibers and cortical taste units to each of the 4 conventional taste stimuli in the rabbit. A given unit response was classified as excitation when the evoked discharge rate for the first 5 sec was larger than the average spontaneous discharge + S.D. and classified as inhibition when smaller than the average spontaneous discharge - S.D.. As shown in Table I, responding units were classified into 5 types following responsiveness to each taste quality. Type I shows units increasing their

Table I
Classification of Responses

Chorda Tympani Fibers

Type	S H N Q	Total
I	+ 0 0 0 1 0 + 0 0 1 0 0 + 0 4 0 0 0 + 0	6
II	+ + 0 0 1 + 0 + 0 3 + 0 0 + 1 0 + + 0 2 0 + 0 + 1 0 0 + + 5	13
III	+ + + 0 1 + + 0 + 3 + 0 + + 4 0 + + + 4	12
IV	+ + + + 4	4
V	0	0
	Total	35

Cortical Taste Units

Type	S H N Q	Total
I	+ 0 0 0 2 0 + 0 0 0 0 0 + 0 1 0 0 0 + 2	5
II	+ + 0 0 2 + 0 + 0 0 + 0 0 + 1 0 + + 0 0 0 + 0 + 0 0 0 + + 1	4
III	+ + + 0 0 + + 0 + 2 + 0 + + 2 0 + + + 3	7
IV	+ + + + 4	4
V	- - - - 1 - - 0 - 1 - 0 - 0 1 + 0 - 0 1	4
	Total	24

S: 0.5M Sucrose, H: 0.01M HCl,
N: 0.5M NaCl, Q: 0.02M Quinine-HCl, +: increased response,
0: no response, -: decreased response

firing rate to single taste quality, Type II to double, Type III to triple, Type IV to all the 4 taste qualities, and those units which decreased their firing rate to taste stimulation were classified as Type V. No chorda tympani fibers belonged to Type V. The amounts of chorda tympani fibers and cortical units responding to one, two, three or four of the four taste qualities were 17.1 and 20.8 %, 37.1 and 25.0 %, 34.3 and 33.3 % and 11.4 and 20.8 %, respectively. No obvious difference could be detected between chorda tympani fibers and cortical units.

In the next step, unit activities were examined for random distribution of responsiveness. If the stimulating effectiveness of the 4 taste qualities of the chorda tympani and the cortical units are independent and random, the probability of obtaining responses to any pair of the 4 stimuli would be given by the product of the probability of obtaining responses to each stimulus[16]. The probability of occurrence of responses to individual stimuli can be estimated from the ratio of responsive units to the total number of units tested. Table IIA shows the predicted and observed numbers of units responding to one,

Table II
Distribution of Sensitivities to 4 Taste Stimuli

Chorda Tympani Fibers

A.

Number of Responses	Number of Units Predicted	Observed
1	5.25	6
2	12.52	13
3	12.25	12
4	4.24	4

Cortical Taste Units

Number of Responses	Number of Units Predicted	Observed
1	2.92	5
2	7.80	6
3	9.05	8
4	3.84	5

B.

Response Pairs	Number of Units Predicted	Observed
Suc-HCl	8.74	9
Suc-NaCl	13.87	12
Suc-Quinine	11.32	12
HCl-NaCl	13.12	11
HCl-Quinine	10.70	12
NaCl-Quinine	16.97	17

Response Pairs	Number of Units Predicted	Observed
Suc-HCl	9.21	10
Suc-NaCl	10.62	10
Suc-Quinine	11.33	10
HCl-NaCl	8.13	9
HCl-Quinine	8.68	10
NaCl-Quinine	10.00	11

Suc : 0.5M Sucrose   HCl : 0.01M HCl
NaCl : 0.5M NaCl   Quinine : 0.02M Quinine-HCl

two, three or four of the four taste qualities. There is no significant difference between the two sets of numbers in both chorda tympani and cortical
units judging from Chi-square test. The predicted and observed numbers of the
chorda tympani and cortical units responding to the possible 6 pairs of the 4
stimuli are given in Table IIB. It is noted that the observed values are quite
close to the predicted ones. From these results, it was suggested that sensitivities of chorda tympani and cortical units to the 4 taste qualities are
mutually independent and randomly distributed among chorda tympani and cortical
units, respectively.

Since most chorda tympani fibers in mammals respond to more than one kind
of stimulus, it has been proposed that the stimulus quality is coded by the
response pattern across many neurons. Erickson[17] have suggested that any pairs
of stimuli which show similar response profiles across many neurons produce a
similar taste, and those which give different profiles taste different. In our
final study, we evaluated the interstimulus correlations obtained for chorda
tympani fibers and those for cortical taste units. Figure 3 shows 14 correlation taste profiles of varying taste stimuli across the conventional 4 taste
qualities. Across-neuron correlation coefficients between responses to the test
stimulus and to one of the four stimuli are plotted in ordinate. Calculation
was based on the number of impulses for the first 5 sec after onset of stimulation. Closed circles indicate the values from cortical units and open circles from chorda tympani fibers. Correlation profiles in each test stimulus

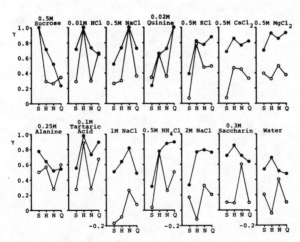

Fig. 3
Correlation taste profiles across the 4 tastes for chorda tympani fibers
(open circles) and cortical taste units (solid circles). S: 0.5M Sucrose,
H: 0.01M HCl, N: 0.5M NaCl, Q: 0.02M Quinine-HCl

at the chorda tympani level are roughly preserved at the cortical level. However, a great difference is that the correlation coefficients for cortical units are much higher than those for chorda tympani fibers. Physiologic meanings of such high correlation magnitudes at the cortical level are unclear. It has been reported by Scott and Erickson[18] and Perrotto and Scott[19] that interstimulus correlations increase at pontine taste area and at thalamus in the rat. Conclusively, the results of the present investigation demonstrate that gustatory impulses undergo several distinct transformations in travelling from the periphery to the final cortical taste area, although some response characteristics are common in the first order neurons and cortical taste neurons.

ACKNOWLEDGEMENT

This study was supported by a Scientific Grant from the Ministry of Education of Japan (No. 144068). We are grateful to Dr. Ryuji Matsuo for his assistance in preparation of the histological material and in behavioral experiments.

REFERENCES

1. Benjamin,R.M.and Burton,H.(1968) Brain Res.7,221-231
2. Benjamin,R.M.,Emmers,R.and Blomquist,A.J.(1968) Brain Res.7,208-220
3. Benjamin,R.M.and Pfaffmann,C.(1955) J.Neurophysiol.18,56-64
4. Burton,H.and Earls,F.(1969) Brain Res.16,520-523
5. Funakoshi,M.,Kasahara,Y.,Yamamoto,T.and Kawamura,Y.(1972) in Olfaction and Taste,Vol.IV,pp.336-342,Wissenschaftliche Verlagsgesellschaft MBH,Stuttgart
6. Ganchrow,D.and Erickson,R.P.(1972) Brain Res.36,289-305
7. Patton,H.D.and Amassian,V.E.(1952) J.Neurophysiol.15,245-250
8. Yamamoto,T.and Kawamura,Y.(1975) Brain Res.94,447-463
9. Burton,H.and Benjamin,R.M.(1971) in Handbook of Sensory Physiology,Vol.IV, Chemical Senses,Part 2,pp.148-164,Springer,Berlin
10. Norgren,R.and Wolf,G.(1975) Brain Res.92,123-129
11. Yamamoto,T.and Kawamura,Y.(1972) Physiol.Behav.9,789-793
12. Welker,C.(1971) Brain Res.26,259-275
13. Giachetti,I.and Mac Leod,P.(1975) in Olfaction and Taste,Vol.V,pp.303-307, Academic Press,New York
14. Benjamin,R.M.(1963) in Olfaction and Taste,Vol.I,pp.309-329,Pergamon,Oxford
15. Nachman,M.and Ashe,J.H.(1973) Physiol.Behav.10,73-78
16. Frank,M.and Pfaffmann,C.(1969) Science 164,1183-1185
17. Erickson,R.P.(1963) in Olfaction and Taste,Vol.I,pp.205-213,Pergamon,Oxford
18. Scott,T.R.and Erickson,R.P.(1971) J.Neurophysiol.34,868-884
19. Perrotto,R.S.and Scott,T.R.(1976) Brain Res.110,283-300

Sensory effects of continuous and repetitive electrical stimulation of the tongue

Z. Bujas

Dep. Psychology, University of Zagreb, 41000 Zagreb, Djure Salaja 3, Yugoslavia

ABSTRACT

Stimulating the human tongue with single and repetitive positive, negative and biphasic, current pulses, the strength-duration and threshold-frequency functions were determined. With an increase in the action time the
sensory effect changes from touch to taste. The temporal summation is pronounced for positive pulses and very limited for negative and biphasic pulses. The stimulation of single papillae shows that the taste quality depends
on the polarity of the electrode rather than the supposed specialization of
papillae. The results suggest that electrochemical processes probably play a
dominant part in provoking taste in anodal stimulation while the cathodal and
biphasic stimuli predominantly act directly on afferent structures.

Inadequate or unusual modes of stimulation of sense organs may be interesting because their effects sometimes can give a better insight into transduction processes in adequate stimulation. Electrical stimulation of afferent
taste structures represents one of such approaches.

The purpose of this paper is to re-examine some relations between different kinds of electrical stimulation of the tongue and their sensory effects.

Rectangular monophasic positive and negative pulses were used as stimuli,
as well as biphasic rectangular pulses, single or repetitive, with different
repetition rates.

In the first experiment with a larger tongue surface, psychophysical
strength-duration functions for single pulses, in the range between 0.025 and
10 msec, were determined. The active electrode was a glass tube, enlarged in
the middle and with a round opening of about 1 cm in diameter, at which the
subject presented his tongue. Above the opening a silver chloride wire was
inserted in glass. Prior to each stimulus, the tube was filled with 0.1 %
solution of NaCl, warmed up to the tongue temperature. The indifferent electrode was a silver chloride wire placed in a bath for the subject's fingers.
During threshold determinations a forced choice procedure was used. Pulse
widths between 0.025 and 10 msec were employed.

Three subjects gave comparable results, both regarding relations between threshold values and action time and regarding the quality of induced sensations on the liminal level and just above.

Fig. 1 shows, for one subject, the strength–duration functions for three kinds of electrical stimulation.

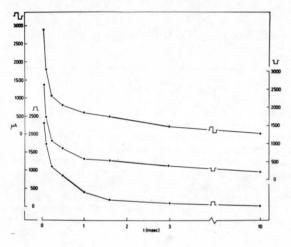

Fig. 1. Strength–duration functions for positive, negative and biphasic single pulses

The temporal summation is similar for three modes of stimulation from 0.025 to 0.5 msec. In this range, different kinds of pulses provoke only tactile sensations. For action times exceeding 0.5 msec, significant differences in thresholds appear, probably due to differences in afferent structures affected by the stimulus. When the action time is longer than 0.5 msec, positive pulses produce sour taste, resulting in a pronounced threshold decrement. Negative and biphasic single pulses provoke tactile sensation up to about 1.6 msec, while taste dominantly appear when the duration is 3 msec or longer.

Fig. 2 shows, for one subject, changes in the percentage of taste occurence for three kinds of pulses as a function of the action time.

All three types of single pulses, when effective, produce the same quality : sour taste. This is the typical quality elicited by anodal stimulation. Sour taste appearing in cathodal stimulation is probably not a cathodal "on" but a cathodal "off" effect.

In the second experiment, conducted also on a larger surface of the tongue, threshold measurements were made for repetitive monophasic and biphasic pulses of 0.025, 0.5, and 1.0 msec in the frequency range between 10 and 450, or 1000 pulses per sec. The subjects having taken part in the first experiment participated also in the second experiment.

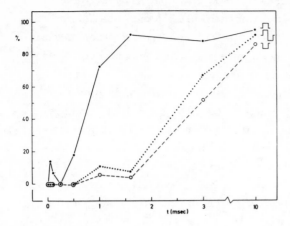

Fig. 2. Percentage of stimuli evoking taste at threshold values of current (ordinate) as a function of pulse duration (abscissa)

In repetitive stimulation, lasting 4 sec, different modes of stimulation produce somewhat different results. For biphasic and negative pulses of short duration the temporal integration exists up to the frequency of about 100 per sec ; after that the thresholds stabilize up to the frequency of about 500 per sec. On the contrary, the higher the frequency, the lower the thresholds for positive pulses. Differences in temporal integration are in agreement with sensory effects. Biphasic and negative pulses, in the quoted frequency range, only produce sensations of vibration, while anodal stimuli produce vibration only at the frequency of 10 and 20 per sec, and almost invariably sour taste at higher frequencies. A decrease of liminal values for cathodal pulses between 500 and 1000 per sec is connected with the appearance of bitter-sweet taste which is chracteristic of the sufficiently long cathode "on" period.

Fig. 3 shows, for one subject, relations between liminal values and the frequency, with the pulse duration of 0.025 msec.

The third experiment was performed on single taste papillae. It was a re-examination of some data published earlier and obtained under somewhat different conditions.

As the stimulating electrode a silver chloride point electrode was used, and a silver chloride plaque attached under the chin served as the indifferent electrode. The subject himself placed the point electrode on single papillae. He did this under the control of a magnifier and looking at a mirror. In each series of observations the subject randomly chose 20 papillae at the tip and the sides of his tongue.

The stimulation of single papillae by repetitive pulses of different form, duration, and frequency yielded varied results. Anodal stimulation of individual papillae, regardless of the pulse duration and frequency, dominantly provokes sour taste. Anodal stimuli were most frequently monosapid, and very efficacious in provoking taste. The dominant taste quality provoked by the cathode was bitter-sweet. Cathodal stimulation proved to be poorly effective in provoking taste sensation. However, both those papillae having reacted with some taste and those having shown no reaction, at the definite cessation of repetitive cathodal stimuli of medium and high frequency, reacted in most cases by a clear sour or sour-sweet taste. Cathodal stimuli were more polysapid than anodal stimuli. Biphasic repetitive stimulation of single papillae differs from the analogous stimulation of a larger surface, primarily because, to a certain extent, it produces taste. In the taste composition of biphasic stimuli there is no clearly dominant taste, and in the majority of cases the effect is a taste mixture.

As an example, Fig. 4 shows the percentage of different taste qualities evoked by stimulating 40 papillae for each of our five subjects. The pulse duration was 0.01 msec at the pulse rate of 1000 per sec. The figure does not give the percentage of reports on three or more tastes, which occured almost only in biphasic stimulation. Regardless of the mode of stimulation, out of 600 stimulated papillae, about 36 % reacted to stimuli by one taste, 18 % by two tastes, and 3 % by three or more qualities.

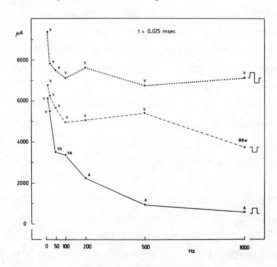

Fig. 3. Threshold-frequency functions. Ordinate : threshold current ; abscissa : number of pulses per sec. A letter at each point marks the sensory effect : V = vibration, A = sour, BSw = bitter-sweet

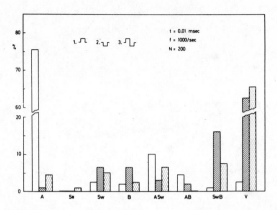

Fig. 4. Occurence of different taste qualities evoked by repetitive stimulation of single papillae. The first open bars represent the effects of anodal stimulation, the lined bars the effects of cathodal stimuli and the dotted bars those of biphasic stimuli. Results of five observers and 200 stimuli.

The results obtained differ from those obtained by von Békésy. While in Békésy's experiments repetitive anodal current provoked different tastes on different papillae depending on their selective sensitivity, our data show that the taste quality depends on the polarity of the active electrode rather than the "individual characteristic" of the stimulated papilla. Papillae differ markedly in their sensitivity to electric current and to taste different substances, but generally they are not specialized in the sense of possessing only one kind of receptors.

Electrical taste is a combined effect of electrolysis of saliva, displacement of ions across the cell membrane, and the direct depolarisation of the end organs or of nerve fibers.

It seems that in anodal stimulation, depending on the electrode types (inert or reversible) electrolysis or displacement of ions, that is electrochemical processes, are dominant factors. Sour taste, which is primarily the result of the excess of H-ions in the vicinity of the anode or of the ionic transfer in or out of the receptor cells, is clear to such an extent that it completely covers the effects of a direct current action. That the anodal stimulation is very similar to adequate chemical stimulation of receptors by acids is corroborated by records of summated neural activity of the rat's chorda tympani. As shown in Fig. 5, the neural response to anodal current is comparable to the neural response to adequate chemical stimulation with HCl solution.

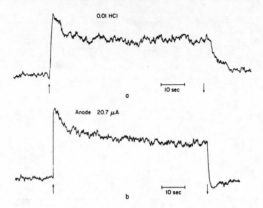

Fig. 5. Summated activity of the rat's chorda tympani evoked by adequate stimulation with 0.01 HCl solution (upper record), and the response to continuous anodal current of 20.7 microampers (lower record)

At cathodal stimulation, chemical processes, seem to participate to a lesser extent than in anodal stimulation. This is all the more probable in the stimulation of single papillae on which cathodal pulses of short duration act directly rather than via receptors. But, even in cathodal stimulation, especially if the action time is relatively long, it is not possible to rule out a certain electrochemical influence. Electrochemical products appear not to bind themselves to the chemical sites on the surface of cell membranes, because cathodal stimulation can produce bitter-sweet taste also in the conditions when these qualities cannot be evoked by adequate chemical stimulation. For instance, potassium gymnemate, which blocks the receptor sites for sweet and partially also for bitter,does not prevent the appearance of these tastes on the cathode "on" and "off". Similarly, adaptation to sweet or bitter substances does not practically affect electrically evoked tastes of these qualities. The explanation of such a by-passing of the first step in chemical stimulation, might be a certain ionic transfer across the cell membrane and the binding of ions to the parts of receptor molecules at the inner side of the membrane.

Biphasic pulses of short duration probably act only directly on the taste afferent structures. This is supported by the fact that with this form of stimulation, taste can be provoked only by a point-electrode, and also that the effect of stimulation is generally polysapid, with no dominant quality. Moreover, in this case, the electrolysis, and displacement of charged particles within the cell and tissue fluids are minimized.

Von Békésy maintained a complete specialization of papillae speaks against the pattern theory, but we have not been able to confirm this argument. Yet, experience from the field of electrical taste does indicate that there is a need for some extension of taste theories. The fact that in electrical stimulation, in some cases, the first step in adequate stimulation can be passed by, should be considered in the attempts to explain how taste is produced and in which way different taste qualities are coded on the periphery of the taste organ.

REFERENCES

Bealer, S.L. and Smith, D.V. (1975)
Physiol. and Behavior 14, 797-799

Békésy, G. (1964) J. Appl. Physiol.
19, 1105-1113

Bekesy, G. (1966) J. Appl. Physiol.
21, 1-9

Bujas, Z. et Chweitzer, A. (1937)
C. R. Soc. Biol. 126, 1106-1109

Bujas, Z. (1970) Rad JAZU 358, 79-96

Dzendolet, E. (1962) Percept. Motor Skills
14, 303-317

Dzendolet, E. and Murphy, C. (1974)
Chem. Senses and Flavor 1, 9-15

Harper, H. W., Jay, J.R. and Erickson, R.P.
(1966) Physiol. and Behavior 1, 319-325

McCutcheon, N.B. and Saunders, J. (1972)
Science 175, 214-216

Pfaffmann, C. (1941) J. Cell. Com. Physiol.
17, 243-258

Pfaffmann, C. (1974) Chem. Senses and Flavor
1, 61-67

Plattig, K.H. (1972) in Olfaction and Taste, Vol. IV,
pp. 323-328, Wissenschaftl. Verlags, Stuttgart

Plattig, K.H. and Innitzer, J. (1976)
Pflügers Arch. 361, 115-120

Rollman, G.B. (1969) Perception and Psychophysics
5, 289-293

Abstracts of Poster Presentations

<u>Functional anatomy of human fungiform papillae.</u> K. Arvidson & U. Friberg
(Dept. of Histology, Karolinska Institutet, S-104 01 Stockholm, Sweden)

In studies on taste perception in man, one factor lacking has been reliable
data concerning the functional anatomy of the taste receptors. Hence we
have studied some basic problems related to the occurrence, structure and
gustatory response of human fungiform papillae.

 <u>First</u>, an SEM study on the surface topography of human fungiform
papillae, obtained by biopsy, was performed. Taste pores occurred in nearly
half of the papillae. The pores were situated on the convex, dorsal surface
of the papillae. Usually they opened in the form of a rounded crater,
slightly elevated above the surface.

 <u>Second</u>, a light microscopic study was done on the occurrence of taste
buds in 182 fungiform papillae. These were obtained at autopsy from 22
individuals, aged 2 days to 90 days, and serially sectioned. Again, the
taste buds were always confined to the dorsal surface of the papillae. The
number of taste buds was found to vary to a considerably greater degree
than has earlier been assumed. Thus, the number of taste buds in a single
papilla varied from 0 to 27. Some 63% of the papillae had no taste buds at
all, 23% had 1-3 buds and the remainder 4 or more buds. The mean number of
taste buds per papilla in a given individual varied from 0 to 9. This
latter variation was not seen to be dependent upon age to any great extent.

 <u>Third</u>, and in view of the above noted variations, a combined psychophysical and light microscopic study was done in order to correlate the
gustatory response to chemical stimulation of a single fungiform papilla to
the presence of taste buds in the very same structure. Thus, the sensitivity
was tested of 110 fungiform papillae, in 31 subjects, to the four basic taste
qualities (salt, sour, sweet and bitter). The subjects were instructed to
respond to a 5-choice card, including 'no taste'. Subsequently each
stimulated papilla was excised, embedded in paraffin, and serially sectioned
for bud counting. In agreement with the above results some 57% of the
papillae had no taste buds and, as expected, gave no taste response. Up to
15 tastebuds were found per bud-bearing papilla. Of the bud-bearing papillae
4% were non-responsive, whereas 13% responded to one, 34% to two, 19% to
three,and 30% to all four taste stimuli. While up to four taste qualities
were perceived upon stimulation of papillae with only one taste bud, there
was in general a positive correlation between the number of taste qualities
identified and the number of taste buds present per papilla.

Correlation of behavioural activity and biochemical status of sodium deficient calves assessed by operant conditioning F.R.Bell and Jennifer Sly

(Department of Medicine, Royal Veterinary College, London, NW1 0TU)

Exteriorization of the parotid duct in ruminants causes continuous loss of saliva and produces sodium deficiency. Calves proved suitable subjects for operant conditioning and learned to push a lever for food or liquid rewards. Sodium deficient calves (n=5) received 10ml 0.5M $NaHCO_3$ rewards on a Variable Interval Schedule (mean 20 sec); the rate of lever pressing increased with the development of sodium deficiency and decreased as sodium balance was restored. The negative correlation between operant activity and the sodium level in parotid saliva proved highly significant ($p<0.001$). Blood samples from 3 calves also demonstrated that the increased pressing behaviour was significantly correlated with a marked fall in blood pH, HCO_3^-, base excess, plasma sodium and osmolality.

When Na^+ deficient calves (n=6) were tested against a range of salts for 10 sessions (5 min/salt), motivation was significantly greater when 0.3M rewards of $LiCl$, Na_2SO_4, $NaHCO_3$, $NaCl$ and $Na\ Ac^-$ were offered than when the reinforcements were KCl, $KHCO_3$, $MgCl_2$, NH_4Cl, Na_2CO_3 or water. Sodium deficient calves also had a significant appetite for $CaCl_2$ and $Ca\ Lact^-$.

The changes shown by operant behaviour, with varying sodium status of the extracellular fluid, suggest that the calves could recognise and discriminate between different levels of sodium deficiency and that the degree of motivation was proportional to the degree of biochemical deficiency as noted by Bell & Sly (1975).

Bell, F.R. & Sly, Jennifer, 1975, Vth Internat. Symp. Olf. Taste, 267.

This work was supported by the Agricultural Research Council.

The flavor chemistry of cat fungiform papillae taste systems James C.
Boudreau, Sensory Sciences Center, University of Texas at Houston

The properties of fungiform papillae taste systems were investigated by
recording single unit pulse potentials from single neurons in the geniculate
ganglion. These neurons were found to be responsive to a wide variety of
water soluble compounds naturally present in vertebrate tissues, such as inorganic ions and a wide variety of nitrogen and nitrogen-sulfur compounds,
including nucleotides. Among the salts, phosphate compounds and $CaCl_2$ are
particularly stimulatory. Certain amino acids (L-cysteine, L-proline, L-
lysine, L-histidine) and peptides (e.g., carnosine), are highly stimulatory
as are the di- and tri- phosphate nucleotides. Nitrogen and nitrogen-sulfur
heterocyclic rings with pKa values greater than 5.0 are often associated
with prominent stimuli. Unresponsiveness or inhibition is associated with
anionic groups, aromaticity, hydrophobicity, amine groups with low pKa
values and most nonacidic oxygen compounds. The chemoresponsive neurons of
the geniculate ganglion are divisible into three distinct functional groups
with differing fiber diameters. These groups are selectively responsive to
different chemical aspects of food solutions, with two of the unit groups
being highly responsive to selected nitrogen compounds. Both unit groups I
and II maximally respond to 5 and 6 member ring N heterocycles, but their
response could be differentiated in terms of the pKa of the active group
and the effect of ring substituents. Group III unit stimuli are less well
defined but large responses may be obtained to nucleotides at concentration
levels at or below those commonly found in animal tissues. This work was
supported in part by NSF Research Grants.

Changes in taste responses of solitary tract neurons during development

R.M. Bradley and C.M. Mistretta, (Dept. of Oral Biology, School of Dentistry, Ann Arbor, MI 48109, USA)

We previously recorded chorda tympani nerve responses during chemical stimulation of the fetal sheep tongue, and reported that over the last third of gestation the response characteristics of the fetal gustatory system are similar to those in lambs and adults. We now report functional changes in the taste system during development, based on electrophysiological records from chemosensitive units in the fetal, lamb, and adult nucleus of the tractus solitarius (NTS). By recording from neurons in the NTS, it has not only been possible to study more single unit responses, but also units in younger fetuses. Responses were recorded from 33 single or few-unit, and 7 multi-unit preparations in 18 fetal sheep aged 84 days of gestation to term (147 days), in 2 lambs, and 2 adults. The responses of these neurons to stimulation of the anterior two-thirds of the tongue with 0.5 M NH_4Cl, 0.5 M KCl, 0.5 M LiCl, 0.5 M NaCl, 0.1 M citric acid, and 0.01 N HCl were compared. We found that: (1) In younger fetuses ($\leqslant$ 105 days), units usually respond to lingual stimulation with NH_4Cl, KCl, and citric acid, but not to stimulation with LiCl, NaCl or HCl. In older fetuses, lambs, and adults, units usually respond to all of these salts and acids. (2) In younger fetuses most units respond to lingual stimulation with NH_4Cl, KCl, and citric acid after a long latency ($\geqslant$ 500 msec), whereas in older fetuses, lambs, and adults, the response latency to stimulation with these three chemicals is usually short (50-200 msec). (3) In younger fetuses the neural discharge of most units adapts completely during lingual stimulation with NH_4Cl; in contrast, units in older fetuses, lambs, and adults do not adapt completely during lingual stimulation with NH_4Cl.

From these data we conclude that: (1) Even as early as 84 days of gestation, when taste buds are structurally immature, it is possible to record chemosensitive responses from the fetal taste system. Thus, the taste system is functional before morphological development of the receptors is complete. (2) However, although the taste system is functional early in gestation, neurophysiological response characteristics change during development. Taste units only gradually acquire short latency, slowly adapting response characteristics, as well as responsiveness to an increasing range of salts and acids. Functional characteristics alter, therefore, as receptors and neural pathways mature morphologically. (3) Units in younger fetuses respond to lingual stimulation with NH_4Cl, KCl, and citric acid; sensitivity to NaCl, LiCl, and HCl appears later, in older fetuses. Therefore, salt and acid responses seem to develop in a particular sequence, not randomly. (Supported by NIH Grant HD 07483.)

Two classes of amino acid taste fibers and receptors in the catfish   John
Caprio and Don Tucker, (Department of Zoology and Physiology, Louisiana
State University, Baton Rouge, Louisiana 70803 and the Department of Biolo-
gical Science, Florida State University, Tallahassee, Florida   32306, USA)

Single unit analysis of in vivo barbel nerve preparations from the channel
catfish (Ictalurus punctatus) revealed that gustatory fibers can be classified into at least 2 categories, alanine-best responding and arginine-best
responding fibers. Gustatory single fiber responses to amino acid concentration series were more variable than observed for the whole nerve bundle
(Caprio, Olfaction & Taste V) and thresholds ranged between 10^{-4}M and 10^{-11}M.
The impulse rate of the majority of both fiber types increased exponentially
with logarithmic increase of concentration, similar to the whole nerve preparation, and some fibers responded over 7 log units of stimulus concentration
(mean, 4.7 $\pm$ 1.4; n=26). Amino acid specificities of individual units were
used to characterize the fiber types. The alanine-best taste fiber responded
with highest frequency to L-alanine and its esters, but also responded to all
the amino acids tested at 10^{-4}M or 10^{-3}M. The order of stimulus effectiveness was similar to that for the whole nerve response, except that the unit
response to arginine was less than predicted from the whole nerve activity.
The arginine-best taste fiber, however, was highly specific and responded
primarily to L-arginine, L-arginine methyl ester, D-arginine, and slightly
to L-alanine. Cross-adaptation studies provided additional evidence for the
existence of 2 types of amino acid receptors, alanine and arginine receptors.
The present evidence suggests that alanine-best and arginine-best responding
taste fibers innervate taste cells containing primarily alanine and arginine
receptors, respectively. These studies also provide evidence that primary
carboxyl esters of amino acids bind to the same receptor as the parent free
amino acid, and therefore an ionically charged carboxyl group is unnecessary
for amino acid-receptor binding.

Gustatory nerve discharges in sodium deficient rats R.J. Contreras & M.
Frank, (The Rockefeller University, New York, N.Y. 10021, USA)

Many species exhibit a craving for salt in sodium need. This appetite is an
innate response which is specific to the taste of sodium salts. Richter suggested that sodium deprived rats increase their intake because their taste
receptors become more sensitive to NaCl. Since the response of the whole
chorda tympani nerve to threshold and suprathreshold concentrations of NaCl
was unaltered with sodium deficiency, Richter's hypothesis was superceded by
hypotheses involving central mediation. But, a recent single fiber study has
shown a specific decrease in responses to .1 M NaCl after deprivation. To
clarify the effects of 10 days of sodium deprivation, the activity of the rat
chorda tympani (whole nerve and single fiber) in response to concentration
series of NaCl, sucrose, HCl, and quinine hydrochloride was recorded and
analyzed without knowledge of the animal's deprivation state. Whole nerve
recordings showed a decrease in median response to NaCl with deprivation.
This difference was statistically reliable only at .1 M NaCl, when 10 sodium
deprived (E) and 10 control (C) animals' nerves were compared. No differences in response to sucrose, HCl, or quinine were observed. There was also
an effect of deprivation on single fiber sensitivities to NaCl. The vari-
ances of responses to NaCl (.1 and .3 M) differed, with the sodium replete
animals showing greater response variability. There were no consistent differences in responses to the other three compounds. When fibers from both E
(n = 60, from 21 nerves) and C (n = 73, from 23 nerves) were divided in half
on the basis of greater or lesser responsivity to .1 M NaCl, it was shown
that the more sensitive units from sodium deprived animals responded less to
NaCl. Thus, there was a reduction in chorda tympani sensitivity to suprathreshold concentrations of NaCl after sodium deprivation.

TASTE PRIMARIES. R. Erickson, A. Johnson, S. Kaufmann, D. Macdougall, Georgette Somjen, D. Woolston. Psychology Department, Duke University.

The concept of taste primaries has been used at at least 5 levels; psychophysical, neural coding, neural organization (e.g. fiber types?), receptors and stimuli. Discoveries at one level may have powerful heuristic or validating relationships with other levels. However, use of the idea of primaries at any one level may not have simultaneous implications for all levels.

In taste, at the psychophysical and coding levels, the neural relationships, as given in across-fiber patterns (AFP) have been shown to accurately describe the psychophysical relationships. The neural and psychophysical measures do not require, but may conveniently use, taste primaries. If psychophysical primaries are used, they may be arbitrary in number and not describe the structure of the taste sensation (by analogy, any color may be described in terms of 3, 4 or 5 color "primaries", although the sensation is singular) nor describe the neural or stimulus organization (computor analysis of 38 stimuli and 59 neurons by "hierarchial cluster analysis" gave no evidence of groups). Fiber types would be necessary for sensation types only if the "best stimulus" identified the sensation resulting from activity in a labeled neural line (LL), and that assumption has not been supported. Thus, neither LL nor AFP require fiber types, nor would fiber types distinguish between them. Psychophysical synthesis, however, is consistent only with the AFP position; in studies of mixtures of sucrose and NaCl, and NaCl and $MgCl_2$, the taste system appeared to synthesize, as in color.

Relationships between the organization at stimulus, receptor and neural levels could be straight-forward, although primary groups could exist independently at any level.

NSF (BNS75-22692), Army (14195-L).

Renewal of taste bud cells in rat circumvallate papilla. A. I. Farbman, (Northwestern University, Chicago, Ill., U.S.A.)

This study was done to determine the rate of renewal of the 2 taste bud cell types in rat circumvallate papilla. Dark and light cells can easily be distinguished morphologically in 2-3 μ thick sections of taste buds fixed in a buffered aldehyde mixture, post-fixed in buffered OsO_4 and embedded in plastic (Epon & Araldite). A single dose of ^{3}H-thymidine was administered intraperitoneally to weanling male rats (0.5 μc/gm body weight) between 9:00 and 10:00 PM. Data from a previous study indicated that the maximum number of taste bud precursor cells would be in S-phase of the cell cycle at this time of day. In the first experiment, 2 animals were killed each day at 10:00 AM, beginning at 1.5 days after injection and continuing through 14.5 days; thereafter, animals were killed every other day until 25.5 days. In a second experiment, this was repeated, with 3 animals for each time period. Data from the two experiments were pooled. Circumvallate papillae were excised and processed as above for autoradiography (Kodak NTB-2 emulsion; exposure time 3 weeks). Every other section was discarded to avoid counting a labeled cell nucleus twice in adjacent sections (nuclei are about 5 μ in diameter). A minimum of 5 silver grains over a nucleus was used to identify a labeled cell. For each time period, the number of labeled cell nuclei was counted in 200-450 taste buds and plotted as the ratio of labeled cells/ taste bud vs. time after injection of ^{3}H-thymidine. A total of 5,967 taste buds was counted.

The total number of labeled cells (dark plus light) reached major peaks at 6.5 days (1.4 cells/bud), 13.5 days (1.0 cells/bud) and 20.5 days (0.67 cells/bud). On the ascending slope of the first peak, there was a shoulder at 3.5 days. The curve for the number of labeled <u>dark</u> cells/taste bud was essentially parallel to that for total cells. The number of labeled <u>light</u> cells/taste bud reached a plateau at 4.5-6.5 days (maximum value = 0.31 labeled cells/bud) and slowly declined to about 0.1 cells/bud at 25.5 days.

The data suggest that dark cells are renewed every 6.5-7.5 days, thus confirming a previous estimate based on a degeneration study (Farbman, J. Embr. Exp. Morphol., 22:55, 1969) in which the life of dark cells in rat fungiform papilla taste buds was estimated to be about 7 days. The shoulder on the ascending slope of the first major peak may suggest that there is more than one population of dark cells. Light cell renewal time was difficult to estimate quantitatively, but this cell type was labeled at a much slower rate than dark cells and is assumed to have a significantly longer life span.

(Supported by USPHS grant #NS-06181).

Taste development and sweetener preference in the puppy Fay Ferrell, (Department of Biological Science, Florida State University, Tallahassee, Fl., 32306 USA)

Preweanling beagle puppies as young as three and one-half weeks were trained using two-bowl tests to indicate their preferences for flavors presented in soft-moist dogfood and in solution. Lactose and fructose were the sugars most highly preferred by preweanlings. Puppies receiving exposure to any palatable sugar demonstrated an enhanced preference for other palatable sugars used in later tests. In an attempt to determine the course of maturity of the puppy taste system, the fungiform and circumvallate papillae of fetal and postnatal tongues were examined. Mature taste buds with open pores were found in both types of papillae during the final third of gestation and were numerous by birth. Evidence of large, multipored buds similar to those described by Bradley and Cheal (1976) in the epiglottis of the fetal sheep were observed in the circumvallate and fungiform papillae of fetal puppies of 47 and 54 days gestational age (term 63 days). Integrated responses were obtained from the chorda tympani nerves of beagle and mixed breed pups ranging in age from a few hours to 36 days. In every animal examined, fructose elicited a significantly higher neural response than any other sugar. For comparison, the kitten, a carnivore usually found to be indifferent to sugars in behavioral tests, was examined. Absolute magnitude of the integrated chorda tympani response to sugars compared to a 0.1 or 0.05 molar NH_4Cl standard was noticeably lower in the kitten than in the puppy, and maltose and xylose were the most effective sugars. These contrasts observed between kittens and puppies suggest that the receptor sites for sugars vary between the two species. Findings indicate the need for employing a large number of sweeteners before drawing conclusions concerning a species' ability to respond to sweet compounds.

Developmental features of the human fetal tongue: scanning electron microscopic studies Donald Ganchrow, (Department of Anatomy and Embryology, Hebrew University-Hadassah Medical School, Jerusalem, Israel)

The development of papillary structures on the surface of the tongue was studied in a series of human fetuses aborted spontaneously, or by saline induction, in whom no pathology was detected. Tissue was prepared for SEM by glutaraldehyde or neutral buffered formalin fixation, dehydration, critical point drying and coating with gold. At 8 wk. developmental age the anterior tongue is relatively undifferentiated. In the area of the foramen caecum appear beginnings of raised structures, some of which show the circumvallate-like shape, without surrounding trenches; two of these show apparent openings at the papillary center, usually not seen in mature circumvallate papillae (CVP). Between 10-13 wk. fungiform (FP) and filiform (FiP) papillae differentiate on the dorsal and lateral tongue. Polygonal, scale-like epithelial cells with prominent nuclei comprise the papillary surface and reach to edges of pores; partially desquamated cells, in formation, may erroneously suggest pore openings. Higher magnification reveals a pleated configuration of epithelia, as described for adult human tongue biopsies (Arvidson, '76). Not all FP have discernible pores. From within FP flowery formations reminiscent of gustatory "microvilli" (or exudates of the papillary interior?) project through the "pore"; these projecting structures are also seen with the light microscope (H and E, and Bodian stains). Inner walls or floors of some FP pores contain openings of unknown function. Foliate papillae also are evident at 10 wk. CVP are entrenched and the mature papillary pattern seems consistent by 15-24 wk. Openings in the tongue dorsum, anterior and posterolateral to CVP, contain projections not unlike those of papillary pores and resemble cryptae of tonsillar tissue (Saito et al, '75). Do these early "pores" and "villi" represent a stage prior to final development of the taste bud receptor itself?

Peripheral distribution of facial gustatory neurons M.M. Gomez,
E.H. Lubarsky, and I.J. Miller, Jr., (Dept. of Anatomy, Bowman Gray School
of Medicine, Winston-Salem, No. Carolina, USA.)

The rat geniculate ganglion sends afferent axons to innervate about 100 taste
buds on the anterior tongue and about 110 on the palate via the chorda
tympani (CT) and greater superficial petrosal (GSP) nerves, respectively.
The CT sends a branch to the foliate papillae, 2 posterior branches to 25
taste buds near the intermolar eminence, a mid-region branch to 25 taste buds,
and 4 parallel branches to the remaining 50 receptors on the tongue tip. The
GSP gives a branch to the posterior palate which has 45 taste buds per side
and sends 2 branches through the palatine foramen rostral to the nasoincisor
duct with 35 taste buds and caudal to the Geschmacksstreifen (35 taste buds).
The electron microscope has been used to count the number of axons in the
major divisions which distribute fibers to each receptor field. Cranial
nerves VII and VIII were sectioned in the internal auditory meatus in order
to degenerate fibers of central origin from the periphery. Control GSP
nerves contained 626 (28%) myelinated and 1637 (72%) unmyelinated, or 2263
total. The deefferented GSP nerves had 460 (28%) myelinated and 1189 (72%)
unmyelinated fibers for 1649 total. Control CT nerves contained 1017 fibers
with 545 (54%) myelinated and 472 (46%) unmyelinated, while a deefferented
CT had 444 (76%) myelinated and 140 (24%) unmyelinated for a total of 584
fibers. Thus, there are 4-6 myelinated axons per ipsilateral taste bud on
both tongue and palate, but there are 18 fold more unmyelinated profiles in
the GSP than CT. Since the total number of axons exceeds the number of
ganglion cell bodies (1721), there must be intermingling of other nerve
fibers or collateral branching among afferents near the ganglion. Physiological studies of the GSP must be undertaken to determine if functional differences exist among the two major populations of facial nerve taste buds.
(Supported in part by NIH Grant NS 10389)

Discriminative responses to taste in chronic decerebrate rats H. J. Grill,
(The Rockefeller Univ., 1230 York Ave., New York, N. Y., U.S.A.)

One or two bottle preference tests constitute the primary methodology for
determining acceptance or rejection of tastes. These tests require organisms
to initiate drinking and, therefore, can not be applied to preparations which
do not eat or drink spontaneously. The taste reactivity test, a new method
for assessing responses to taste stimuli, circumvents this shortcoming. A
50 μl taste stimulus is injected directly into the oral cavity of a freely
moving rat and the immediate response videotaped for frame by frame analysis.
Each of the sapid stimuli used (4 concentrations of sucrose, NaCl, HCl, and
QHCl) generated a stereotyped response derived from a lexicon of four mimetic
(oral musculature) and five body response components in all rats examined.
For example, sucrose elicited a response sequence beginning with low amplitude mouth movements, followed by tongue protrusions, swallowing, and then
lateral tongue movements. In contrast, quinine (3 x 10^{-5}M and above) was
rejected from the mouth by a response pattern that began with gaping and proceeded through as many as five body responses. The taste reactivity test was
used to determine the capacity of brainstem structures to integrate ingestion
and rejection responses. Both chronic decerebrate and thalamic rats were examined repeatedly, and their taste responses compared with intact rats. Decerebrates executed the same mimetic response components, and very similar
response sequences as intact rats. Based on these similarities, it appears
that discriminative responses to taste result from integrative mechanisms
complete within, or caudal to, the midbrain. In thalamic rats mimetic responses associated with ingestion were completely absent; all taste stimuli
elicited a quinine-like rejection sequence. Since decerebrates have the capacity of intact rats to execute both ingestion and rejection response sequences, it seems that mechanisms rostral to the midbrain suppress ingestion
and/or release rejection in thalamic rats (Grill & Norgren, Brain Res., in
press).
Supported by NIH AM 02360 and GM 1789.

The effect of miraculin on the response of single taste fibres in the Rhesus monkey. G. Hellekant, Brouwer J.N., Van der Wel H., Ninomiya Y., Hard C. and Glaser D. (Department of Physiology, Veterinarhogskolan, S - 750 07, Uppsala, Sweden).

Miraculin seems to offer a possibility to shed some light on the problem of the coding of taste information from the periphery to the CNS, because after miraculin psychophysical observations demonstrate that the neural information must have changed in such a way that acids, instead of eliciting only a sour sensation, elicit a sour and sweet sensation. It is implicit that the basis for this changed sensation must be a change of the neural activity in the taste fibres from the tongue. The problem is only where and how ?

In the experiments to be reported, behavioural as well as electrophysiological observations have been made in 12 Rhesus monkeys. During the behavioural experiments the monkeys were offered different acids in a two-bottle choice before and after miraculin. A change of their behaviour from rejection to preference of the acids was observed to be caused by miraculin. After the behavioural experiments the neural response from the chorda tympani proper nerves of the monkeys was recorded both in summated recordings and in single or few fibre preparations.

The summated recordings showed an enhancement of the response to acids after miraculin. The fibre preparation showed that only fibres which responded to sweet substances increased their activity to stimulation with acids after miraculin. Fibres, which responded to acids or any other stimuli except the sweet ones, were not affected by miraculin. This pattern seemed consistent among the 20 fibres which were tested with regard to the effect of miraculin. The most extreme was observed in one preparation which contained two fibres, whose impulses were of different amplitude and therefore distinctly different. One of them must, according to its response before miraculin, be classified as a sweet fibre, because it did not respond to any of the four acids, the salt or the quinine tested, but gave a very strong response to the five sweet stimuli which consisted of such chemically different substances as sucrose, aceto-sulfame, aspartame, monellin and thaumatin. The other fibre in the preparation must be classified as an acid fibre. The striking observation was that after miraculin the sweet fibre responded strongly to the acids, while the other one responded to the acids in the same way as it had done before miraculin.

It seems to us that our observations support the idea that information of the quality of a taste stimulus is mediated by the type of fibre while information on the strength of a stimulus is mediated by the frequency of impulses in the fibre. These finding supports the concepts of "fibre specificity" by Zotterman and "labelled lines" by Pfaffmann.

Taste stimulation and feeding behavior in fish: Effects of amino acids and
betaine I. Hidaka, (Faculty of Fisheries, Mie University, Tsu, Mie, Japan)

Various chemicals are effective in stimulating the lip chemoreceptors of the
puffer (Fugu pardalis).[1] Their effects on the feeding behavior of the fish
were studied by applying them in starch pellets. The starch pellet by itself,
made by suspending starch in a small amount of water and heating it above 80°C
(to obtain α-starch), was not taken by the fish but it was taken when stimulants such as clam extracts were added to it. Thus, some lip-stimulative
substances in starch were accepted, while others were rejected.   NaCl, to
which the lip chemoreceptors show a low sensitivity,[1] was not accepted; when
added at 2 M to clam extracts, it depressed the feeding response weakly or
did not affect it at all.   Sucrose, ineffective for the lip chemoreceptors,[1]
appeared indifferent. Alanine, glycine, proline and betaine were individually
accepted. Mixtures of the 4 substances were accepted much better, suggesting
some synergistic interactions among them.   The effects of binary mixtures of
amino acids plus betaine on the lip chemoreceptors were studied. An enhancement of the facial nerve response was yielded by mixing alanine and betaine
and other pairs of amino acids plus betaine; the summated whole nerve response
to a mixture of alanine and betaine, for example, was larger in magnitude
than the sum of the responses to alanine and betaine applied separately. The
results obtained suggested that the enhancement of the response by some of the
above pairs may be ascribed to the synergistic interaction between the two
substances applied together. Some pairs showed a depression of the response.

1) Hidaka, I., and Kiyohara, S., 1975. In "Olfaction and Taste V", ed. by
    Denton, D.A., and Coghlan, J.P., Academic Press, New York, pp. 147-151.

Nerve-epithelium interactions during taste bud and papilla development

C.M. Mistretta and R.M. Bradley, (Dept. of Oral Biology, School of Dentistry, Ann Arbor, MI 48109, USA)

To study interactions between nerves and epithelia during taste bud and papilla development, autogenous cross-grafts of external cheek skin and dorsal anterior tongue mucosa (epidermis and dermis) were made in 12 sheep fetuses aged 52-107 days of gestation (term = 147 days). Grafts were transplanted during sterile surgical procedures and fetuses were then replaced in utero. Fetuses were delivered and perfused close to term; therefore, grafts remained in situ for 37 to 80 days before the tissue was dissected and prepared for light microscopy. In the youngest fetal age at time of grafting (52 days), the tongue epithelium contains immature fungiform papillae and presumptive taste buds; cheek skin contains immature wool follicles. At 107 days the lingual fungiform papillae contain 1-2 taste buds with well defined pores, and cheek skin contains well developed follicles and a few wool fibers.

On examination of histological sections, we found that all grafts had continued to differentiate at the transplant site, had acquired character- istics of the adult epithelium, and had become innervated. Cheek skin grafted to the anterior tongue was characterized by mature wool follicles, wool fibers, and cornified surface layers. No fungiform papillae or taste buds were found in these grafts.

Tongue epithelium transplanted to the external cheek contained mature filiform papillae covered with several layers of cornified cells. In tongue grafts made in fetuses aged 98-107 days, no fungiform papillae or taste buds were found. Thus, immature fungiform papillae and taste buds that were initially present, degenerated and did not re-form. However, in each graft of tongue epithelium made in fetuses aged 52-67 days, several structures that resembled fungiform papillae were present. Furthermore, in some of these early grafts, two-three papillae contained a structure resembling an immature taste bud.

We conclude that: 1. Tongue epithelium and cheek skin cross-grafted during fetal development continue to differentiate at new sites, and become innervated. 2. Tongue nerves do not induce fungiform papilla or taste bud development in grafted, fetal cheek skin. 3. Structures resembling fungiform papillae and a few immature taste buds develop in fetal tongue epithelium grafted to external cheek, if the tongue tissue is transplanted early enough in development. Therefore, these preliminary results indicate that nerves and epithelia interact differently at different stages of development in the process of taste bud and papilla differentiation. As yet, though, we have no indication of whether any functional taste buds are present in these grafts. 4. Development of fungiform papillae (as well as taste buds) seems to proceed under specific neural and epithelial influences. 5. During later stages of gestation, it appears that taste buds and fungiform papillae will not develop in grafted, non-lingual epithelium innervated by lingual nerves, or in grafted, lingual epithelium innervated by non-lingual nerves. (Supported by Nat. Inst. Dent. Res., NIH Grant DE 04491.)

Phosphatases in the taste organs of frog and rabbit H. Nomura, N. Kono and
N. Asanuma, (Dept. of Oral Physiol., Matsumoto Dent. Coll., Shiojiri, Japan)

Several kinds of phosphatases, such as alkaline and acid phosphatases and ATP-
ase, have been demonstrated histochemically in foliate and circumvallate papillae in mammals, each of which showing different localization. These phosphatases probably have important roles in transduction process of taste stimulation or for the maintenance of taste buds. In frog, information about such
phosphatases is as yet lacking. The present study, therefore, was carried out
to get some information about such phosphatases in the taste organ of frog.
The experiments were carried out histo- and biochemically on both frog's tongue and rabbit's foliate papilla. Histochemical examination of frog's tongue
revealed ATPase and alkaline phosphatase activities being located on the
superficial layer of the tongue, while acid phosphatase activity being in the
epithelial layer. The properties of the ATPase and alkaline phosphatase were
also examined biochemically. Biochemical studies were carried out with intact
tongue as well as with homogenate. The results were as follows: (1) ATPase is
divalent cation-dependent, but alkaline phosphatase is not, (2) alkaline phosphatase has optimum pH around pH 9.6, but ATPase does not, (3) ruthenium red,
PCMB, quinacrine hydrochloride and NEM do not inhibit ATPase activity in intact tongues, (4) both the phosphatases are highly heat-resistant.
Adenyl cyclase, 3',5'-nucleotide phosphodiesterase, ATPase, alkaline and acid
phosphatase and 5'-nucleotidase activities were examined on rabbit's foliate
papilla histochemically. Among these phosphatase activities, ATPase, adenyl
cyclase and 3',5'-nucleotide phosphodiesterase activities were shown to be localized at the taste cavity. This finding seems interesting, because it suggests that adenyl cyclase-cyclic AMP system may have a role in the transduction processes of taste stimulation.

Location of pontine relay neurons projecting to VPMm in the rat by means of horseradish peroxidase   Hisashi Ogawa and Taketoshi Akagi, (Department of Physiology, Kumamoto University Medical School, Kumamoto, 860, Japan)

After injection of 0.02-0.03 μl of horseradish peroxidase (HRP, Sigma VI) into the medial VPM (VPMm) and the adjacent structures of 40 albino rats weighing 300-450 g, by means of 1 μl Hamilton syringe, retrogradely labelled neurons were observed in the pons and in the rostral medulla.

Injection of HRP into the medial tip of VPMm labelled the small-sized fusiform neurons in the bilateral marginal nucleus of the brachium conjunctivum (BCM). But many more neurons were labelled in the ipsilateral BCM than in the contralateral one, and in the dorsal part of BCM than in the ventral one. Some labelled neurons were found inside the brachium conjunctivum itself.

When HRP was injected into the medial third of VPMm, sparing the medial tip, HRP-labelled neurons were found bilaterally in BCM. Many more neurons were labelled in the ipsilateral nucleus, but about the same number of labelled neurons were located in the ventral part as in the dorsal part of the nucleus and, moreover, more widely distributed in the rostrocaudal extent. Some labelled neurons were also located contralaterally in the supratrigeminal nucleus (SV) and in the dorsal part of the principal nucleus of the trigeminus (PV).

By injecting HRP into the lateral half of VPMm and the medial tip of the ventrobasal complex, HRP-labelled neurons were observed contralaterally in SV and PV, and in the contralateral region encompassed by the motor nucleus of the trigeminus dorsally, by PV laterally, and by the superior olivary nucleus ventrally. Only a few labelled neurons were located bilaterally in BCM as well as ipsilaterally in SV and PV.

None of the neurons in the solitary tract nucleus on either side to the injection site in VPMm were labelled, whether HRP was injected into the medial part of VPMm or into the lateral part.

The effect of temperature on the turnover of taste bud cells in channel
catfish Randie Raderman-Little, (Florida State University, Tallahassee,
Florida 32306 USA)

There are many similarities between the taste receptors of mammals and some
lower vertebrates. The taste buds of catfish provide an excellent model for
the study of taste bud cell maintenance and renewal. This study examines the
structure and dynamics of the taste buds on the barbels of channel catfish
(Ictalurus punctatus). Light microscopy, transmission electron microscopy
and scanning electron microscopy were used to examine the internal and surface morphology of the taste bud cells. A new method for observing the
inner cell surfaces of the taste buds was described.

Groups of channel catfish, held in and acclimated to 14°, 18°, 22°, and
30°C water were injected intraperitoneally with 3μC/gram body weight of ^{3}H-
thymidine (6.7 ci/mmol). Barbels were sampled at various times after
injection and prepared for light microscope autoradiography. The number of
labelled cells per center cross section of taste bud was counted for each
sample. Results show that epithelial cells surrounding the taste buds in
the barbel divide and some of their daughter cells migrate into the taste
buds. By graphic analysis, an approximate average turnover time or life span
of taste bud cells was obtained for each temperature studied. The average
life span as well as the time spent inside the taste buds was highly
temperature dependent. The average life span of these cells at 14°, 18°,
22°, and 30°C was on the order of 40, 30, 15, and 12 days, respectively.

Semi-continuous labelling studies were done by repeated daily injection.
Light and dark cells were distinguished by their staining characteristics
and by their contour in the basal region of the bud as seen in Araldite
embedded 1μm sections. Results showed that both light and dark staining
cells were labelled, indicating that light and dark cells are renewed.

A model of neural taste adaptation in the rat David V. Smith, (Dept. Psych., Univ. Wyoming, Laramie, Wyo., 82071, USA)

The rate of stimulus change is an important determinant of the magnitude of the transient portion of the integrated chorda tympani response and of the initial impulse frequency in single chorda tympani fibers of the rat (Smith, D. V., & Bealer, S. L., Physiol. Behav., 1975, 15, 303-314), both being a power function of the rate of stimulus onset. In addition to this rate-sensitive component, the rat chorda tympani response to NaCl shows a slow exponential decay over time (Smith, D. V., Steadman, J. W., & Rhodine, C. N., Am. J. Physiol., 1975, 229, 1134-1140). Following adaptation to NaCl there is a period of postexcitatory depression, first described in the cat by Hellekant (Acta Physiol. Scand., 1968, 74, 1-9). The magnitude of this postexcitatory depression is dependent upon the concentration of the adapting stimulus (Smith, D. V., & Bealer, S. L., Sens. Processes, 1976, 1, 99-108) and upon its duration. Responses of the rat chorda tympani nerve to NaCl were obtained after adapting the tongue to NaCl for varying periods of time. Longer adapting durations produced greater reductions in the magnitude of both the phasic and tonic portions of the response to a subsequent test stimulus. Both portions of the response recovered slowly with the presentation of a distilled water rinse. The reduction in the tonic portion of the response with increasing adapting duration followed the time course of the slow exponential decay in the response to the adapting stimulus and the time course of the recovery from postexcitatory depression was the reverse of this slow exponential. The phasic portion of the response recovered more rapidly than the tonic component. Compounds that do not produce a prolonged slow adaptation in the rat chorda tympani response (e.g., HCl) do not produce a postexcitatory depression that is dependent upon adapting duration (Plock, S. E., master's thesis, University of Wyoming, 1977). The slow adaptation to NaCl stimulation, but not to HCl stimulation, is also seen in the rat taste receptor potential (Ozeki, M., J. gen. Physiol., 1971, 58, 688-699). Although most receptor potential studies have used rates of solution flow that are much too slow to produce transient responses even in the first-order nerve, it has recently been shown that the receptor potential of the frog does not exhibit a phasic response, even at fast rates of stimulus onset (Balnave, P. A., doctoral dissertation, Duke University, 1976; Sato, T., Experientia, 1976, 32, 1426-1428). The rise time of the receptor potential, however, is proportional to the rate of solution flow (Sato, T., Experientia, 1976, 32, 1426-1428). This lack of a phasic response in the taste receptor cell suggests that the receptor potential is not proportional to the rate of stimulus binding, as predicted by a recently proposed rate theory of gustatory stimulation (Heck, G. L., & Erickson, R. P., Behav. Biol., 1973, 8, 687-712). Taken together, these various data suggest a model of the probable sequence of events leading to the first-order neural response. The taste receptor potential is proposed to be proportional to the number of occupied receptor sites minus the magnitude of a slowly building adaptive process. This adaptive process declines equally slowly during the rinse period, producing the prolonged period of postexcitatory depression. The response of the chorda tympani nerve is proposed to be sensitive to the amplitude of the receptor potential and to its rate of change, i.e., the first-order nerve adds a derivative to the taste receptor input. Thus, the rate sensitivity of the chorda tympani nerve can be accounted for under an occupation model (Beidler, L. M., J. gen. Physiol., 1954, 38, 133-139) of taste receptor stimulation.

(Supported by NINCDS Grant NS10211 and Research Career Development Award NS00168)

CO_2 responses of exteroceptors in the minnow (Pseudorasbora parva)

S. Yamashita and K. Yoshii, (Biol. Inst., Coll. Lib. Arts, Kagoshima Univ., Kagoshima 890, Japan)

CO_2 responses of exteroceptors in the southern top-mouthed minnow (Pseudorasbora parva) were recorded from the ramus maxillaris, the ramus mandibularis and the ramus buccalis, which are major branches of the infra-orbital nerve, and from the ramus palatinus facialis. The r. maxillaris, the r. mandibularis and the r. palatinus showed spontaneous discharges of extremely low frequency and spike heights were less than 40 μV. The threshold concentration for the stimulation with a solution of CO_2 was about 4×10^{-5} M and concentration-response curves obtained from three nerves well fitted with each other. The responses depended on the concentration of free CO_2 rather than H^+, HCO_3^- and CO_3^{2-} in total CO_2 content. Responses produced by test solutions, which were the same in total amount of CO_2 but different in pH values, depended not only on the concentration of free CO_2 but also on that of bicarbonate ion. On the other hand in the r. buccalis spontaneous discharges occurred in fairly high frequency and the largest spike height attained about tenfold that in other three nerves. Excitatory responses were followed by inhibitory responses during the stimulation of the upper snout region with CO_2 solution. Threshold concentrations for excitatory and inhibitory responses were about 7×10^{-4} M and 3×10^{-4} M, respectively. Both the responses and the duration of the inhibition depended directly on the concentration of free CO_2 in total CO_2 content. Many terminal buds were identified on upper and lower lips and the palate which are innervated by the r. maxillaris, the r. mandibularis and the r. palatinus, respectively. Many pit organs and few terminal buds which are innervated by the r. buccalis were located on the upper snout region.

CHEMORECEPTION IN INVERTEBRATES

Abstracts of Poster Presentations

Insect sensillum specificity and structure: an approach to a new typology

Helmut Altner[1]

Institut für Zoologie, Universität Regensburg, D-84 Regensburg, GFR

ABSTRACT

Insect sensilla are usually classified according to their external morphology. A comparative investigation using a technique for marking individual sensilla leads to a system based on structural features correlated with function. Three main categories are distinguished :(1) NP(no pore)-sensilla, which are either mechano-sensitive or hygro- and thermosensitive. These subgroups can be distinguished by the structure of their dendrites. (2) TP (terminal pore)-sensilla, which contain gustatory units alone or together with a mechanoreceptor. (3) WP(wall pore)-sensilla, which occur as 2 main types :single-walled (SW)-sensilla having pore tubules, and double-walled (DW)-sensilla having spoke canals and secretion as stimulus conducting systems. SW-sensilla contain olfactory units. In DW-sensilla, olfactory and/or thermo-and hygrosensitive units are found. The olfactory receptors of SW-sensilla and of DW-sensilla most probably differ in sensitivity.

INTRODUCTION

Insect hair and peg sense organs are generally classified according to their external morphology. The outline and the size of the cuticular outer structures as well as whether or not the sensory pegs are set in pits within the cuticle have been used as criteria. The nomenclature, still used today, was introduced by Schenk[27]. This author coined the terms :sensilla chaetica, trichodea, basiconica, styloconica and ampullacea. Only few types have been added, e.g. sensilla campaniformia by Berlese[6]. The suggestion by Snodgrass[31],"... that a truer classification of both hair and peg sense organs, and one probably more coincident with their function might be based on the internal structure ... rather than on the form of the external part, if the state of our knowledge would permit " (p. 44), has not yet led to a new system of classification, though attempts were made to assemble new criteria. Slifer [29,30], basing her system on Dethier[12], discriminates between thick-walled chemoreceptors, which as a rule have a single opening, and thin-walled chemoreceptors, whose walls are perforated by many small openings. While the former are contact chemoreceptors, the latter should be considered to be excited by olfactory stimuli. Since the same names are used for sense organs which differ in function, as well as significantly in structural features, an improved classification is necessary. This is especially true for coeloconic, basiconic, and trichoid sensilla.

This paper shows that sensilla containing chemo-, hygro-, and thermosensitive cells can be distinguished on the basis of their individual structure, and that the properties of the stimulus-conducting structures might indicate differences in sensitivity among olfactory sensilla.

Any generalization in this field gains its strength from the number of different sensilla which have been investigated on a morphological and physiological basis. Since populations of sensilla of the same type are rare, one has to try to mark sensilla after electrophysiological recording for ultrastructural investigation.

MATERIAL AND METHODS

Experiments were performed on adult cockroaches (Periplaneta americana) and stick insects (Carausius morosus). We marked individual sensilla using a simple technique : inserting a cactus needle at a defined point near the sensillum investigated after recording. The needle can easily be used for orientation in scanning as well as in transmission electron microscopic preparations.

RESULTS AND PROPOSAL FOR AN IMPROVED TYPOLOGY

Using the marking technique mentioned above, a conspicuous correlation of structural features with physiological properties of sensilla was found in the cockroach antenna. Eight physiologically distinguishable sensillum types can be characterized by experiments in which the specific sensitivity of the sensory cells in each is tested using pure chemical substances as stimuli. In four of these types, units were found with a specific sensitivity for short chain n-alcohols. Using the substance to which a maximal reaction was found as a key word, these sensilla can be called pentanol-, hexanol-, octanol-, and alcohol-terpene-sensillum. In the same way, others can be designated as butyric acid-, hexanoic acid-cold-, amine-, and cold-moist-dry-sensillum (Sass,[24,25], Altner et al.[4],).

A structural investigation of these physiologically defined
types demonstrated two interesting facts :(1) sensory cells sensitive
to temperature are included in both double-walled pegs with pores
and spoke canals filled with secretion material (hexanoic acid-cold-
sensillum, Fig. 1), and in pegs without pores (cold-moist-dry-sensillum).
In pegs with pores, thermosensitive units are combined with olfactory
cells. In pegs without pores they are combined with hygrosensitive
units :a moist air cell and a dry air cell. (2) Cells sensitive to
alcohols and terpenes occurred exclusively in single-walled sensilla
with wall pores and pore tubules, whereas cells with a marked
sensitivity for fatty acids and amines were only found in double-walled
hairs with spoke canals.

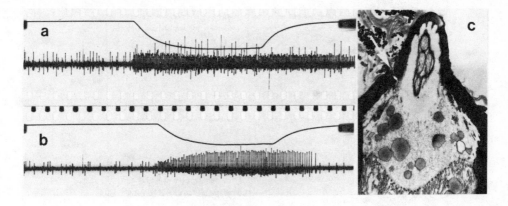

Fig. 1 a-c. Reactions of units in a hexanoic acid-cold-sensillum
to stimulation with hexanoic acid (a) and cold air (b). (c) Oblique
section through the basis of a sensillum of this type. Cuticular lesion
caused by electrode insertion is shown (arrow). (c,b courtesy of H.Sass)

Thus, differences in the pore structures correlate with those
in physiological properties because stimuli are transmitted to the
dendritic membranes through these pores which can be regarded as part
of the stimulus transmitting system.

In Periplaneta antennal sensilla two systems are developed,
both widespread among insect sensilla (Tab. 1) :(1) pore tubules,
which are formed together with the cuticular outer structure by the
trichogen cell during development. (2) Secretion material, which
is found in the spoke canals connecting the receptor lymph space
around the dendrites with the outside world. This material is most

probably secreted by the tormogen cell. It appears as droplets within the receptor lymph space, above the membranes of this cell. It can be derived from the structural properties of the droplets that they contain lipids. The material is most probably transported to the spoke canals.

These stimulus-conducting structures might differ in their affinity for odorous substances. Thus, the selectivity of the dendritic membranes might be paralleled by a selectivity of the stimulus-conducting structures. Both parts of the system may be equally balanced, so that knowing the properties of one part could allow predictions regarding the properties of the other one.

morphological type		physiological properties
	pore tubules as stimulus conducting system	4 types, sensory cells with specific sensitivity for short-chain n-alcohols
	secretion filled spoke canals as stimulus conducting system	3 types, sensory cells with specific sensitivity for short-chain n-acids or amines, one type with cold receptor
	no pores	1 type, sensory cells sensitive to temperature (cold) and humidity (dry, moist air)

Table 1. Antennal sensilla in Periplaneta :morphological types and their physiological properties. (courtesy of H. Sass)

In the antenna of Carausius we find a sensillum with a combination of one temperature- and two humidity-sensitive units. This sensillum lacks pores. From its external morphology it would be designated as "coeloconic" (Fig. 2). Thus coeloconic sensilla either contain hygro- and thermoreceptive sensory cells such as in Carausius, in Aedes (McIver,[19] Davis and Sokolove,[10])and in Locusta (Waldow[38]), or are equipped with olfactory units such as in Locusta (Boeckh[8],). A similar situation exists regarding other sensillum types, especially basiconic and trichoid sensilla. Basiconic sensilla for example may or may not have pores. The pores, when present, may lead either into

pore tubules (single-walled) or into spoke canals (double-walled).
Consequently, the units included differ in modality and sensitivity.

A classification system which uses the pore system as the
primary criterium for discrimination seems advantageous. Table
2 gives a proposal, distinguishing between 3 main categories :
NP-sensilla which do not possess pores, TP-sensilla with a terminal
(or subterminal) pore system, and WP-sensilla with wall pores. These
main groups are further subdivided according to functionally relevant
criteria.

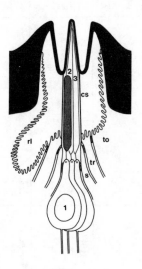

Fig. 2. Diagrammatic representation of a "coeloconic" sensillum
without pores in <u>Carausius</u> comprising one thermosensitive and two
hygrosensitive cells (1-3). cs cuticular sheath, rl receptor lymph
cavity, s sheath cell, tr trichogen cell, to tormogen cell.

NP-sensilla which contain hygro- and thermoreceptors seem
to be rather seldom. In <u>Periplaneta</u> and <u>Carausius</u> they do not occur on
all antennal segments (Schafer and Sanchez,[26] ;Altner,[2]). Most NP-
sensilla are mechanosensitive. They are characterized by a flexible
socket and a tubular body within the dendrite.

TP-sensilla as contact chemoreceptors in most cases possess
a flexible socket and a mechanosensitive unit besides the gustatory
elements. In some cases, however, the socket is rigid and hence only
gustatory units are present. This is true for sensilla of the
hypopharyngeal organ (Moulins,[22,23])as well as for sensilla in the

morphological properties		sensitivity	usual designation	important references
"NP"	socket flexible: dendrite: 1 sensory cell: dendrite with tubular body	hair	mechanosens.	S. chaetica	Thurm 1964, 1965, 1968
		cupola	mechanosens.	S. campaniformia	Thurm et al., 1975; Moran et al., 1976
no pores	socket inflexible 3–4 sensory cells (1 dendrite folded or lamellated)	surface peg	thermosens. and hygrosens.	S. basiconica	Periplaneta antenna (Yokohari et al., 1975; Loftus, 1976)
		peg in pit		S. coeloconica	Carausius antenna (Altner et al., 1977b)
"TP"	socket flexible 2–20 sensory cells: 1 dendrite with tubular body, dendrites not branched	hair, peg	gustatory and mechanosens. (contact chemoreceptor)	S. chaetica, S. trichodea, S. basiconica, S. styloconica	Hansen and Heumann, 1971
terminal pore (thick walled)	socket inflexible 2–9 sensory cells, dendrites not branched	peg	gustatory	–	Periplaneta maxillary palp (Altner, unpubl.)
		cupola	gustatory	–	Blabera hypopharyngeal organ (Moulins, 1968, 1971)
"WP" wall pores (thin walled)	single-walled; pore tubules (or similar structures); 1–40 sensory cells, dendrites branched or not branched	hair, peg	olfactory[1)2)]	S. basiconica, S. coeloconica, S. trichodea	Slifer, 1967; Schneider and Steinbrecht, 1968; Kaissling 1971, 1974; Steinbrecht, 1973
		plate	olfactory	S. placodea	
(socket inflexible[1)])	double-walled, spoke canals with secretion; 2–4 sensory cells, dendrites not branched	surface peg	olfactory[3)] and thermosens.	S. basiconica	Periplaneta antenna (Sass, 1977; Altner et al., 1977a); Locusta antenna (Boeckh, 1967; Steinbrecht, 1969)
		peg in pit	olfactory[3)] thermosens. and hygrosens.	S. coeloconica	Locusta antenna (Waldow, 1970)

1) In Apterygota WP-sensilla sometimes with flexible socket and 1 mechanosensitive cell (tubular body) (Altner and Ernst, 1974).
2) Special sensitivity for short-chain n-alcohols (Altner et al., 1977a).
3) Special sensitivity for short-chain n-acids or amines (Altner et al., 1977a).

Table 2. Morphological and physiological properties of sensilla common in insects.

maxillary palp of cockroaches.

Here the sensilla are crowded together within a field comprising about 2600 pegs. The whole cuticle of the field is flexible and held convex by hemolymph pressure, making it elastic when it comes into contact with the substrate. The contact with the substrate is not controlled individually, but rather by a single chordotonal organ. The fact that neighbouring contact chemoreceptors with flexible sockets standing on a rigid cuticle contain just one more dendrite (which is mechanosensitive) shows that the type occurring within the sensillum field has developed by reduction. The advantage gained by the reduction of the mechanosensitive elements is a higher density of gustatory elements and thus a better spatial resolution, a density of about 200 000 sensory cells/mm^2, is achieved (Altner,[1] and unpublished results).

WP-sensilla such as those we have investigated are wide-spread. The differences in sensitivity we have found are in agreement with data from other investigators. Boeckh[9] mentions that in Locusta, sensory cells in "basiconic" sensilla - these are single walled and have pore-tubules - react only to alcohols and not to fatty acids. Cells sensitive to fatty acids were found in the Locust in "coeloconic" sensilla (double-walled with spoke canals). Our hypothesis is further supported by the findings of Bernard[7] and Davis and Sokolove[11] and, at least partly, by those of Kaib[15].

Hawke and Farley[14] showed that there are differences in the chemical properties of the stimulus conducting structures by observing that such structures react differentially to solvents.

CRITICISMS REGARDING TYPOLOGY

It has to be kept in mind that our proposal is based on limited knowledge. With regard to the WP-sensilla which show the highest variability, a review of all data on insect sensilla available shows that the two types distinguished by us (single-walled with pore tubules ; double-walled with spoke canals and secretion, Fig. 3 a,b) are common and found in most insect groups. It should be realized, however, that there are types which do not fit into this bipartite scheme. One of them is characterized by an irregularly formed wall which can be regarded to be an intermediate between the types mentioned (Fig. 3c). The pores within the wall are underlaid by a material which seems to have a tendency to assemble into tubule-like structures. Clear-cut pore tubules are not found. Such sensilla, containing olfactory units, occur in the stick insect. Structurally similar sensilla have been observed in beetles (Meinecke,[20]). Deviations from the main "standard" sensilla can particularly be expected to occur in phylogenetically isolated groups of insects (Apterygota, see Table 2) and in species adapted to special environments, such as water.

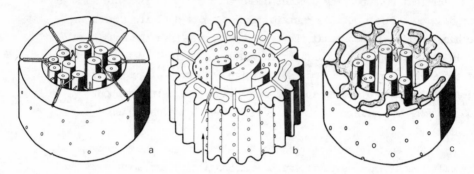

Fig. 3 a-c. Comparison of the structure of WP-sensilla.

Moreover, we are ignorant about the chemical composition of pore tubules and secretion products filling pore canals. Although appearing identical in electron micrographs, such stimulus-conducting structures or materials may well differ in composition and properties.

These limitations, on the other hand, do not render the proposed system impracticable. They must be seen as inherent to all attempts to press evolutionary diversity into a system of a few clearly defined categories.

[1]Supported by DFG grant A156/7

REFERENCES

 1. Altner, H.(1975) Cell Tiss. Res. 165, 79-88.
 2. Altner, H.(1977) Verh. Dt. Zool. Ges. -in press-
 3. Altner, H. and Ernst, K-D.(1974) Pedobiologia 14, 113-122.
 4. Altner, H.; Sass, H. and Altner, I.(1977a) Cell Tiss. Res. 176, 389-405.
 5. Altner, H.; Tichy, H. and Altner, I.(1977b) -in preparation-
 6. Berlese, A.(1909) Gli Insetti, Soc. Editrice Libraria, Milano.
 7. Bernard, J.(1974) These, Universite de Rennes, 1-285.
 8. Boeckh, J.(1967) Z. Vergl. Physiol. 55, 378-406.
 9. Boeckh, J.(1974) J. Comp. Physiol. 90, 183-205.
10. Davis, E.E. and Sokolove, Ph.G.(1975) J. Comp. Physiol. 96, 223-236.
11. Davis, E.E. and Sokolove, Ph.G.(1976) J. Comp. Physiol. 105, 43-54.

12. Dethier, V.G.(1953) in Insect Physiology, ed. K. Roeder, pp 544-576, Wiley, New York.
13. Hansen, K. and Heumann, H.-G.(1971) Z. Zellforsch. 117, 419-442.
14. Hawke, S.D. and Farley, R.D.(1971) Tissue and Cell 3, 649-664.
15. Kaib, M.(1974) J. Comp. Physiol. 95, 105-121.
16. Kaissling, K.-E.(1971) in Handbook of Sensory Physiology, IV/1, ed. L.M. Beidler, pp 351-431.
17. Kaissling, K.-E.(1974) in Biochemistry of Sensory Functions, ed. L. Jaenicke, pp 243-273, Springer, Berlin-Heidelberg-New York.
18. Loftus, R.(1976) J. Comp. Physiol. 111, 153-170.
19. McIver, S.B.(1973) Tissue and Cell 5, 105-112.
20. Meinecke, C.-Ch.(1975) Zoomorphologie 82, 1-42.
21. Moran, D.T.; Rowley, J.C. III; Zill, S.N. and Varela, F.G.(1976) J. Cell Biol. 71, 832-847.
22. Moulins, M.(1968) J. Ultrastruct. Res. 21, 474-513.
23. Moulins, M.(1971) Z. Vergl. Physiol. 73, 139-166.
24. Sass, H.(1976) J. Comp. Physiol. 107, 49-65.
25. Sass, H.(1977) J. Comp. Physiol. -submitted-
26. Schafer, R. and Sanchez, Th.V.(1973) J. Comp. Neurol. 149, 335-354.
27. Schenk, O.(1903) Zool. Jahrb. Abt. Anat. Ontog. Thiere 17, 573-618.
28. Schneider, D. and Steinbrecht, R.A.(1968) Symp. Zool. Soc. Lond. 23, 279-297.
29. Slifer, E.H.(1967) in Insects and Physiology, ed. J.W. Beament, J.E. Treherne, pp 233-245, Oliver and Boyd, Edinburgh.
30. Slifer, E.H.(1970) Annu. Rev. Entomol. 15, 121-142.
31. Snodgrass, R.E.(1926) Smithsonian Miscell. Collections 77, No. 8, 1-80.
32. Steinbrecht, R.A.(1969) in Olfaction and Taste III, ed. C. Pfaffmann, pp 3-21, Rockefeller Univ. Press, New York.
33. Steinbrecht, R.A.(1973) Z. Zellforsch. 139, 533-565.
34. Thurm, U.(1964) Science 145, 1063-1065.
35. Thurm, U.(1965) Cold Spring Harb. Symp. Quant. Biol. 30, 75-82.
36. Thurm, U.(1968) Symp. Zool. Soc. Lond. 23, 199-216.
37. Thurm, U.; Stedtler, A. and Foelix, R.(1975) Verh. Dt. Zool. Ges. 67, 37-41.
38. Waldow, U.(1970) Z. Vergl. Physiol. 69, 249-283.
39. Yokohari, F.; Tominaga, Y.; Ando, M. and Tateda, H.(1975) J. Electron. Micr. 24, 291-293.

Central olfactory pathways and plasticity of responses to odorous stimuli in insects

Claudine Masson

Laboratoire de Neurobiologie Sensorielle, EPHE, CENFAR, BP No. 6, F 92260, Fontenay aux Roses, France

ABSTRACT
      An overview of recent functional anatomical data leads us to propose a schematic description of the olfactory information flow from the first order neurons (in the antenna) to the higher centers of the brain (deutocerebrum and mushroom bodies), in order to consider in neurobiological terms the possible steps of the plasticity of the responses to odorous stimuli.

Early observations by ethologists as well as more recent learning experiments (48) show that insects can selectively and consistently associate chemical clues and visual patterns for initiating an adequate behavioural response. Such capacities imply that simultaneously presented sensory inputs finally reach a unique central system where the incoming information is actually linked to the relevant effector program. Other obvious implications are long lasting information storage and plasticity of the link between input and output.

      Although a great deal of data have already been collected concerning the description of behavioural sequences, anatomical features and neurophysiological responses, they are far from exhaustive and one is limited in their interpretation, especially as regards CNS functioning as a whole.

1. FIRST RELAY OF THE AFFERENT ANTENNAL PATHWAY : THE DEUTOCEREBRUM

      Most cephalic olfactory and mechanical information is collected by the primary neurons of specialized sensilla along the antennae, and reaches the first central relay by the axons of the antennal sensory nerve. Structural organization of the sensory lobe is strongly correlated with the antennal sensory function. In the ant *Formica fusca* which uses mainly olfactory and tactile senses, 18.1 % of the total brain volume is occupied by the sensory antennal lobe versus only 9.9 % by the visual system ; on the contrary, the antennal lobe of the "visual" dragonfly occupies 1.3 % versus 80 % for the optic neuropile (12).

      The antennal sensory system (afferents, glomeruli, interneurons, efferents) is characterized by a large convergence. In the cockroach *Periplaneta americana* (6,9) there are 120,000 afferent fibers, 125 glomeruli, 750 interneurons and only 250 efferent processes in the tractus olfactorio-globularis (T.O.G.).

1.1. Deutocerebral afferents and efferents

The primary axons of the different antennal sensory modalities are combined to form one, or two sensory antennal nerves. There are no contacts between the parallel fibers which reach separately the CNS. The antennal chemical modality is represented by olfaction and contact chemoreception. In a primitive insect, *Periplaneta americana*, 50,000 olfactory fibers, 45,000 gustatory and 25,000 mechanical and other fibers have been counted (5) ; and, in a social insect, *Camponotus vagus*, 35,000 chemical mainly olfactory with some hundreds of gustatory fibers, and 25,000 mechanical exteroceptive as well as proprioceptive fibers (24). Degeneration experiments, silver impregnations (11, 4, 33, 9), and procion yellow injection (45) show that the bulk of antennal sensory fibers end in the ipsilateral sensory lobe of the deutocerebrum, and that they subdivide in several compact bundles at their entrance in the deutocerebral neuropile (57).

The T.O.G. (and more precisely the antenno-glomerular tract of the T.O.G.) represents the main efferent bundle of the sensory lobe (700 fibers in *Locusta*) and connects it with the corpora pedunculata (C.P.) (12, 33, 53,9)

Apart from a few exceptions (4, 11, 23) these efferents are essentially ipsilateral. In numerous insect brains, the fibers go to the C.P. either in the ipsilateral calyx, or in the calyx and α-lobe (18, 10, 33, 23, 53, 9). The deutoneurons processes are also traced into the lateral protocerebral lobe between the deutocerebrum and the optic lobe (9) : these findings are further documented by electrophysiological responses in this area to antennal olfactory stimulation (6).

Some other efferents are traced in the anterior sub-glomerular part of the tritocerebrum (lobus glomeratus) near the place where the palp contact chemoreceptors are also ending (9, 20).

1.2. Intrinsic organization and functional implications

The large convergence of the system (about 100,000 afferents for only 250 efferents) induces the formation of glomeruli in the deutocerebral neuropile ; they are very similar to the homologous structures in the olfactory bulb of vertebrates (36). In the cockroach *Blaberus craniifer*, we have recently demonstrated a true bilateral symetrical pattern of the glomeruli suggesting a non-random organization (28).

The bundles of afferents are assigned to groups of glomeruli (23, 9).

Localized sections of the antenna (33, 44) and differential histochemical staining correlated with electrophysiological recording (24, 25, 27) suggest that these grouping glomeruli represent a spatial segregation of chemical and mechanical sensory modalities. In *Musca*, a specific chemical projection among glomeruli has also been reported (44).

Whether a glomerulus, or a group of glomeruli, represents a functional unit remains an unanswered question ; in this way, it would be useful to explore them as "identified glomerulus" by comparison with "identified neurons" (16).

It is clear now that the first order neuron branches end in the cortical layer of the glomeruli where they connect to the centrally located post-synaptic efferents (42, 4, 33, 23, 9).

Dense sub-units inside glomeruli suggest microglomeruli (25, 27) similar to those described in the olfactory bulb of vertebrates (21).

The endings of one afferent can be seen spreading to as many as three different glomeruli. Up to eight different deutoneuron branches originate in one average glomerulus (9) ; conversely one deutoneuron is connected to up to six different glomeruli. The deutoneuron somata are clustered in a few limited areas peripheral to the deutocerebral neuropile ; one counts 7,000 of them in the bee (54), 1,200 in the cockroach and 950 in the locust (9). By comparison with the few hundreds of efferents in the T.O.G., these figures demonstrate that most of them (2/3 in *Periplaneta*) are interneurons whose processes are overlapping large areas of the sensory lobe, up to five glomeruli each (9). Pre-and post-synaptic sites in the same terminal branches suggest self-inhibitory loops (42).

The high degree of convergence which characterizes deutoneurons is not distributed in correlation with chemical selectivity of antennal fibers, it is rather a random process as it is clearly shown by electrophysiological findings (5, 52). Such a random convergence is obviously needed to increase the signal-to-noise ratio, and takes advantage with the highest possible effectiveness of probabilistic summation of single unit temporal pattern of firing. Moreover, randomness of connections minimizes the distorsion of the spatial pattern of incoming information.

Once "clean" information has been conveyed in a reduced pool of deutoneurons there is still a need to make it "sharper" and to protect it against intensity variations. This function is achieved by the local neuronal network which is responsible for inhibition. Interneuron branches take part in glomerular synaptic connections in opposite directions ; the same ending is altogether post-synaptic in excitatory junctions and pre-synaptic in inhibitory ones (42, 56, 3, 5).

They are therefore able to simultaneously generate self-inhibition which narrows the dynamic range of glomerular output and stabilizes it against large variations of input intensity, and lateral inhibition which enhances the intensity contrast between adjacent glomeruli.

Such a huge inhibition would have, if alone, the disavantage of lowering too much the intensity level of the output. The convergence of many excitatory glomerular outputs onto the same deutoneuron should fortunately have an opposite effect.

2. SECOND RELAY OF THE AFFERENT ANTENNAL PATHWAY : THE CORPORA PEDUNCULATA
(Fig.1)

Symetrically located in both sides of the brain and typically subdivided into calyx, pedunculus, α and β-lobe, the corpora pedunculata (C.P.) were first described in the bee (8).

Their size and shape are positively correlated with the prevalence of sensory antennal input in functional, behavioural and social performances of the insect (53, 14). A reduced C.P. is thus correlated with reduced sensory deutocerebrum (1, 35, 18). Among all anatomical descriptions, few are available in specific techniques, and few have been made with the goal of a detailed description of connectivity (11, 15, 34, 40, 41, 53,13, 44). Presently,their function is still not well established with adequate physiological experiments (17).

2.1. Afferent and efferent organization

The major input fibers come from the two bundles of the T.O.G.. One coming from the deutocerebrum ("antennal-glomerular tract") ; the other, partly from the anterior part of the tritocerebrum, partly from the sub-oesophageal ganglia : "tritocerebral tract" (18).

Degeneration experiments, silver impregnation (18, 49, 41, 53, 9), procion yellow injection (45) and electrophysiological recordings (50, 29, 30, 46) have demonstrated that the bulk of efferent deutoneurons forms the larger bundles of the T.O.G. (700 fibers in *Locusta* (9) versus 1,200 in the whole T.O.G.); some processes of primary antennal neurons are directly connected with the C.P. (33, 45).

The other T.O.G. bundle is composed by processes coming from the lobus glomeratus of the tritocerebrum which receives its inputs mainly from the contact chemoreceptors of the maxillary palps (300 fibers in *Locusta*). Similarly

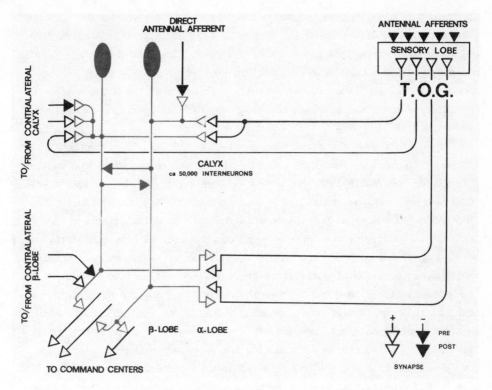

Figure 1. Intrinsic,afferent and efferent synaptical organization of
the second relay of the afferent antennal pathway.

to the antennal afferents, direct inputs from labral sensory cells into the
C.P. have been demonstrated by cobalt chloride injections in locusts (20, 55).

A tract connects calyces and β-lobes on both sides of the brain (49, 34,
46, 44).

The efferent system originates from β-lobe which is connected with the
main motor command center implied into motor programming triggered by antennal and buccal chemical input.

There are processes to the ipsilateral motor lobe of deutocerebrum, to
ipsi- and contralateral side of sub-oesophageal ganglia (33).

2.2. Interneurons, synaptic organization, functional implications

The fiber system of C.P. consists of intrinsic processes of the globuli-cells bodies (interneurons) of the calyx which make contacts with extrinsic fibers in calyx and α and β-lobe(53, 44). The development of the C.P. is
due to an increase of the globuli-cells number and of their dentritic arbo-
rizations in the calyx (54).

In the calyx, only a few hundreds of afferents diverge on the numerous processes of globuli-cells (2.10^5 to 5.10^5) (32, 41, 44). In the calyx, the cell-bodies are organized in groups of different sizes and send their parallel grouping processes of different diameters (0.1 to 1 µm in *Acheta*) in the pedunculus where each fiber is symetrically decussated in the α and β-lobe ; the inter-neuronal system has a conspicuously orderly spatial organization (22, 41, 14).

Fine studies of the nerve endings (10, 34, 39, 41, 53, 44) demonstrate that some fibers form feed-back loops in the calyx. Interneuron processes are directly or indirectly inter-connected in such a reciprocal way that every input sensory fiber is potentially connected with every output fiber. That only a limited number of possible connections are actually effective, means that some selective process must take place. Moreover if some plasticity could be evidenced, the same process should account for it. This device realizes the final integration of qualitative chemical information into its output.

Contrasting with α and β-lobe, the calyx lacks any visible spatial patterning, it looks like if every incoming T.O.G. fiber had an equal chance to connect numerous intrinsic neurons. This would result in loosing the qualitative features while evenly distributing the summated intensity information. Such a non-specific activation of the whole C.P. properly damped by inhibition should result in strengthening the activation pattern in α and β-lobes through excitatory synaptic cooperation in every involved neuron.

The motor output lasts usually longer than the sensory input. This implies that some re-entry plays a role in refreshing the trigger input. This function is quite in accordance with the anatomical findings (10, 42) which describe reciprocal excitatory synapses between T.O.G. fibers and intrinsic neurons in the α-lobe. If the commissure between calyces on both sides was reciprocally inhibitory, it would be in the right place to account for orientation behaviour by respect to concentration gradient of odorant.

For BULLOCK and HORRIDGE (7), plasticity is the "ability to be modified "or changed. Usually plasticity is an inferred property (mechanism unspeci-"fied) of a nervous system which can make an adaptive change in activity".

The plasticity of neurons has been examined as a function of complex stimulus sequences derived from learning paradigms (19).

Chemical synapses are the best candidates for explaining plasticity of neuronal networks : as a result of previous activity, they can undergo short-term alterations of functional effectiveness : these changes, lasting from minutes to hours, can be regarded as a form of information storage.

Habituation is certainly the simplest and most common form of plasticity and, KANDEL (19), assumes that it is possible to establish in theory " a hierarchy of learning using habituation as a basic building block... Habituation is learning to recognize, and ignore as familiar, recurrent external or internal stimuli" and provides therefore a quite attractive interpretation of learning processes as a gradual elimination of all but the reinforced responses (not stimuli).

Keeping these assumptions in mind, a second view on the olfactory brain should help us to decide whether its functional plasticity is diffusely distributed or restricted to a particular area (Fig.2).

The deutocerebrum is a highly convergent structure with only partial overlapping of adjacent fiber synaptic fields. Virtually no change can consequently occur in its connectivity and it looks rather a wired logic with a constant output to input relationship.

The C.P. are, on the contrary, a highly divergent - highly convergent structure, with a densely interwoven fiber network resulting in a fully versatile output to input correspondence, provided some device selects the appro-

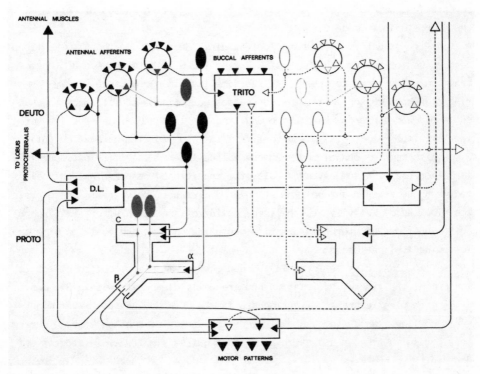

Figure 2. Schematic representation of the functional implications of the afferent antennal information flow.

priate combination of synapses among countless equiprobable possibilities. There is however a striking difference in this respect between the calyces and the α and β-lobes : the calyces display a fully integrative and non-specific organization whereas α and β-lobes look like a switch-board with a perpendicular input and a parallel output.

As the inputs to calyx and α-lobe are synchronous duplicates, one is tempted to assume that the non-selective facilitation generated by calyx strengthens only these synapses which are simultaneously activated by these inputs throughout the α and β-lobes.

Regular spatial arrangement of fibers in α and β-lobes is a tremendous improvement : it increases the probability of similar but not identical inputs resulting, in direct relation to the amount of similarity, in one and the same output, and this is really close to intelligent behaviour !

Some experimental evidences clearly support the idea that neuronal plasticity is relevant to insect olfactory behaviour and that it is mainly located in C.P..

In fact, there are few experiments of local lesions at the CNS level, nevertheless some of them (51, 31) seem to show a trend in the direction of the proposed above model.

After olfactory discrimination training, sectioning either T.O.G. fibers between deutocerebrum and calyx of C.P., or T.O.G. fibers between deutocerebrum and α-lobe does not result in the same loss in performance : only severing of fibers connected with α-lobe causes performance to fall back to chance level, and suggests that the memory trace is in the C.P. and requires an input via the α-lobe or a signal out from the lobe for its activation (51).

With simple conditioned response a true lateral specifity of odour information has been demonstrated (31) :the conditioned response was only elicited when the trained antenna was stimulated. Furthermore, direct and reversible blocking of activity by localized cooling of the brain after training results in a loss of stored information, depending on time and position, with the following implications :

– no plasticity is found in the deutocerebrum, since cooling effect is maximum at the time of stimulation and gradually disappears within 2-3 min.

– no plastic change either occurs in the C.P. during this first minute since cooling results in chance level performance. Information storage during this period must be in a dynamic form and requires simultaneous integrity of deutocerebrum and C.P..

– plastic changes responsible for olfactory learning start in the α-lobe of the C.P. by the end of the first minute following reinforced C.S. presentation, and need about 5 minutes to be completed.

Knowing where and when the plastic changes associated with olfactory learning occur, the next question concerns the discriminatory power of the system. Other experiments (47) bring conclusive evidence in this respect : provided enough reinforcement is given, a bee always succeeds in discriminating odours in associative learning irrespective to their quality proximity.

As far as plastic behaviour refers to habituation processes, preliminary data on group responses of gregarious cockroach, *Blaberus craniifer*, to an attractive odour (congener) and to an aversive one (cumarin) give some indications on the time course of extinction phenomena. Not reinforced responses to aversive stimulus fall back to chance level within one week whereas attractiveness needs more than two weeks to decrease significantly (26).

Supported by CNRS : ERA 623 and RCP 349

REFERENCES
(1) BALDUS, K.(1924) Z. Wiss. Zool., 121, 557-620
(2) BOECKH, J.(1974) J. Comp. Physiol., 90, 183-205
(3) BOECKH, J.(1975) Proceedings IUSSI, Symposium Dijon, 155-172
(4) BOECKH, J.J., SANDRI, C., AKERT, K. (1970)Z. Zellforsch. Mikrosk., Anat., 103, 429-446
(5) BOECKH, J., ERNEST, K.D., SASS, H., WALDOW, U.(1974) in Olfaction and Taste V (Denton ed.) 239-245
(6) BOECKH, J., ERNEST, K.D., SASS, H., WALDOW, U.(1976) Verh. Dtsch. Zool. Ges., (G. Fisher ed.) 123-139
(7) BULLOCK, T.H., HORRIDGE, G.A.(1965) in Structure and Function in the Nervous System of Invertebrates, Sans Francisco-Freeman
(8) DUJARDIN, F.(1850) Ann. Sci. Nat.(Zool.) 14, 195-206
(9) ERNST, K.D., BOECKH, J., BOECKH, V.(1977) Cell. Tiss. Res.,176, 285-308
(10) FRONTALI, N., MANCINI, G.J.(1970) Insect Physiol., 16, 2293-2301
(11) GOLL, W.(1967) Z. Morph. Tiere, 59, 143-210
(12) HANSTROM, B.(1928) in Vergleichende Anatomic des Nervensystems der wirbellosen Tiere, Berlin, Springer
(13) HONEGGER, F. W., SCHURMANN, F.W.(1975) Cell Tissue Res., 159, 213-225
(14) HOWSE, P.E.(1974) in Experimental Analysis of Insect Behaviour (Barton Brown, ed.) 180-194
(15) HOWSE, P.E., WILLIAMS, J.L.D.(1969) Proc. VI Congr. IUSSI, Bern, 59-64
(16) HOYLE, G.J.(1975) Exp. Zool., 194, 51-73
(17) HUBER, F.(1974) in Physiology of Insects IV, 4-101 (Rockstein ed.)
(18) JAWLOWSKI, H.(1963) Acta Anat., 53, 346-359
(19) KANDEL, E.R.(1976) Cellular Basis of Behaviour (Freeman ed.) 548 p.
(20) KLEMM, N.(1976) Progress in Neurobiology, 7, 99-169
(21) LAND, L.J., SHEPHERD, G.M.(1974) Brain Research, 70, 506-510
(22) MASSON, C.(1970) Z. Zellforsch.. 106, 220-231
(23) MASSON, C.(1972) Z. Zellforsch., 134, 31-64
(24) MASSON, C.(1973) These Doctorat Etat. Univ. Provence 8303, 332 p.
(25) MASSON, C.(1974) Proceedings ECRO Congress, Orsay
(26) MASSON, C., POUGALAN, M.(1976) Proceedings ECRO Congress, Reading
(27) MASSON, C., STRAMBI, C.(1977) J. of Neurobiology (in press)
(28) MASSON, C., CHAMBILLE, I., ROSPARS, J.P. unpublished

(29) MAYNARD, D.M.(2962) Amm. Zoologist, 2, 79-96
(30) MAYNARD, D.M.(1967) in Invertebrate Nervous System, their significance for mammalian neurophysiology (Wiersma ed.) 231-255
(31) MENZEL, R., ERBER, J., MASUHR, T.(1974) in Experimental Analysis of Insect Behaviour (Barton Brown, ed.) 195-217
(32) NEDER, R.(1959) Zool. Jb (allg. Zool. Physiol.) 77, 411-464
(33) PARETO, A.(1972) Z. Zellforsch., 131, 109-140
(34) PEARSON, L.(1971) Phil. Trans. R. Soc., 259, 477-516
(35) PFLUGFELDER, O.(1937) Zoologica, 93, 1-102
(36) PINCHING, A.J., POWELL, T.P.S.(1971) J. Cell Sci., 9, 347-377
(37) POWER, M.E.(1946) J. Comp. Neurol., 85, 485-517
(38) RALL, W.(1970) in The Neurosciences, 2nd Study Program (Schmitt ed.) 552-565
(39) SCHURMANN, F.W.(1971) Brain Res., 26, 169-176
(40) SCHURMANN, F.W.(1972) Z. Zellforsch., 127, 240-257
(41) SCHURMANN, F.W.(1973) Z. Zellforsch., 145, 247-285
(42) SCHURMANN, F.W., WECHSLER, W.(1970) Z. Zellforsch., 108, 563-581
(43) SHEPHERD, G.M.(1970) in the Neurosciences, 2nd Study Program (Schmitt ed.), 539-552
(44) STRAUSFELD, N.J.(1976) Atlas of an Insect Brain, Springer, Berlin
(45) SUZUKI, H.(1974) J. Insect Physiol., 21, 831-847
(46) SUZUKI, H., TATEDA, H.(1974) J. Insect Physiol., 20, 2287-2299
(47) VARESCHI, E.(1971) Z. Vergl. Physiologie, 75, 143-173
(48) Von FRISCH, K.(1967) The Dance language and orientation of bees, Belknap Press, Harvard, 566 p.
(49) VOWLES, D.M.(1965) Q.J. Microsc. Sci., 96, 239-255
(50) VOWLES, D.M.(1961) in Current Problems in Animal Behaviour (Thorpe and Zangwill ed.) 5-29
(51) VOWLES, D.M.(1964) J. Comp. Physiol. Psych., 58, 105-111
(52) WALDOW, U.(1975) J. Comp. Physiol., 101, 329-341
(53) WEISS, M.J.(1974) J. Morph., 142, 21-69
(54) WITTHOFT, W.(1967) Z. Morph., Tiere, 61, 160-184
(55) WILLEY, R.B.(1961) J. Morph., 108, 219-261
(56) YAMADA, M.J.(1971) J. Physiol., (Lond.) 214, 127-143
(57) a) in bee and cockroach, some afferents reach directly the motor lobe (33, 45, 9) where direct synaptic contacts between sensory and motor fibers, without intermediate interneuron, occur thus permitting mono-synaptic reflexes ;
b) others go directly to the first thoracic ganglia (33) ;
c) some fibers can reach directly the protocerebrum, either near the giant ocellar fibers, or in the calyx of C.P. (45, 9).

Further data on the topography and physiology of central olfactory neurons in insects

J. Boeckh, V. Boeckh, A. Kühn

Institut für Zoologie, Universität Regensburg, Regensburg, GFR

INTRODUCTION.

In certain insects as e.g. in Periplaneta americana the antennal
olfactory receptor cells are - according to their odor spectra
- grouped in a limited number of receptor cell types (Sass,
1976, and this vol.). Recently, it could be demonstrated that
functionally defined types are localized in defined morphological types of antennal sensilla (Altner et al. 1977, and this
vol.). This fortunate situation allows one to record purposely
and reproducibly from cells of certain properties, and gives
hope that, finally, one gets a complete picture of receptor
activity in the whole olfactory organ for **every** odor tested.
A similar knowledge of morphological identity on the one hand,
and physiological property on the other hand, is lacking at the level
of the central olfactory pathways. Here, conventional as well
as experimental neuroanatomy together with neurophysiology revealed a rather coarse and preliminary picture of connections
and pathways in the parts of the brain which are connected to
antennal inputs (for summary see Ernst et al., 1977, and Masson
this vol.).

For a combined morphological and electrophysiological identification of constituents of neuronal pathways dye injection
methods have been useful tools during the last decade. In the
case of the insect olfactory pathway, pheromone inputs seem to
be most suited for such an investigation: Firstly, a defined
and biologically significant odor can be presented which is an
efficient stimulus for a great number of receptor cells, and
which gives rise to considerable central activity. Secondly,

the only populations of central olfactory neurons which - until
now - can be defined as reaction types with predictable and homogeneous odor spectra are (1) the type Ia neurons in males of
Periplaneta americana, responding to odors from female colonies
(Boeckh et al., 1976, Waldow, 1977), and (2) certain neurons in
the deutocerebrum of male saturniid moths responding to the female lure substances (see below).

TOPOGRAPHY OF A SPECIFIC OLFACTORY PATHWAY.

From Sass (this vol.) we know that in male cockroaches receptor
cells for female odors are housed in a defined antennal sensillum type with single walls and pore-tubule-systems (cf.
Altner, this vol.). After cutting a number of these sensilla
and immersing the stumps in 6 % $CoCl_2$, cobalt precipitates can
be observed in certain regions of the deutocerebrum, especially
in a "macroglomerulus" of the dorsolateral portion of the deuto
-cerebrum (fig. 1).
This glomerulus was described by Jawlowski (1954) as specialty
of the deutocerebrum of adult male Periplaneta americana.

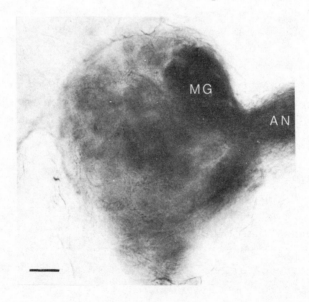

Fig. 1. Periplaneta americana ♂, left hand deutocerebrum, frontal view. Cobalt stain invaded the brain from the cut stumps
of sensilla of ipsilateral antenna, housing receptors for female odors. AN, antennal nerve; MG, "macroglomerulus"; bar
length 100 μm.

Schaller (1977) could correlate the size and the occurrence of this glomerulus with the development of the sensilla which house receptors for female odors. The cobalt probably was taken up by the cut processes of the sensory cells underlying the cut sensilla, and transported via the cells'processes to the deuto-cerebrum. It looks, therefore, as if the "macroglomerulus" is the (or one) site of primary projection from sensilla housing receptors for the female odors.

As Waldow has shown (1977), type Ia neurons in the male deuto-cerebrum respond to odors from female colonies. After injection of 30 % $Co(NO_3)_2$ from a microelectrode during or after record-ing extracellularly from such a neuron, cobalt precipitates again in the "macroglomerulus", indicating that the cobalt was transported via the cell's process from or near the recording site towards the terminal (and other) regions of the neuron. Figure 2 shows the result of the procedure. Only one neuron was observed in the recording but several took up the dye into their somata and processes.

It is not clear whether all these neurons are of type Ia or which one might be the neuron which was observed in the recor-ding. All of them, however, seem to project into the "macroglo-

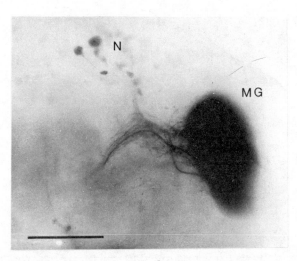

Fig. 2. Periplaneta americana ♂, left hand deutocerebrum, fron-tal view. Marking of "macroglomerulus" with cobalt dye injec-ted via microelectrode recording from a type Ia neuron.
MG, "macroglomerulus"; N, somata of neurons; bar length 100 /um

merulus", which clearly is the site of connection between receptor cells for female odors and type Ia neurons. After intensification of the cobalt stain using Timm's method according to Tyrer and Bell (1974), one can trace processes of type Ia neurons into the tractus olfactorio-globularis right into the calyces and the lateral protocerebral lobe (fig. 3). These regions have been described as terminal areas of deutocerebral neurons by Ernst et al. (1977), but only by injection the final proof could be accomplished. Further details about the connections of these neurons remain to be studied.

THE ROLE OF SPATIAL CONVERGENCE.

One of the most simple modes of connections between receptor cells and central neurons in the olfactory pathway of insects

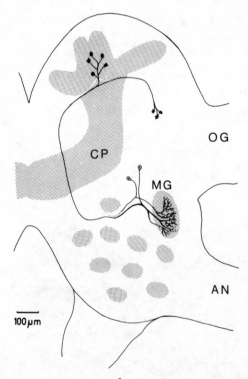

Fig. 3. Periplaneta americana ♂. Camera lucida drawing of left hand half of the brain, frontal view. Staining with cobalt injected via microelectrode recording from a type Ia neuron. AN, antennal nerve; CP, corpus pedunculatum; MG, "macroglomerulus"; OG, optic ganglia.

is the spatial convergence by which a high number of receptors
is connected to a low number of relay neurons (Boeckh, 1974).
In Periplaneta americana more than 150.000 olfactory receptors
are connected to less than 250 neurons leaving the deutocerebrum (Boeckh et al., 1975). Another example for such a convergence is in certain male saturniids where the majority of antennal olfactory receptor cells are designed to receive female
pheromone odors (Schneider et al., 1964, Kaissling, 1974).
There are neurons in the deutocerebrum of such a saturniid
moth, Antheraea pernyi, and also in A. polyphemus, the dendrites of which embrace a whole region of neuropil in the deutocerebrum near the entrance of the antennal nerve (fig. 4). This
might be another example for a "macroglomerulus". The neurons
are in very low number and respond very sensitively to pheromone odors. Kaissling (pers. comm.) and Zack (this vol.) report
that the antennal receptor cells of A. pernyi respond significantly to 10^{-4} /ug of trans-6,cis-11-hexadecadienal at the
stimulus source, which is one of the major components of the
female lure gland. Deutocerebral neurons respond already at
10^{-6} /ug at the odor source (fig. 5). At this concentration only a few receptor cells of the whole set will fire a few impul-

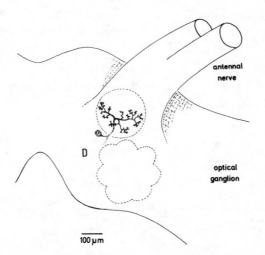

Fig. 4. Antheraea pernyi ♂. Camera lucida drawing of the brain,
frontal view, after cobalt injection via microelectrode recording from a neuron responding to female pheromone compound.
D, deutocerebrum.

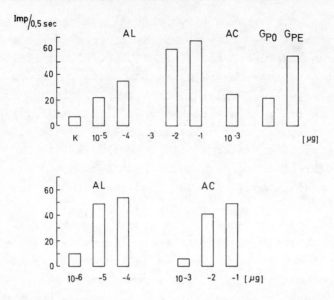

Fig. 5. Antheraea pernyi ♂. Reactions of two deutocerebral neurons to different concentrations of trans-6,cis-11-hexadecadienal (AL), the corresponding dienylacetate (AC), a female lure gland of the same species (G-PE), and of a closely related species (A. polyphemus, G-PO). Stimulus strength given as amount of substance at odor source. K, control stimulus.

ses altogether (Kaissling, pers.comm.). Apparently, such a deuto-cerebral neuron collects inputs from many receptor cells and hence responds with considerable excitation at such a low concentration. In this aspect the deutocerebral olfactory neurons of insects work similar to the wide field neurons in the visual pathway which collect inputs from many visual cells allowing a safe detection of low intensity stimuli at the central level.

REFERENCES.

Altner, H., Sass, H., Altner, I. (1977) Cell Tiss. Res. 176, 389-405
Boeckh, J. (1974), J. comp. Physiol. 90, 183-205
Boeckh, J., Ernst, K.D., Sass, H., Waldow, U. (1975), in Olfaction and Taste V, pp. 239-245 Academic Press, New York.
Boeckh, J., Ernst, K.D., Sass, H., Waldow, U. (1976), Verh. Dtsch. Zool. Ges. 1976, 123-139
Jawlowski, H. (1954), Ann. Univ. M. Curie-Slodowska, Lublin, 8 C, 403-434
Kaissling, K.E. (1974), in Biochemistry of Sensory Functions, pp. 243-273, Springer-Verlag, Heidelberg

Sass, H. (1976), J. comp. Physiol. 107, 49-65
Schaller, D. (1977), Ph. D. Thesis, Naturwiss. Fak. Univ.Wien
Schneider, D., Lacher, V., Kaissling, K.E. (1964), Z. vergl.
Physiol. 48, 632-662
Tyrer, N.M., Bell, E.B. (1974), Brain Res. 73, 151-155
Waldow, U. (1977), J. comp. Physiol. 116, 1-17

Gustatory sensing of complex mixed stimuli by insects

V. G. Dethier

Department of Zoology, Morrill Science Center, University of Massachusetts, Amherst, MA 01003, USA

ABSTRACT

Gustatory stimuli encountered in nature are seldom pure compounds. For plant feeding insects especially they are complex mixtures. Perception of these involves integration both at the peripheral and central level. Peripheral factors affecting perception of mixtures are: number and kinds of specifically different receptors, band width of each receptor, character of each tuning curve, absolute threshold and rate of adaptation, and synergism and inhibition. Different insects have different kinds and numbers of receptor primaries. A comparison of the electrophysiological responses of various caterpillars and the blowfly to leaf saps reveals that the majority of caterpillar receptors are activated by most saps and most fly receptors are inactive. In almost all cases a salt receptor is responsive. These results lend support to a pattern hypothesis of perception. The relative silence of the fly receptors is explained in terms of specificity and band widths of receptors.

INTRODUCTION

From the beginning, investigations of the gustatory senses have been shaped, and to a degree, constrained by the concept of four primary taste qualities as perceived by man. Thus, experimenters have invariably used, in addition to water, four compounds that evoke the classical four tastes: a salt, an acid, a sugar, and quinine. Only more recently has the list of pure compounds been extended [23,30].

This approach has served well for identifying the number of different kinds of receptors and for studying transducing mechanisms. In nature, however the gustatory stimuli encountered are seldom pure compounds. For most animals natural stimuli are extraordinarily complex solutions. Accordingly the results of investigations involving pure compounds, even when they are naturally occurring components of food, do not reflect the true sensory capacity of an animal. They may provide an exaggerated picture in the sense that they overemphasize the role of labeled lines in gustatory perception or a diminished one in the sense that by implication they oversimplify complexities of peripheral and central integration.

The complexities of the perception of mixtures is strikingly disclosed by comparing the responses of insects that can detect the same pure compounds but respond differently to mixtures. To this end a comparative electrophysiological study has been made of the blowfly Phormia regina and several species of lepidopterous larvae especially the eastern tent caterpillar, Malacosoma americanum.

DETERMINANTS IN THE SENSING OF MIXTURES

The sensing of mixtures depends upon a multiplicity of peripheral and central factors. Unfortunately analyses of central phenomena are still beset with great technical difficulties. It appears that little progress will be made until central interneurons can be monitored electrophysiologically as Boeckh and Suzuki are now doing with the olfactory system or until computer analyses can be made of the total integrated sensory input to the central nervous system[2-4,31,32]. This presentation is concerned with peripheral events only.

At the peripheral level sensing capacity is determined by: the number and kinds of specifically different receptors, the band width of each receptor, the character of each tuning curve, the absolute threshold and the time course (adaptation) of response, the capacity of the receptor to engage in synergistic and inhibitory interactions with multiple compounds. Some of these parameters have been discussed elsewhere , and will be alluded to only briefly here[12,23,30].

NUMBER AND KINDS OF RECEPTORS

As soon as one looks beyond terrestrial vertebrates it becomes apparent that the variety of gustatory receptors is considerable. Insects possess many qualitatively different kinds. All species examined have receptors sensitive to salt[11]; many have water receptors; sugar receptors are common; however, beyond these basic types no generalization is possible. The commercial silk worm (Bombyx mori) has three receptors for salts, one for deterrents (miscellaneous compounds evoking aversive reactions), one for sucrose and glucose, one for glucose alone, one for inositol, and one for water[15]. Larvae of the cabbage butterfly (Pieris brassicae) have two receptors for salt, one for glucosinolates (mustard oil glycosides), one for glucotropaeolin and sinalbin, one for sugars, one for amino acids, one for anthocyanins, and one for deterrents[23,24,25]. The tobacco hornworm (Manduca sexta) has two receptors for salt, one for deterrents, one for salicin, one for sugars, and two for inositol. Tent caterpillars (Malacosoma americanum) have receptors for salts, sugars, inositol, amino acids, and water (?). The leaf-feeding beetle,

<u>Chrysolina brunsvicensis</u>, has, in addition to other receptors, one that is specific for hypericin[19]. <u>Phormia</u> <u>regina</u> has two salt receptors, a sugar receptor, and a water receptor. Thus, in the six species combined there are twelve qualitatively different receptors. This means that more and different compounds can be sensed than a universal application of the concept of four taste primaries would allow.

BAND WIDTHS

Although the receptors mentioned in the preceding paragraphs are designated by specific names, they are usually not restricted in their sensitivities to the categorizing compounds. The action spectra or band widths vary from very narrow specificities to broad sensitivities. Some of the reported differences in band widths may be spurious and represent differences in the band widths of the experiments rather than of the receptors themselves. Nevertheless, even our incomplete knowledge indicates that many of the differences are real.

The water receptor of <u>Phormia,</u> for example, has a very narrow specificity. Some investigators have suggested that it is actually a receptor sensitive to low (<0.1 M) concentrations of salts because these are what it encounters in nature. However true this may be, the cell is a water receptor in that pure water is an adequate stimulus. Triply distilled deionized water with a conductivity of less than one micromho stimulates maximally as does also 99.8% D_2O of comparable purity. The conclusion that ions supplied endogenously are required to depolarize the neuron does not negate the fact that this receptor and only this receptor responds to ambient water. (It also responds to some non-physiological compounds, e.g. the anesthetic halothane[10].)

Sugar receptors are less rigidly specific. Generally they respond to several sugars, sugar derivatives, and some amino acids. Within this spectrum, however, there is a high level of specificity. Particular molecular structures, as, for example, pyranoside and furanoside configurations, may be limiting.

Glucosinolate receptors are characterized by rather narrow band widths restricted to compounds in or related to this particular glycoside category[17, 24,33]. The hypericin and salicin receptors appear to be restricted to their signature compounds, but extensive analyses of band widths have not been made.

Salt receptors and deterrent receptors have broad band widths. The former respond not only to many salts but to organic acids, some amino acids, and some glycosides. The latter respond to a wide variety of unrelated compounds including acids, glycosides, alkaloids, and terpenes.

In general, as we have come to realize, specificity, that is, band width, is a relative character and attention must be paid to its finer details.

TUNING CURVES

Points of maximal sensitivity in response spectra can be compared quantitatively and qualitatively. In the first instance two receptors could be sensitive to exactly the same range of compounds, sucrose, fructose, and glucose, for example; yet, one could be maximally sensitive to fructose and the other to glucose.

In the second instance the family of compounds to which each receptor responds might be entirely different except for one compound to which each is maximally sensitive. A comparison of the sugar receptors of Phormia and man illustrates this point. Only the latter are sensitive to saccharin, cyclamates, and monellin.

ABSOLUTE SENSITIVITY AND ADAPTATION

There are many examples of differences in thresholds among receptors that are similar in other respects. Stimulus fractionation accomplished by having one receptor which responds to low concentrations and another to high concentrations of the same compound, adds another dimension of discrimination to the sensory system.

Less attention has been paid to the effect of adaptation on discrimination. Under continuous stimulation, as usually occurs during feeding, different compounds induce different rates of adaptation in a receptor, and different receptors do not adapt at the same rate to a given compound. Rates of adaptation are particularly important when considering sensory coding and discrimination as Schoonhoven has so clearly described[25].

PERIPHERAL INTERACTIONS

Considerable interaction of stimuli is possible at the peripheral level. Both synergism and inhibition involving individual receptors have been demonstrated. Mannose inhibits fructose at the sugar receptor of Phormia; glucose and fructose act synergistically. Inhibition occurs between salicin and caffeine at the salicin receptor of Manduca[25].

Other types of interactions involve enhancement of the stimulating effectiveness of sucrose on Phormia when NaCl is present[6], inhibition of the water receptor by ions above a critical concentration[20], and by osmotic effects of non-electrolytes[13], inhibition of the sugar receptor by high concentrations of salt and of the salt receptor by high concentrations of sugar. Synergistic interactions involving amino acids and sugars and sinigrin and sugar have been demonstrated behaviorally[17], but the site of action, whether peripheral or central has not been identified.

REACTIONS TO MIXTURES

When a population of receptors is stimulated with pure single compounds, all of the aforementioned phenomena interact to generate complicated multi-fiber patterns of activity. When the stimulus is a mixture of compounds, the complexity of the interaction is enormously increased as the following two cases illustrate.

Responses of Caterpillars to Leaf Saps   Leaf saps are among the most complex natural chemical mixtures known. In addition to water, carbohydrates, salts and amino acids they contain an extraordinary variety of secondary substances[1,24]. When caterpillars bite leaves, the gustatory receptors of the maxillae and epipharynx are bathed in these mixtures. In the majority of cases more than one, often three or four, cells in each of the two maxillary and epipharyngeal sensilla, respond[5,7,28]. Tomato sap, the preferred food of Manduca, generally stimulates three cells in each sensillum of that species although considerable variation from one larva to the next is usual[27]. Cherry and apple, the preferred foods of Malacosoma, also stimulate three and sometimes four maxillary cells in that species.

Considering the fact that the two maxillary sensilla of caterpillars have different complements of receptors and that the total number of receptor species ranges from six to eight, the results of electrophysiological tests (note that each sensillum is tested individually) indicate that plant saps may stimulate the entire complement. When fewer than eight cells respond, it is difficult to ascertain which. In only a few instances is it known which component or components of the sap constitute the stimulus. One cell that responds in nearly every case is that one which, when tested with pure compounds, responds preferentially to salt[7]. This is not surprising considering the ionic composition of the saps. On the other hand, the universal presence of water does not always cause water receptors to respond because ions and non-electrolytes are often sufficiently concentrated to inhibit them. Similarly carbohydrates can pass undetected because of inhibition by other compounds.

The Response of Phormia to Foods and Non-Foods   The mixtures that the blowfly normally encounters are nectars, fermenting plant and fruit juices containing carbohydrates, salts, amino acids, esters, aldehydes, et cetera and decomposing proteinaceous material containing amino acids, fatty acids, peptides, salts et cetera. To all of these the gustatory responses consist of activity of one to four cells[8].

Although the blowfly does not feed on leaf saps, it is instructive to examine electrophysiologically its responses to these mixtures because our knowledge of its gustatory system is so extensive. Altogether 59 species of plants representing 35 families were tested on the labellar hairs. The plants were chosen to include gymnosperms, mono- and dicotyledons, plants containing toxic compounds, and those with high cencentrations of aromatic chemicals.

Surprisingly, 83% of the species stimulated only the classical salt receptor. Salt and water cells responded to 10.2% of the species, three cells to 5.1%, and four cells to 1.7%. With one exception (Rumex Acetosella) the salt cell responded in every case.

GENERAL CONSIDERATIONS

Three observations emerge from these studies. First, the responses of all insects to their foods and to materials that they might normally be expected to encounter in searching for food (e.g., non-host plants for caterpillars) involve the activity of many or all of the receptors comprising the gustatory complement. Second, activity of the salt cell is almost universal. Third, the response of the blowfly to leaf saps is generally not multineuronal.

1. At first glance it is not surprising that many kinds of receptors respond to foods containing mixtures of compounds. This fact together with the behavioral observation that different foods can be discriminated lends further support to the hypothesis that meaning is embodied in the total sensory pattern. There is much to support this idea, but it is not without its weaknesses [7,8]. At a very elementary level the experimenter can relate patterns to behavior by assuming that all positive (e.g., sugar, water, etc.) and all negative (e.g., deterrents) add simply. Thus, an unacceptable mixture may be made acceptable by adding an excess of sugar, and an acceptable mixture may be rendered unacceptable by adding a deterrent. It is clear from the preceding paragraphs that the situation is incredibly more complex. Not only the patterns themselves but also the factors that influence their generation await further analysis.

2. The ubiquity of the salt response may simply be a heritage from a primitive common chemical sense. Its necessity for protecting osmotic balance in the body fluids of insects is questionable [11]. It could play a significant role in the sensing of mixtures. If sensory patterns are distinctive codes, the code is going to change as the participating receptors adapt differentially and as the concentration of a mixture changes. In either of these circumstances a leaf sap could become a qualitatively different "taste" and be confused with another sap unless some compensating mechanism exists. It is

tentatively suggested that an omnipresent salt receptor could play such a
compensatory role by modifying a central set point as its own frequency of input changed with concentration or adaptation. Conceivably this could be accomplished by differential raising and lowering of central excitatory and
central inhibitory states.

  3. The "blindness" of the gustatory system of <u>Phormia</u> to the richness of
many leaf saps is not surprising because the fly does not encounter
leaf saps in nature though it is surprising considering the kinds and specificities of its receptors. It is sensitive to a considerable number of compounds[8,14,29]. The comparative silence of its system to plant saps indirectly provides some understanding of the active responses of caterpillars to
these saps.

REFERENCES

1. Bernays, E. A. and Chapman, R. F. (1967) Deterrent chemicals as a basis of
  oligophagy in <u>Locusta</u> <u>migratoria</u> (L.), Ecol. Ent.1, 1-18

2. Boeckh, J. (1974) Die Reaktionen olfaktorischer Neurone im Deutocerebrum
  von Insekten im Vergleich zu den Antwortmustern der Geruchssinneszellen,
  J. Comp. Physiol. 90, 183-205.

3. Boeckh, J. (1976) What can neurophysiology tell us about olfaction? In
  Structure-activity Relationships in Chemoreception (G. Benz ed.) pp.
  171-183, IRL, London

4. Boeckh, J. Ernst, K. D., Sass, H. and Waldow, U. (1975) Coding of odor
  quality in the insect olfactory pathway. In Olfaction and Taste V (D. A.
  Denton and J. P. Coghlan eds.), pp. 239-245, Academic Press, New York

5. de Boer, G., Dethier, V. G. and Schoonhoven, L. M. (1977) Chemoreceptors
  in the preoral cavity of the tobacco hornworm, <u>Manduca</u> <u>sexta</u>, and their
  possible function in feeding behavior, Ent. exp. appl. (in press)

6. Broyles, J. L., Hanson, F. E. and Shapiro, A. M. (1976) Ion dependence of
  the tarsal sugar receptor of the blowfly <u>Phormia</u> <u>regina</u>, J. Insect
  Physiol. 22, 1587-1600

7. Dethier, V. G. (1973) Electrophysiological studies of gustation in lepidopterous larvae. II Taste spectra in relation to food-plant discrimination. J. Comp. Physiol. 82, 103-134

8. Dethier, V. G. (1974) The specificity of the labellar chemoreceptors of
  the blowfly and the response to natural foods, J. Insect Physiol.20,
  1859-1869.

9. Dethier, V. G. (1976) The importance of stimulus patterns for host-plant
  recognition and acceptance, Symp. Biol. Hung. 16, 67-70

10. Dethier, V. G. (1976) Anesthetic stimulation of insect water receptors,
  Proc. Nat. Acad. U.S.A. 73, 3315-3319

11. Dethier, V. G. (1977) The taste of salt, Amer. Sci. (in press)

12. Dethier, V. G. (1978) Manheimer Lecture, Univ. Penn. Phila. (in press)

13. Evans, D. R. and Mellon, DeF. (1962) Electrophysiological studies of a water receptor associated with the taste senilla of the blowfly, J. Gen. Physiol. 45, 487-500

14. Goldrich, N. R. (1973) Behavioral responses of *Phormia regina* Meigen to labellar stimulation with amino acids, J. Gen Physiol. 61, 74-88

15. Ishikawa, S., Hirao, T. and Arai, N. (1969) Chemosensory basis of host-plant selection in the silkworm, Ent. exp. appl. 12, 544-554

16. Jermy, T. (1966) Feeding inhibitors and food preferences in chewing phytophagous insects, Ent. exp. appl. 9, 1012

17. Ma, W.-C. (1969) Some properties of gustation in the larva of *Pieris brassicae* L., Ent. exp. appl. 12, 584-590

18. Peters, J. H. (1968) Genetic factors in relation to drugs, Ann. Rev. Pharmacol. 8, 427-452

19. Rees, C. J. C. (1969) Chemoreceptor specificity associated with choice of feeding site by the beetle *Chrysolina brunsvicensis* on its foodplant *Hypericum hirsutum,* Ent. exp. appl. 12, 565-583

20. Rees, C. J. C. (1972) Responses of some sensory cells probably associated with the detection of water. In Olfaction and Taste IV (D. Schneider (ed.) pp. 88-94, Wiss. Verlag MBH, Stuttgart

21. Schoonhoven, L. M. (1967) Chemoreception of mustard oil glucosides in larvae of *Pieris brassicae*. Koninkl. Nederl. Akad. Wetenschappen Amstersam Proc. Ser. C, 70, 550-568

22. Schoonhoven, L. M. (1969) Amino-acid receptor in larvae of *Pieris brassicae* (Lepidoptera), Nature (London) 221, 1268

23. Schoonhoven, L. M. (1969) Gustation and foodplant selection in some lepidopterous larvae, Ent. exp. appl. 12, 555-564

24. Schoonhoven, L. M. (1972) Plant recognition by lepidopterous larvae, Symp. Roy. Ent Soc. London, 6, 87-99

25. Schoonhoven, L. M. (1972) Secondary plant substances and insects. In Structural and Functional Aspects of Phytochemistry (V. C. Runeckles and T. C. Tso eds.), pp. 197-224, Academic Press, New York

26. Schoonhoven, L. M. (1976) On the individuality of insect feeding behavior, (in press) Tours, France

27. Schoonhoven, L. M. (1976) On the variability of chemosensory information (in press)

28. Schoonhoven, L. M. and Dethier, V. G. (1966) Sensory aspects of host plant discrimination by lepidopterous larvae, Arch. Neerl. Zool. 16, 497-530

29. Shiraishi, A. and Kuwabara, M. (1970) The effects of amino acids on the labellar hair chemosensory cells of the fly, J. Gen Physiol. 56, 768-782

30. Staedler, E. (1976) Sensory aspects of insect plant interactions, Proc. XV internat. Congr. Ent. Washington, D.C. 228-248

31. Suzuki, H. (1975) Convergence of olfactory input from both antennae in the brain of the honeybee, J. Exp. Biol. 62, 11-28

32. Suzuki, H., Tateda, H. and Kuwabara, M. (1976) Activities of antennal and ocellar interneurons in the protocerebrum of the honey-bee, J. Exp. Biol. 64, 405-418

33. Wieczorek, H. (1976) The glycoside receptor of the larvae of Mamestra brassicae L. (Lepidoptera, Noctuidae), J. Comp. Physiol. 106, 153-176

Evolutionary potential of specialized olfactory receptors

Ernst Priesner

Max-Planck Institut für Verhaltensphysiologie, D-8131 Seewiesen, GFR

ABSTRACT

Response spectra of lepidopterous pheromone receptors reflecting their chemical specificities are considered with respect to (i) stepwise alterations between taxonomically closely-related species, and (ii) characteristics for higher taxa. There is a close formal similarity between certain structure-response relationships and the structural strategies of the receptors in their evolutionary transitions to new key compounds. The data are viewed in terms of a recent acceptor model.

INTRODUCTION

The olfactory systems of insect species are noted for their distinct types of odour specialist[1,2] cells of relatively uniform chemical specificities. Studies of these receptors are increasingly contributing to our understanding of basic chemoreception phenomena, e. g., the physicochemical mechanisms underlying the specificities of single olfactory cells[3-5], or the events in the sensory transduction of the chemical stimulus into the cellular response[6,7]. Here I will consider some aspects of interspecific, evolutionary alterations in homologous odour specialist receptors, affecting their chemical specificities.

For certain pheromone systems there is little doubt that the receptors have undergone such stepwise, interspecific changes. In a number of moth families the magnitude of interspecific electroantennogram responses to the female sexual pheromones has been shown[8-10] to decrease gradually with the degree of taxonomic separation (highest responses obtained within genera, and the lowest between different subfamilies). On the other hand, recent chemical analysis has revealed (i) the nature of the basic type of pheromone and the range of its modification for particular higher taxonomic groups, and (ii) distinct differences in the structures of pheromone molecules between taxonomic neighbours, suggesting evolutionary steps which have been preserved in these species. Both of these features will here be considered in terms

of chemical receptor specificity. Examples will be taken from the pheromone
receptor cells in the sensilla trichodea of male Lepidoptera.

RECEPTOR KEY COMPOUNDS

As in other insects, the sexual pheromones of lepidopterous species are
usually composed of several active components[11,12]. Correspondingly, several
types of receptors cells with respect to their key compounds may regularly be
found combined within a male sensillum trichodeum[6,9,13-19]. These multicomponent systems apparently can differentiate a broad variety of species-specific
signals by minute shifts in component proportions[12,20,21]. Here, those interspecies differences in these signals are considered which are reflected by
the altered molecular structures of certain components. Such alterations may
occur in the functional end group of the molecule, the length of certain chain
segments, or the number, position, and configuration of olefinic double bonds
(Fig. 1). However, as I will point it out, different moth families seem to use
different structural strategies in these stepwise, molecular modifications.

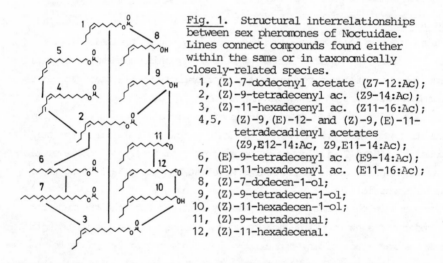

Fig. 1. Structural interrelationships
between sex pheromones of Noctuidae.
Lines connect compounds found either
within the same or in taxonomically
closely-related species.
1, (Z)-7-dodecenyl acetate (Z7-12:Ac);
2, (Z)-9-tetradecenyl ac. (Z9-14:Ac);
3, (Z)-11-hexadecenyl ac. (Z11-16:Ac);
4,5, (Z)-9,(E)-12- and (Z)-9,(E)-11-
      tetradecadienyl acetates
      (Z9,E12-14:Ac, Z9,E11-14:Ac);
6, (E)-9-tetradecenyl ac. (E9-14:Ac);
7, (E)-11-hexadecenyl ac. (E11-16:Ac);
8, (Z)-7-dodecen-1-ol;
9, (Z)-9-tetradecen-1-ol;
10, (Z)-11-hexadecen-1-ol;
11, (Z)-9-tetradecanal;
12, (Z)-11-hexadecenal.

Little is known of evolutionary capabilities of certain receptors often
quoted as paradigms of extreme specialization. In Bombyx mori, receptors for
bombykol[22] and those for the corresponding aldehyde, (E)-10,(Z)-12-hexadeca-
dienal (bombykal), seem to concur within each male sensillum trichodeum[23].
In Antheraea saturniids, a dienic acetate (Fig. 2a) and the corresponding aldehyde, both identified pheromone components[16], act on respective specialist
receptors[6,7,18]. Evolutionary modification of the Antheraea acetate has probably given rise to the isovalerate (Fig. 2b) peculiar to the phylogenetically-

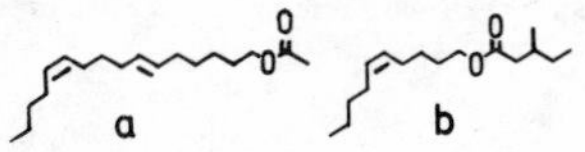

Fig. 2. Sex pheromones of Saturniidae.
a, (E)-6,(Z)-11-hexadecadienyl acetate;
b, (Z)-5-decenyl isovalerate.

advanced saturniid genus Nudaurelia[8,23]; twelve further pheromone structures indicated[8] in this subfamily, all related to the Antheraea components, await final identification.

RESPONSE SPECTRA REFLECTING RECEPTOR SPECIFICITY

The chemical specificity of an olfactory receptor cell is described by the set of dose-response curves to effective compounds[3-7,25]. Here, all statements refer to a standard level of cell excitation, given by the amplitude of the slow receptor potential to 0.001 µg of the single receptor key compound. For each analogue and receptor, the relative efficacy is thus presented by a single value indicating the stimulus amount (µg) required to elicit this standard response[26,27]. The total set of these values obtained on a given receptor is its response spectrum.

For the receptors for long-chain, olefinic pheromones discussed here, up to several hundreds of systematic, stepwise modifications may be required[26,27] to determine the similarities and differences in the chemical specificities between species, to define structure-response characteristics for higher tax-onomic groups, and to draw conclusions about acceptor interaction. In Fig. 3 are shown some relevant lines in the structural modification of (Z)-7-dodec-enyl acetate (Z7-12:Ac), the female pheromone of the cabbage looper moth, Trichoplusia ni[28]. The compound is the maximally effective stimulant for type A cells in sensilla trichodea of the T. ni male antenna; efficacy values to 130 analogues have been reported for this receptor[8,26,27,29].

The response spectra of male pheromone receptors to a set of (Z)-alkenyl acetates are presented (Table I) for this species, three additional noctuids, and one tortricid species (S. laricana). In these compounds the chain is alt-ered from dodecenyl to hexadecenyl, and the (Z)-double bond is shifted from position 5 to the penultimate carbon, all by 1-carbon steps. The receptor key compound (effective at 0.001 µg) is respectively Z7-12:Ac, Z7-14:Ac, Z9-14:Ac and Z11-16:Ac for the Noctuidae species, all being typical noctuid pheromones (see Fig. 1); and (Z)-8-tetradecenyl acetate (Z8-14:Ac) for Spilonota larica-na, a pheromone structure so far only known for this tortricid genus[30].

With each species, starting from the key compound the response gradually decreases both upon shifting the double bond from the optimum position and

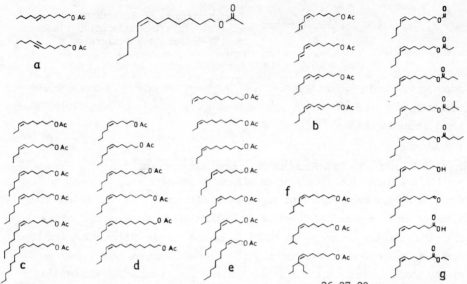

Fig. 3. Some stepwise modifications of Z7-12:Ac used[26,27,29] in studying receptor specificity. a, E-isomer and acetylene; b, dienes; c,d, altered chain segments $\underline{n}$ and $\underline{m}$; e, Z-isomers; f, side chains; g, altered end group.

upon altering the length of the chain. However, with the noctuids, elongating or shortening by two CH_2 groups invariably displaces the preferred position for the (Z) double bond by two carbons (e. g., from Z7-12:Ac to Z9-14:Ac, and further to Z11-16:Ac) such that the number of CH_2 groups in the apolar end alkyl part ($\underline{n}$ in $\underline{I}$)

$$CH_3-(CH_2)\underline{n}-CH=CH-(CH_2)\underline{m}-O-COCH_3 \qquad (\underline{I})$$

remains the same as in the natural pheromone (Table I). All receptors for monounsaturated alcohol and ester pheromones in Noctuidae test species so far showed this relationship[26,27]. In contrast, for $\underline{S}$. laricana the optimum for the (Z) double bond throughout all the five steps in chain length is always position 8 (Table I). Within certain Tortricidae subgroups all test species tended to follow this Spilonota pattern[31]. Basic differences in the receptor specificities between the two families (which use pheromones of a common structural type) are also apparent in the responses to stereoisomers[26], or to alkyl-branched chains[27], not treated here.

Closely correlated with these response characteristics, presumed steps in the chain length of pheromone molecules between Noctuidae species (Fig. 1) are preferentially those at the $\underline{m}$ part (with $\underline{n}$ kept constant). There is evidence that all three congeners, Z7-12:Ac, Z9-14:Ac, and Z11-16:Ac, may be pheromone

Table I. Response spectra of pheromone receptors of five lepidopterous species to 40 acetates, altered in chain length (12 to 16) and in position (5 to 14) of a double bond. Values indicate equipotent stimulus amounts in a half log scale (0.0056 to 0.018 μg are given as 0.01; 0.018 to 0.056 μg, as 0.03; etc.).

	Tricho-plusia ni	Syngrapha variabilis	Cucullia umbratica	Chersotis multangula	Spilonota laricana
Z5-12:Ac	0.01	0.03	0.03	0.3	1
Z6-12:Ac	0.01	0.1	0.1	0.3	1
Z7-12:Ac	0.001	0.03	0.01	0.1	0.3
Z8-12:Ac	0.01	0.1	0.03	0.3	0.03
Z9-12:Ac	0.03	0.1	0.03	0.3	0.3
Z10-12:Ac	0.1		0.1		1
Z5-13:Ac	0.03	0.03	0.03	0.3	
Z6-13:Ac	0.03	0.03	0.03		0.3
Z7-13:Ac	0.01	0.01	0.01	0.1	0.1
Z8-13:Ac	0.01	0.03	0.01	0.03	0.003
Z9-13:Ac	0.03	0.03	0.01	0.1	0.1
Z10-13:Ac	0.1	0.1	0.03	0.3	0.1
Z11-13:Ac	0.1		0.1	0.3	0.3
Z5-14:Ac	0.1	0.01	0.03	0.3	0.3
Z6-14:Ac	0.1	0.01		0.3	0.3
Z7-14:Ac	0.03	0.001	0.01	0.1	0.03
Z8-14:Ac	0.03	0.01	0.01	0.03	0.001
Z9-14:Ac	0.01	0.01	0.001	0.01	0.03
Z10-14:Ac	0.1	0.1	0.01	0.03	0.1
Z11-14:Ac	0.1	0.1	0.03	0.1	0.1
Z12-14:Ac	0.3	0.3	0.1	0.3	0.1
Z5-15:Ac	0.3		0.3	0.3	1
Z6-15:Ac	0.3	0.03		0.3	1
Z7-15:Ac	0.1	0.01	0.1	0.1	0.3
Z8-15:Ac	0.1	0.01	0.03	0.1	0.01
Z9-15:Ac	0.03	0.01	0.01	0.03	0.03
Z10-15:Ac		0.03	0.01	0.01	0.1
Z11-15:Ac	0.1	0.1	0.03	0.01	0.3
Z12-15:Ac	0.3		0.1	0.1	1
Z13-15:Ac		0.3	0.3	0.3	1
Z5-16;Ac	1	0.3	0.3	0.3	1
Z6-16:Ac	1		1	0.3	
Z7-16:Ac	0.3	0.1	0.3	0.1	1
Z8-16:Ac	0.3	0.1	0.3	0.1	0.03
Z9-16:Ac	0.1	0.01	0.1	0.03	0.1
Z10-16:Ac	0.3	0.1	0.03	0.01	
Z11-16:Ac	0.1	0.03	0.01	0.001	0.3
Z12-16:Ac	0.3	0.1	0.1	0.03	0.3
Z13-16:Ac	1	0.3	0.1	0.1	0.3
Z14-16:Ac		1	0.3	0.3	1

components in species of the same noctuid genus[32]. This type of pattern is unknown for any group of Tortricidae, which are evolutionarily more conservative in the distance between the -C=C- double bond and the functional end group (segment m in I). These few examples may point to the as yet undiscussed close interrelationship between the specific structure-response characteristics of specialized odour receptors, and their structural strategies in the evolutionary transitions to new key compounds.

ACCEPTOR MODELS

As with other types of pheromone receptors[5-7,33,34] it is tacitly assumed that a homogeneous population of olfactory acceptors generated each of the response spectra. The graded stimulus amounts of a spectrum are thus viewed as reflecting the probabilities for the different analogues to activate the same single species of molecular acceptor.

Acceptor interaction by these flexible ligands could conceivably be initiated by the acetate group assuming that this polar group orients the molecule to the binding site[35,36] where it may complex with an amino acid residue. This initial nucleation complex could then be followed by conformational rearrangements of the partly bound chain, leading to complete binding of the remaining segments to appropriate subsites[37]. A physico-mathematical model has recently been used[5,34,38] to simulate this 'cooperative multiposition interaction'. The model is based on the cooperative attachment of stimulant compounds to 3 to 5 subsites in spatial correspondence to electronically pronounced positions of the receptor key compound in its minimum energy conformation. The 40 alkenyl esters of Table I all have the same pronounced positions (the terminal CH_3- group, the -C=C- double bond, the acetate group) but at different distances. The values for electron polarisabilities and dipole moments at the corresponding acceptor subsites have been calculated[5,34,38] by fitting Boltzmann statistics with the sensory efficacies for such a set of test compounds. A model defined as such was able to predict the relative efficacies for various further test compounds in close correspondence to experimental (electrophysiological) data[5,34,38].

Would this model also account for the interspecific variety in chemical receptor specificity observed experimentally? - including (i) the structure-response relationships specific to certain higher taxonomic groups, (ii) the transitions to new key compounds, and (iii) the distinct differences in response spectra (not treated here) observed[26,27] between receptors which share the same key molecule. By modifying the number of binding positions, their geometrical arrangement, their polarisabilities and dipole moments, and their steric accessibilities, the model was varied stepwise[39,40] to accomodate these specificities. Response spectra of certain receptors for different, homologous key compounds (as in the four noctuid examples of Table I) could be closely simulated by spatially re-arranging electronically equivalent acceptor positions. Evolutionary steps in the functional end group of key molecules, and certain distinct differences between receptors for the same key compound, so far were best approached by keeping the geometry of the interacting positions constant while changing electronic data for one of them[39,40] (As yet, the model does not differentiate between an alteration in the electronic setup of the actual acceptor and the steric accessibility to its interacting positions). Finally, in terms of the model, the differential structure-response relationship discussed here for certain Noctuidae vs. Tortricidae species is due to differential penetration of the interacting potential field of the π electron cloud of the -C=C- double bond into that of its acceptor counterpart[40].

CONCLUSION AND PERSPECTIVE

Results of this modelling support the concept of an acceptor site which could have undergone a multitude of evolutionary, stepwise modifications, reflected by the chemical specificities of the receptor cells. The pheromone receptors of male moths, discussed here, are distributed over tens of thousands of species in an apparent continuum. By applying the present techniques to broader sets of species of known taxonomic relationships, current work is directed at determining closer segments of the phylogenetic sequence in the chemical specificities of these receptors.

ACKNOWLEDGEMENTS

I wish to thank Drs. H. Arn, H. J. Bestmann, C. Descoins, D. Hall, M. Jacobson and S. Voerman for providing test compounds; W. Baltensweiler and A. N. Kishaba for insect species; W. A. Kafka, L. Williams and C. Zack for critical comments; and Miss D. Thomas for excellent technical assistance.

REFERENCES

1. Schneider,D. (1969) Science 163, 1031-1037.

2. Schneider,D. (1971) in Gustation and Olfaction (Ohloff,G. & Thomas,A.F. eds.), pp. 45-60, Academic Press, London & New York.

3. Schneider,D. (1971) Naturwissenschaften 58, 194-200.

4. Kafka,W.A. (1970) Z. vergl. Physiol. 70, 104-143.

5. Kafka,W.A. (1974) Ann. N. Y. Acad. Sci. 237, 115-128.

6. Kaissling,K.E. (1974) in Biochemistry of Sensory Functions (Jaenicke,L. ed.), pp. 243-273, Springer Verlag, Berlin.

7. Kaissling,K.E., this symposium.

8. Priesner,E. (1968) Z. vergl. Physiol. 61, 263-297.

9. Priesner,E. (1973) Fortschr. Zool. 22, 49-135.

10. Priesner,E. (1975) Z. Naturforsch. 30 c, 676-679.

11. Silverstein,R.M. & Young,J.C. (1976) in ACS Symposium Series No. 23, pp. 1-29.

12. Roelofs,W.L. & Cardé,R. (1977) Ann. Rev. Entomol. 22, 377-405.

13. O'Connell,R.J. (1972) in Olfaction and Taste IV (Schneider,D. ed.), pp. 180-186, Wiss. Verlagsges., Stuttgart.

14. O'Connell,R.J. (1975) J. gen. Physiol. 65, 179-205.

15. den Otter,C.J. (1976) Abstract, 2nd ECRO Congress, Reading.

16. Kochansky,J., Tette,J., Taschenberg,E., Cardé,R., Kaissling,K.E. & Roelofs,W.L. (1975) J. Insect Physiol. 21, 1977-1983.

17. Saglio,P., Priesner,E., Descoins,C. & Gallois,M. (1977) C. R. Acad. Sci. Paris Ser. D 284, 2007-2010.

18. Zack,C., this symposium.

19. van der Pers,J., this symposium.

20. Karandinos,M.G., Tumlinson,J.H. & Eichlin,T.D. (1977) J. Chem. Ecol. 3, 57-64.

21. Cardé,R., Cardé,A.M., Hill,A.S. & Roelofs,W.L. (1977) J. Chem. Ecol. 3, 71-84.

22. Kaissling,K.E. & Priesner,E. (1970) Naturwissenschaften 57, 23-28.

23. Kaissling,K.E. & Bestmann,H.J., personal communication.

24. Henderson,H.E., Warren,F.L., Augustin,O.H.P., Burger,B.V., Schneider, D.F., Bishoff,P.R., Spies,H.S.C. & Geertsma,H. (1973) J. Insect Physiol. 19, 1257-1263.

25. Sass,H. (1976) J. comp. Physiol. 107, 49-65.

26. Priesner,E., Jacobson,M. & Bestmann,H.J. (1975) Z. Naturforsch. 30 c, 283-293.

27. Priesner,E., Bestmann,H.J., Vostrowsky,O. & Rösel,P. (1977) Z. Natur-forsch., in press.

28. Berger,R.S. (1966) Ann. Entomol. Soc. Amer. 59, 767-771.

29. Gaston,L.K., Payne,T.L., Takahashi,S. & Shorey,H.H. (1972) in Olfaction and Taste IV (Schneider,D. ed.), pp. 167-173, Wiss. Verlagsges. Stuttgart.

30. Arn,H., Städtler,E. & Rauscher,S. (1975) Z. Naturforsch. 30 c, 722-725.

31. Priesner,E., unpublished results.

32. Steck,W., Underhill,E.W., Chisholm,M.D., Bailey,B.K., Loeffler,J. & Devlin,C.G. (1977) Canad. Entomol. 109, 157-160.

33. Schneider,D., Kafka,W.A., Beroza,M. & Bierl,B. (1977) J. comp. Physiol. 113, 1-15.

34. Kafka,W.A. (1975) in Structure-Activity Relationships in Chemoreception (Benz,G. ed.), pp. 123-135, IRL, London.

35. Beets,M.G.J. (1973) in Transduction Mechanisms in Chemoreception (Poynder,T.M. ed.), pp. 129-143, IRL, London.

36. Dodd,G.H. (1975) in Structure-Activity Relationships in Chemoreception (Benz,G. ed.), pp. 1-9 and 55-61, IRL, London.

37. Burgen,A.S.V., Roberts,G.C.K. & Feeney,J. (1975) Nature 253, 753-755.

38. Kafka,W.A. & Neuwirth,J. (1975) Z. Naturforsch. 30 c, 278-282.

39. Kafka,W.A., this symposium.

40. Kafka,W.A. & Priesner,E., in preparation.

Aspects of chemoreception in marine crustacea

Barry W. Ache

Department of Biological Sciences, Florida Atlantic University, Boca Raton, FL 33431, USA

ABSTRACT

Antennular chemoreceptors in the spiny lobster are characterized as low threshold, amino acid-sensitive cells with possible restricted response spectra. The projection of this afference to the protocerebral lobes is verified physiologically and characterized as lacking apparent sensitivity to spatiotemporal parameters of antennular stimulation. These findings are discussed relative to our understanding of crustacean chemosensitivity.

INTRODUCTION

As stated at this group's last meeting (12), knowledge of crustacean chemosensory physiology is limited. Little new information has accrued since the frequently-cited studies of Case (4) and Laverack (11). The paucity of data reflects in part the logistical problems of recording from small, labile cells in a highly conductive medium. Crustaceans, like other arthropods, however, are candidate model systems for neurobiological research and their chemosensory competence is well established from behavioral studies. The organizational similarities of the crustacean "olfactory" pathway to that of vertebrates (16) and the aquatic vs terrestrial habitat difference that contrasts most Crustacea with the Insecta add comparative interest to analyses of crustacean chemosensory physiology.

Research to date focuses attention on the paired antennular filaments, the pereiopod dactyls, and the mouthpart appendages as sites of chemosensitivity in crustaceans. Our laboratory has been using the spiny lobster, Panulirus argus, as a model system to study antennular chemosensory organization in crustaceans, extending the earlier work of Maynard (17) on the chemosensory competence of this organism. This paper summarizes what we know of the peripheral organization of antennular chemosensitivity in the spiny lobster and presents new results describing central connections made by antennular chemoreceptors responsive to amino acids.

METHODOLOGY

Primary afferent chemoreceptor activity is recorded from excised, saline-perfused antennular filaments using conventional extracellular recording techniques. Fifty microliter aliquots of potential stimulant solutions flow over the preparations as a 2-3 sec duration stimulant pulse in a carrier flow of reagent grade artificial seawater that continuously washes the filament. Responses of chemosensory cells, identified as such by their sensitivity to temperature-, pH- and osmotically-controlled stimulant solutions and their insensitivity to mechanical stimulation, are quantified directly from photographed records and/or counted electrically to generate post-stimulus time histograms. These procedures are detailed in (3).

Central neural activity is recorded from essentially intact preparations, maintained viable by continuous intrapericardial saline perfusion following initial blood replacement with saline. The supraesophageal ganglion-optic tract-protocerebral (eyestalk) ganglia complex is exposed to allow direct access for extracellular recording from optic tract neurons. The antennular filaments extend into a 4-channel olfactometer which carries 50 µl aliquots of stimulant solutions over the filaments as 2-3 sec duration stimulant pulses similar to those used in the excised preparation. In selected trials, a continuous stimulant flow from a linear mixing device provides an ascending concentration profile of stimulant to single filaments. Activity in units responsive to antennular stimulation is quantified directly from photographed records. These procedures are detailed in (2).

RESULTS: PERIPHERAL

Low molecular weight (MW) substances are adequate stimulants for lateral filament chemoreceptors. The capacity of extracts of eight potential food organisms to stimulate these chemoreceptors resides in molecular constituents of <10,000 MW (3). Further analysis delimits the stimulatory capacity of one of these extracts, pink shrimp, to molecular constituents of <1,000 MW,

with the amino acid component accounting for most (67%), but not
all, of this fraction's stimulatory capacity (10). No single
amino acid at its extract concentration equals the ability of
all 19 component amino acids to stimulate these receptors.
Taurine, glutamic acid, and lysine, however, each elicits a mean
response greater than 70% that of the total amino acid component
and, as such, represent physiologically adequate stimulants for
further analysis of the antennular chemosensory system (10).

Chemoreceptors in viable preparations show consistently low,
concentration-dependent sensitivity to amino acid stimulation,
with typical thresholds between 10^{-8} and 10^{-9} M for taurine, the
most stimulatory amino acid in shrimp extract (Fig. 1). Units

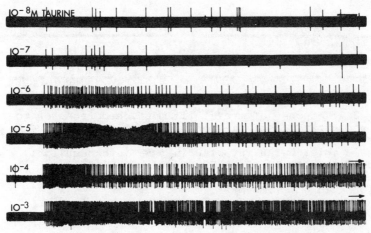

Fig. 1 - Responses of lateral filament chemoreceptors to 2-3 sec duration taurine stimulation at
graded concentrations. Ten and 16 sec deleted from
end of 10^{-4} and 10^{-3} M traces, respectively. Time
mark, 1 sec.

with slowly decaying responses typified by Fig. 1 occur on both
the medial and lateral filaments; those on the lateral filament,
however, do not appear uniquely confined to the aesthetasc tuft
(6). Phasic, more rapidly decaying units appear to predominate
in the aesthetasc region (6). Whether these represent functionally discrete receptor sub-populations remains to be determined.

The response specificity of the amino acid-sensitive units
has not been rigorously determined. At higher stimulant concentrations (e.g. 10^{-2} M, applied), unit specificity appears rela-

tively broad. At 10^{-6}-10^{-5} M, however, responses of taurine receptors on both lateral and medial filaments decrement markedly
to slight variations in taurine's structure. Only two of eight
taurine analogs tested in preliminary experiments stimulate
cells responsive to taurine (Fig. 2) (7).

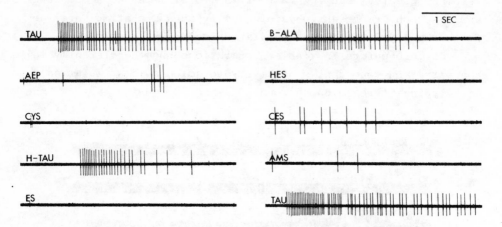

Fig. 2 - Response of medial filament chemoreceptor to
2-3 sec duration stimulation with taurine (TAU) and 8
taurine analogs. AEP, aminoethylsulfonic acid; CYS,
cysteic acid; H-TAU, hypotaurine; ES, ethanesulfonic
acid; B-ALA, B-alanine; HES, hydroxyethanesulfonic
acid; CES, chloroethanesulfonic acid; AMS, aminomethy-
sulfonic acid. Time mark, 1 sec.

The lateral filament "flicks' spontaneously at a mean frequency of 45 flicks/min and increases up to 2-fold on amino acid
stimulation (20), raising the question of flicking's potential
effect on chemoreceptor activity. For most receptors, flicking
does not modify the pattern of response they exhibit during
static chemostimulation, indicating it does not gate-on the
chemosensory response in an all-or none fashion nor affect the
stimulus-receptor interaction per se (20). Receptors can be
phasically recalled on flicking after initial adaptation,
suggesting that flicking enhances the organism's temporal aware-
ness of its odor environment, a competence likely of maximum
value in changing odor environments.

RESULTS: CENTRAL

Neurons responsive to antennular chemostimulation ascend
the optic tract from the supraesophageal ganglion towards the

protocerebral (eyestalk) ganglia, verifying physiologically the early anatomical evidence for this projection. Fibers responsive to antennular stimulation with taurine show characteristic concentration-dependent responses that adapt more rapidly than first order afferents at comparable concentrations (Fig. 3). Two aspects of receptor field organization characterize this system.

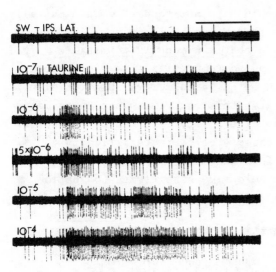

All units are unilateral, but connections are not limited to lateral filament chemoreceptors; 39% receive medial filament input while 22% receive both lateral and medial filament input. Secondly, 22% of the total units surveyed get contralateral filament input. Most units surveyed appear unimodal, although potential multimodality is difficult to eliminate. Those fibers responding to multimodal (visual, distributed tactile) stimulation typically receive contralateral chemosensory input.

Fig. 3 - Response of central neurons to antennular stimulation with 2-3 sec duration taurine pulses at peak concs. shown. Time mark, 1 sec.

Two observations indicate that spatio-temporal parameters of chemosensory integration do not occur antecedent to the protocerebral ganglia. Stimulating lateral filaments as pairs with varying delay (0-2 sec) between stimulus applications does not modify the pattern nor the latency of the response of presumptive unilateral units, suggesting that spatially summated input is not critical to the excitation of the optic tract neurons surveyed. The effect (i.e., the absence of any observable response modification) is independent of stimulating sequences. Secondly, stimulating ipsilateral, lateral filaments with continuous stimulation of ascending concentration profile from a linear mixing device does not elicit a pattern or intensity of response that cannot be matched by stimulation of homogeneous

concentration profile within 0.5 - 1.0 log concentration steps
of the gradient maximum, suggesting that temporally summated
input by itself is not critical to the excitation of the optic
tract neurons surveyed. The possibility that the phasic responses produced by flicking elicit a pattern of input critical to
the excitation of eyestalk neurons has yet to be tested. Tentatively, it can be concluded that the protocerebral ganglia
(the medulla terminalis?, see 16) are not receiving any spatially
or temporally integrated input from the brain proper. These
results support the hypothesis that the medulla terminalis
is responsible directly for spatio-temporal analysis of antennular chemosensory input as suggested by selective ablation of
this ganglion (18, 19). Towards this end, units can be isolated
in the tract carrying descending activity elicited by antennular
chemostimulation. These responses, of characteristically
regular frequency but not of prolonged duration (Fig. 4), are
presently being analyzed for selective sensitivity to spatio-
temporal parameters of antennular chemoreception.

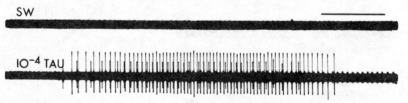

Fig. 4 - Response of descending optic tract neurons to
taurine (10^{-4} peak conc.) stimulation of the contralateral medial antennular filament. Stimulus applied
at start of trace. Time mark, 1 sec.

DISCUSSION

     Amino acids are clearly adequate stimuli for the crustacean
antennular system (1, 10, 11, 13, 21) but, as evidenced behaviorally in Homarus (e.g. 14) and physiologically in P. argus,
amino acid responses do not likely describe the total feeding-
related chemosensory afference mediated by these receptors.
Conversely, multiple types of information can be extracted from
amino acid elicited afference if amino acids stimulate functionally discrete classes of antennular chemoreceptors as suggested
by P. argus studies. The low threshold to amino acids (taurine)
supports the suspected distance or "olfactory" role of antennular chemoreceptors (9) and implicates amino acids as stimuli

controlling the initial food-finding component(s) of feeding
behavior when spatio-temporal discrimination of the organism's
odor environment is presumably important. That "key" amino
acids as taurine in P. argus (hydroxyproline in Homarus (21)?)
dominate overall amino acid sensitivity, possibly via "odor
specialist" receptors, is worthy of further analysis. While
possibly reflecting sampling bias, selective sensitivity to
particular amino acids may reflect an adaptation of the organism
to overcome environmental chemical "noise." The emerging
evidence for distributed antennular chemosensitivity (6, 8)
requires caution in assigning antennular chemosensitivity to
aesthetasc hairs. While aesthetascs are undoubtedly chemosensory, and responsive to amino acid stimulation, further
characterization of aesthetasc chemosensitivity per se is in
order.

Functional studies of central connectivity in crustacean
chemosensory systems are virtually nonexistant (but see 5).
Such studies are feasible, however, as evidenced by the P.
argus preparation. Our results support the contention of
Maynard (17, 18, 19) that the eyestalk ganglia, specifically
the medulla terminalis, are associated with spatio-temporal
processing of antennular chemosensory information. The exact
mechanism(s) by which the protocerebral ganglia modulate this
afference remains to be determined and likely is complex considering the multimodal nature of the information projecting
to this area. Without correlated anatomical and latency
analyses, the position of optic tract neurons in the olfactory
system cannot be rigorously defined. If the unimodal fibers
project directly from the olfactory lobe of the supraesophageal
ganglion as suggested by anatomical studies (16), they likely
represent processes of first-order chemosensory interneurons,
further analysis of which should provide insight into connectivity patterns within the ganglion's glomerular neuropile, an
organizational feature also characteristic of the vertebrate
olfactory bulb (15).

Supported by a grant from the Whitehall Foundation. I
thank Z. Fuzessery for permission to summarize unpublished
data. Dr. W.E.S. Carr, Z. Fuzessery, B. Johnson and R. Price

participated in these studies.

REFERENCES

1. Ache, B. (1972) Comp. Biochem. Physiol. 42, 807-811
2. Ache, B. and Fuzessery, Z. (In Preparation)
3. Ache, B., Fuzessery, Z. and Carr, W. (1976) Biol. Bull. 151, 273-282
4. Case, J. (1964) Biol. Bull. 127, 428-446
5. Field, L. (1974) J. Comp. Physiol. 92, 397-414
6. Fuzessery, Z. (Submitted for Publication)
7. Fuzessery, Z., Carr, W. and Ache, B. (In Preparation)
8. Fuzessery, Z. and Childress, J. (1975) Biol. Bull. 149, 522-538
9. Hazlett, B. (1971) J. Anim. Morph. Physiol. 18, 1-10
10. Johnson, B. and Ache, B. (In Preparation)
11. Laverack, M. (1964) Comp. Biochem. Physiol. 13, 301-321
12. Laverack, M. (1975) In, Olfaction and Taste V, pp. 141-146, Academic Press, N.Y.
13. Levandowsky, M. and Hodgson, E. (1965) Comp. Biochem. Physiol. 16, 159-161
14. Mackie, A. (1973) Mar. Biol. 21, 103-108
15. MacLeod, P. (1971) In Hdbk. Sensory Physiology IV, 1, pp. 182-204, Springer-Verlag, Berlin
16. Maynard, D. (1967) In Invertebrate Nervous Systems, pp. 231-255, U. Chicago Press
17. Maynard, D. and Dingle, H. (1963) Z. Vergl. Physiol. 46, 515-540
18. Maynard, D. and Sallee, A. (1970) Z. Vergl. Physiol. 66, 123-140
19. Maynard, D. and Yager, J. (1968) Z. Vergl. Physiol. 59, 241-249
20. Price, R. and Ache, B. (1977) Comp. Biochem. Physiol. 57A, 249-253
21. Shepheard, P. (1974) Mar. Behav. Physiol. 2, 261-273

Abstracts of Poster Presentations

Structure-activity relationship of the lactic acid-sensitive neurons on the mosquito antenna Edward E. Davis, [SRI International (Stanford Research Institute) Menlo Park, CA, USA]

The grooved-peg sensilla on the antennae of the mosquito Aedes aegypti has two lactic acid-sensitive neurons--one excited by and one inhibited by lactic acid (LA).[*] The investigations reported here were undertaken to define the specificities of these LA-sensitive neurons. The responsiveness-- as characterized by changes in the extracellularly recorded spike frequencies-- of the neurons to chemicals more or less structurally related to LA was examined. The constitution and configuration of the compounds were systematically altered, principally by use of 2- to 4-carbon aliphatic acids with α or β -OH, =O, -SH, -NH$_2$, -CH$_3$, or -Br substitutions. Other 2- to 4-carbon aliphatic alcohols and aldehydes with and without similar α or β substitutions were also tested. The optimum configuration was found to be a 3-carbon mono-carboxylic acid with a side group in the α position. Of the α substitutions tested, -OH > -Br > -SH > =O, -NH$_2$, -CH$_3$, -H in eliciting a change in spike frequency. Thus, the receptor site for LA on both types of LA-sensitive neurons appears to be relatively specific for LA. These electrophysiological results correspond well with the behavioral results reported by Carlson et al.[†] At very low stimulus intensities, D(-)LA appeared to be slightly more effective than L(+)LA in evoking a change in spike frequency; as the stimulus intensities were increased, however, L(+)LA continued to elicit a response that was proportional to the stimulus intensity, whereas D(-)LA did not. This finding that the neurons are sensitive to both the D(-)- and L(+)- isomers of LA is similar to Kafka's finding[†] that the steric configuration of the odor molecule is of secondary importance in determining the specificity of the receptor.

This work was supported in part by Grant AI 10954 from the National Institutes of Health.

[*]E. E. Davis and P. G. Sokolove. J. comp. Physiol. 105, 43-54 (1976).

[†]D. A. Carlson, N. Smith, H. K. Gouck, and D. R. Godwin. J. Econ. Entomol. 66, 329-331 (1973).

[†]W. A. Kafka. Z. vergl. Physiol. 70, 105-143 (1970).

Olfaction in the southern pine beetle, *Dendroctonus frontalis* Zimm. (Col.:
Scolytidae). J. C. Dickens, (Forstzoologisches Inst. der Universität, 78 Freiburg i. Br., DFR) and T. L. Payne (Dept. Entomology, Texas A & M Univ., College Station, USA)

Electroantennogram and single unit recordings in conjunction with a technique
involving the differential adaptation of antennal olfactory acceptors were
used to elucidate the receptor system of Dendroctonus frontalis for insect-
and host-produced volatiles. Previous experiments indicated that response intensity of acceptors for both insect- and host-produced compounds were similar. Thus, the relative interaction of the various odors with the antennal
acceptors could be calculated from the degree of adaptation by one compound
prior to stimulation with a second compound. Among the odors tested frontalin
(a (3.2.1) bicyclic ketal) adapted response to all other compounds and thus,
was considered capable of interacting with acceptors for all of the compounds.
Odors produced by one sex interacted with a larger percentage of the acceptors
in the opposite sex. The oxygen containing insect-produced odors ((3.2.1)
bicyclic ketals and keto- or hydroxy- (3.1.1) bicyclic terpenoids) interacted
with a larger percentage of the acceptors than the hydrocarbon host tree compounds ((3.1.1) bicyclic terpenes). Steric hindrance by the exo-ethyl group
was noted when responses of the acceptors to exo- and endo-brevicomin were
compared. Responses of single units to the enantiomers of exo-brevicomin indicated a chiral acceptor. Therefore, interaction of molecules with the acceptors could be influenced by changes in geometrical and optical isomerism as
well as oxygen content and ring structure. Morphological and electrophysiological studies revealed 2 olfactory sensillum types, sensilla basiconica and sensilla trichodea II, on the antennal club responsive to both the bark beetle
pheromones and host compounds.

<u>Structure and function of the chemoreceptor sheet in Aplysia</u> B. Jahan-Parwar, The Worcester Foundation for Experimental Biology, Shrewsbury, MA 01545, U.S.A.

<u>Aplysia</u> can locate food from a distance by chemoreceptors on its anterior tentacles. A sensitivity study of afferent units from various regions suggests that the Tentacular Cup Mucosa (TCM) is the most sensitive chemoreceptor region on the tentacle (Jahan-Parwar, Am. Zool. 12: 525, 1972). This hypothesis was supported in the present study by systematically recording chemically evocked potentials from various tentacular surface areas. The largest response was obtained from the TCM. The response, which was sharply reduced in the other regions, was a monophasic negative potential whose amplitude increased with the concentration of the chemical stimulus. This response, which probably represents the summated chemoreceptor generator potential, will be referred to as electrotentaculogram (ETG). An examination of the TCM with a scanning electron microscope revealed the presence of extremely long cilia on the sensory surface. The cilia occurred in unidirectionally oriented lumps altenating with bare ("naked") patches which carried few groups of short microvilli and mucous droplets. The density of the long cilia was sharply reduced outside the sensory area.
Sections from the sensory mucosa were then examined with a transmission electron microscope for receptor cells. Neuroepithelial cells were absent. However, microtubule filled cytoplasmic processes were found penetrating the basal lamina and extending between the columnar epithelial cells. Some of these processes which originated from cells, probably neurons beneath the epithelium, reached the epithelial surface and protruded slightly from it. This distal end appeared somewhat enlarged and was always ciliated. These subepithelial cells that send microtubule filled and ciliated processes to the sensory surface are probably chemoreceptor cells. The number of these cells reduced drastically outside the TCM. This is consistent with the electrophysiological findings. (Supported by PHS Grant NS-11452).

Structure and function of the palps of Gryllus bimaculatus(Insecta, Orthoptera) Ulla Klein, (Max-Planck-Institut Verhaltensphysiol., 8131 Seewiesen, BRD)

Gryllus bimaculatus has well developed maxillary and labial
palps, which seem to be primarily a contact receptor system in
contrast to the antennae, which function mainly as distance
chemoreceptors.
The palps are used for palpating the ground while walking (in
special coordination with leg and antenna movements) as well as
to test the food before and during eating. The information perceived by the palp receptors is involved in the sequence of co-
pulatory behaviour and seems to be necessary for the control of
grooming, e.g. cleaning of the antennae.
The maxillary palp consists of 5 segments moveable against each
other by one muscle each. The pliable cuticle at the tip of the
last segment is supported by lymphatic pressure. In this region
nearly 5ooo receptors are distributed, whose afferent axons
combine into 2 nerve fibres. According to TEM and SEM studies
3 of the 9 different sensilla types appear to be of olfactory
function (about 25o sensilla). The majority (nearly 31oo sensilla) consists of another 3 types, which look like gustatory
pegs. The last 3 types are mechanoreceptors, about 16oo hairs
and dome sensilla.
No difference in the sensilla pattern of the palp tip could be
found between maxillary and labial palps or between male and
female. Except for one gustatory peg, all receptor types are
also present on the antenna, but in different proportions.
In addition to the morphological results further evidence for
the chemoreceptive function of some of the receptors comes from
successful electro-antennogram measurements and single cell recordings from gustatory hairs on the maxillary palp.

The influence of very small currents on the reception and transduction of
chemical stimuli in insect contact chemoreceptors. J.J.de Kramer,
J.N.v.d.Molen, (Zool.Lab. afd.Fysiologie, Leiden, Nederland)

Flies are able to taste with hairs on their legs. Experimental results
about the transduction- and amplification-processes are rare. Generally an
electrical transduction hypothesis is accepted. Current-stimulations are
necessary to elucidate the mechanisms involved.

A current-clamping amplifier was developed to investigate the influence of
small (10-300 pA pp) sinusoidal currents on the spike train; frequencies
used were 1, 2, 5 and 10 Hz. D-hairs were stimulated with these currents,
and simultaneously with 109 mOsm meatjuice.

The effect is basically that spikes tend to appear exclusively when di/dt
is positive. This effect increases in time, and depends both on current-
strength and frequency. 10 pA is well above threshold; **5 Hz is the most
effective of the frequencies tested.**

**In the literature an electrical threshold for eliciting spikes of 3000 pA is men-
tioned.** As the effect measured is expressed by grouping the spikes,
primarily evoked by the chemical stimulus, we presume that the current-
stimulation exerts its influence *before* transduction and amplification
take place.

A provisional hypothesis is presented. The dendritic membrane may act as a
current-source, being effective when - as a consequence of chemical stimulation - the membrane conductivity increases. The small current change
causes conformational changes in microtubular structures. These chain-mole-
cules can be responsible for transduction. In the region of the basal bodies
amplification takes place and action potentials are generated.

The fact that grouping appears more pronounced in the course of adaptation
is consistent with the rate-theory.

Odorant deposition onto insect antennal sensilla R. W. Mankin, M. S. Mayer, and P. S. Callahan, (Department of Entomology and Nematology, University of Florida and Insect Attractants, Behavior and Basic Biology Research Laboratory, Agricultural Research Service, USDA, Gainesville, Florida 32504)

A model has been developed that quantifies the deposition of odorant onto specific antennal sensilla. It includes elements of diffusion, deposition and filtration theories and calculates the stimulus in terms of molecules per sensillum, taking into account: (1) sensillar and flagellar morphometry; (2) the fraction of sensilla sensitive to the odorant; (3) odorant concentration; and, (4) airspeed and related dynamic parameters.

The model is experimentally verified for *Trichoplusia ni* and *Porthetria dispar* using ^{3}[H]-(Z)-7-dodecenyl acetate. The results are compared with the deposition of SO_2 onto adsorbing surfaces (Chamberlain 1966) and with other models for pheromonal deposition onto the antennae of *Bombyx mori* (Kaissling 1971, Adam and Delbrück 1968). The new model is more applicable than previous models to insects with non-plumose antennae.

Adam, G. and Delbrück, M. 1968. pp. 198-215 In A. Rich and N. Davidson (eds.) Structural Chemistry and Molecular Biology. Freeman & Co., San Francisco.

Chamberlain, A. C. 1966. Proc. Roy. Soc. (London) A290, 236-265.

Kaissling, K.-E. 1971. pp. 350-431 In L. M. Beidler (ed.) Handbook of Sensory Physiology, Vol. IV, Chemical Senses I, Olfaction. Springer-Verlag, New York.

Olfactory receptor-responses to behavioral synergists. H.Mustaparta, M.E. Angst and G.N.Lanier, College of Environmental Sciences and Forestry, SUNY, Syracuse, USA and Institute of Biology, University of Odense, Denmark.

Pheromones of the bark beetle genus Ips are structurally similar to host attractants which have been implicated as their precursors (Hughes 1973,1974, Brand 1975). In field test compounds of the pheromone mixture and host odours act synergistically as attractants (rev. Bordon 1974, Lanier and Burkholder 1974). This raises the general question of whether these substances which are similar in structure and have the same behavioral effect, act on the same or separate groups of olfactory cells. We have recorded responses from single olfactory cells in two species, Ips pini and I.paraconfusus Lanier. Eleven compounds were tested, including pheromones and host terpenes. The cells obtained in both species could be placed in the same groups, specialized to: 1. the aggregation pheromone ipsdienol of both enantiomers (Silverstein et al 1966, Stewart 1975, Lanier et al 1972) 2. ipsenol, the aggregation synergist in I.paraconfusus, however, aggregation inhibitor in I.pini (Birch and Wood 1975, Birch and Light 1977) 3. cis-verbenol, trans-verbenol and verbenone. Cis-verbenol is a synergist in I.paraconfusus and trans-verbenol is present in the frass of I. pini. Both are aggregation synergists in several bark beetle species. A few other cells responded selectively to the host terpene, myrcene, the precursor for ipsenol/ipsdienol, but no cells so far responded significantly to α-pinene, the precursor of trans/cis-verbenol. In conclusion, the same main type of olfactory cells are found in both species, I.pini and I.paraconfusus. These are highly specialized to one or a very few related compounds of the pheromone and host odour mixture.Compounds which act synergistically on the behavior activate separate groups of cells. This indicates the behavioral synergistic effect, like the inhibition (Mustaparta et al in press) in these species,is a result of a central nervous, integration, where signals from separate cells are converging at a later stage of olfactory processing, resulting in an increased attraction.

References:
Birch,M.C. and Wood,D.L. 1975. J.Chem.Ecol. 1:101-113
Birch,M.C. and Light,D.M. 1977. J.Chem.Ecol. In press
Bordon, J.H. 1974 in Birch,M.C. (ed). Pheromones. North Holland Amsterdam
    p. 136-160
Brand,J.M.,Bracke,J.W.,Markovetz,A.J.,Wood,D.L. and Browne,L.E. 1975.
    Nature 254, 136-137
Hughes,P.R. 1973. Z.angew.Ent. 73, 294-312
    ——   1974. J.Insect Physiol. 20, 1271-1275
Lanier,G.N. and Burkholder,W.E. 1974 in Birch,M.C. (ed). Pheromones. North-
    Holland Amsterdam p. 161-189
Lanier,G.N.,Birch,M.C.,Schmitz,R.F. and Furniss,M.M. 1972. Can.Entomol. 104:
    1917-1923
Mustaparta,H.,Angst,M.E. and Lanier,G.N. J.Comp.Physiol.in press
Silverstein,R.M.,Rodin,J.O. and Wood,D.L. 1966. Science 154: 509-510
Stewart,T.E. 1975. Master thesis. SUNY. Environ.Sci. and Forestry, Syracuse

Influence of sex on electrical resistivity of the labellar taste hairs of *Phormia regina* **M..** P. Pietra,
A.M. Angioy, A. Liscia, R. Crnjar, (Inst. of Gen. Physiol., viale Poetto, 1 – 09100 Cagliari,
Italy)

To study the cause of the greater weight increase and O_2 consumption of the female Phormia
as compared with the male of the species (Calabrese et alii,1974), an investigation on the role
of the mucopolysaccharidic substance located at the tip of the chemosensory hairs (Stürckow,
1967; Moulins et alii, 1972) was performed by evaluating changes in the electrical resistivity of
the labellar taste hairs of male and female Phormia when in contact with stimulating salt solutions (equiconductive solutions of NaCl, KCl, LiCl, $CaCl_2$, $BaCl_2$ and $MgCl_2$). This parameter
may provide information on ion diffusion across the mucopolysaccharidic layer. In fact, the
lower the resistivity, the higher the probabilities of contact with the chemosensory membranes
for a given stimulating substance, and thus the greater the effectiveness of that substance. The
results show that in every case labellar taste hair resistivity is significantly higher in males. This
evidence indicates that a greater concentration of the stimulating agents may be reached in the
chemosensory membranes of the labellar taste hairs of the female Phormia. The higher concentration of the stimulating substance may lead to a greater incentive to feed, and explain, to
some extent at least, the greater weight increase and respiratory rate of the female Phormia
vis-à-vis the male.

Calabrese E.J., Stoffolano J. G., J. Insect Physiol., *20*, 383 - 383, 1974.
Moulins M., Noirot Ch., in "Olfaction and Taste IV", p. 49 - 55, D. Schneider ed., Wissenschaf-
tliche Verlagsgesellschaft MBH,1972.
Stürckow B., in "Olfaction and Taste II", p. 707 - 720, T. Hayashy ed.. Pergamon Press, 1967.

CODING OF FOOD AND SEX ODOURS IN PERIPLANETA AMERICANA

Hinrich Sass

Zoologisches Institut der Universität, D-84 Regensburg
Germany

Reactions from male antennal sensory cells responding to food and sex odours were recorded electrophysiologically. Food stuffs and filter papers impregnated with the odour of virgin females and males respectively served as stimulus sources. Odours from "female papers" elicited sexual behaviour in males. After recording, sensilla were labeled by cactus spines and investigated with transmission and scanning electron microscope.

Receptor cells responding to female papers were found only in smooth single walled hairs with pore tubules and a length of about 20 µm. These sensilla comprise more than 50 % of all olfactory hairs in the middle region of the antenna. In the recordings, simultaneous activity of two receptor cells was observed.

Strong responses to food odours occur both in small (ca. 10 µm) smooth walled hairs with pore tubules and in double walled hairs with spoke canals.

Cells responding to food odours can be classified according to their clearly defined reaction spectra (receptor type). All receptors belonging to one type show the same graded sensitivity to the odorants of their spectrum. Each food odour excites the cells of several types. The response pattern varies according to the food stuff and its momentary composition.

References:

Sass, H. (1973) Verh. Dt. Zool. Ges. 66, 198-201
Sass, H. (1976) J. comp. Physiol. 107, 49-65
Boeckh, J., K.-D. Ernst, H. Sass, U. Waldow (1976) Verh. Dt. Zool. Ges. 70, 123-139
Altner, H., H. Sass, I. Altner (1977) Cell. Tiss. Res. 176, 389-405.

Computerised classification of insect taste cell responses. J.N.v.d.Molen,
J.J.de Kramer, J.v.d.Meulen, F.J.Pasveer, (Zool.Lab. afd.Fysiologie, Leiden,
Comp.Centre, Delft, Nederland)

Flies are able to taste with hairs on their legs. The information about
taste substances is enclosed in spike trains.
In order to describe the activity-pattern of one cell in time, the analogue
signal must be digitized. This is realized by peak-discriminator controlled
sampling; advantage of this method is a considerable saving of computer-sto-
rage. The activity-pattern of one cell can be described in detail with only
4 parameters: f_{max} (maximal frequency), t_{fmax} (time of occurrence of f_{max}),
f_∞ (frequency at t_∞) and a (adaptation-rate). a and f_∞ can be derived
if one treates the descending phase of the activity-curve as a hyperbola;
multiplying f with time t results in a straight line: $f.t = a + f_\infty.t$
45 of the 190 taste hairs on the prothoracic leg of *Calliphora vicina*, were
stimulated with a glucose/fructose-mixture, 0.25 M each. Each hair was stimulated once. At least 10 successfull recordings were made from all the
selected hairs. From each recorded spike train the 4 parameters were calculated for the cell firing with the highest rate. For all hairs the mean
activity pattern was calculated ($\bar{f}_{max}$, $\bar{t}_{fmax}$, $\bar{f}_\infty$ and $\bar{a}$). Factor analysis
showed that $\bar{a}$ and $\bar{f}_\infty$ contributed most effectively in a cluster-separation.
Striking coïncidences were found between cluster-content and topography of
the hairs. There are 4 main clusters. Cluster I contains all D-hairs, II is
dominated by ventral B-hairs, III and IV mainly contain lateral and dorsal
B-hairs. Exceptions can partly be ascribed to inaccuracies in the f_∞-deter-
mination, partly to the fact that sharp bounderies may not exist at all.
The number of parameters will increase when other concentrations and taste-
substances will be used; then it will become possible to describe in detail the
information that is sent to the C.N.S.

Reproductive isolation by means of odours in small ermine moths (Lepidoptera: Yponomeutidae) J.N.C. Van Der Pers, (Department of Zoology, Groningen State. University, Haren, The Netherlands).

Eight representatives of *Yponomeuta* occur in the Netherlands. They show different degrees of taxonomic relationship. The classification on morphological characteristics yields two species groups comprising four distinct species and a complex of four closely related forms (the "*padellus*"-complex).
The various forms of this complex are specific as to their larval food plants. Interbreeding is possible, but in the field their populations are reproductively isolated, although all forms are sympatric. The forms are studied as examples of phases of a speciation process.

In four forms of the *padellus*-complex and one distinct species, male and female antennal olfactory receptors are being studied by electroantennography (EAG) and single-cell analysis. From the EAG recordings it appeared that receptors are present on the female antennae which are sensitive to plant odours. These may enable the females to select their host-plant by olfaction. The male antennae were almost non-excitable by plant odours, but they showed a high sensitivity to chemicals which attract males in the field. Single-cell recordings from antennal *sensilla trichodea* revealed activity from two types of cells sensitive to the sex-attractants. The response spectra of these cells in males for these sex-attractants differed characteristically among the various representatives of *Yponomeuta* tested. This indicates that the composition of the respective female sex pheromones of *Yponomeuta* may differ. Moreover, the activity of two cell types suggests that multicomponent sex pheromone systems are utilized.

The investigations are supported by the Foundation for Fundamental Biological Research (BION), which is subsidized by the Netherlands Organization for the Advancement of Pure Research (ZWO).

Central interneurons in the thoracic ganglion, and motor activity in feeding behaviour of the blowfly Calliphora vicina H. van der Starre, (Zool. Lab. afd. Fysiologie, Leiden, Nederland)

Flies are able to taste with hairs on their legs. The axons of the sensory cells run to the thoracic ganglion. Here, they connect with central interneurons. In order to understand the process of taste discrimination it is necessary to localize the interneurons and study the properties of their connections with the sensory cells on the one hand, and with other central cells concerned with motor activity on the other hand. This problem was attacked with axonal iontophoresis of Cobalt ions. After amputation of one or more tarsomeres, prothoracic legs were immersed in 200 mM $CoCl_2$ and a current of 150 μA was applied. After five hours of iontophoresis about five large cell bodies 15 μ wide could be found after precipitation of CoS with $(NH_4)_2S$. They are situated in the frontal region of the ganglion. The electrical activity picked up extracellularly with an isolated Tungsten electrode in this region, when not independent of simultaneously recorded taste stimulation shows either activation or inhibition. A behaviourally acceptable mixture of meat juice and sugar was used. Intracellular recording and more precise localization as well as systematic variation of stimulus quality are envisaged.

The proboscis extension response resulting from adequate taste stimulation is not caused by a pneumatic mechanism. This follows from registrations of the electrical actvity of the musculus retractor fulcri simultaneous with an objective measure of extension. Also, registrations of the internal air-pressure in the cephalic air-sacs of the tracheal system bring out a drop in pressure concurrent with extension and probably caused by passive expansion of the air-sacs. The proboscis response is caused by direct action of head muscles and can thus be measured quantitatively and related to sensory input.

<u>The morphology of insect taste hairs</u>. Fran M. van der Wolk, (Zool.Lab. afd.Fysiologie, Leiden, Nederland)

Flies are able to taste with hairs on their legs. Furthermore these taste hairs can be found on the proboscis.
The typology of tarsal taste hairs can be based on one criterion - the tipshape - leading to the same classification as the five criteria formerly used. Classification on tipshape is as follows:
  A-hairs have a blunt tip, a diamond-shaped pore at the side;
  B-hairs have a sharp tip, an oval pore at the top;
  D-hairs have a sharp tip, a rectangular pore at the side.
No C-hairs were found. Each species investigated shows a characteristic distribution pattern of hairs on the legs.

The pores are morphologically influenced by solutions. Both the type and the osmolarity of the solution are important.
Tarsal and labellar hairs can close the pore. Besides the labellar hairs loose a prong which simply shrinks in.   When dynamic impedance measurements are carried out simultaneously with the recording of spike trains, both spike amplitude and frequency are increased at the moment the impedance decreases.

The two parallel running lumina, dendrite free (DFL) and dendrite containing (DCL), contain vesicles and fluids. The DFL contains also microtubuli and mitochondria close to the base where it has a tight constriction. The constriction is due to the increase in thickness of the DCL tube. Away from the somata runs a two-chambered tube, porous at first but more distally closed. Each chamber contains either one, or 2 - 5 dendrites. These dendrites pass at least through two enveloping cells. The lumina of the enveloping cells seem to terminate under the socket.

The basal-body-tandem at the apex of the soma is surrounded by vesicles that resemble neuro-synaptic vesicles. These vesicles may contain messengers to depolarize the soma membrane.

BIOCHEMICAL ASPECTS OF SUGAR RECEPTION IN THE COCKROACH

Helmut Wieczorek

Fachbereich Biologie der Universität Regensburg

D-8400 Regensburg, Federal Republik of Germany

The close correlation between the distribution of taste hairs and
α-glucosidase activity in the legs and the proboscis of the fly
resulted in the formulation of the hypothesis that the primary
process of insect sugar reception may be the formation of a sugar-
glucosidase complex (Hansen 1974,Review). So far the glucosidase
hypothesis has been restricted to several species of flies. Therefore it was of interest to examine its validity also in insects
rather unrelated to the holometabolous fly.

The maxillary palp of the hemimetabolous cockroach Periplaneta
americana was chosen for corresponding investigations. Its sensilla
field with an enormously high density of taste hairs appeared to
make it a favourable object for localizing biochemical experiments.

The investigation of α-glucosidase activities in the maxillary
palps with in-vivo and in-vitro methods and the comparison of the
results with those obtained in behavioral experiments indicate
that, in accordance with the situation in the fly, α-glucosidases
may also in the cockroach be involved in the processes of sugar
reception. Moreover, complex kinetic phenomena observed in in-vivo
experiments lead to the assumption that sugars may penetrate into
the maxillary palp. Further investigations are necessary to decide
whether any correlation exists between uptake of sugars and chemoreceptive processes.

Sensory adaptation in Saturniid pheromone receptor cells Camilla
Zack,(Max-Planck-Inst. Verhaltensphysiol., 8131 Seewiesen, GFR)

Sensory adaptation was studied electrophysiologically in the pheromone receptor cells of <u>Antheraea polyphemus</u> and <u>A</u>. <u>pernyi</u>. Receptor potentials(RP) and nerve impulses were recorded extracellularly from sensilla trichodea containing 2 cells, each maximally
responsive to one component of the female sex pheromone. A decrease in the response amplitude following a conditioning stimulus (CS) is more evident the stronger the CS, the weaker the test
stimulus (TS), and the briefer the elapsed time between CS and
TS. This is reflected in the adapted response curves which have
a smaller maximum and a steeper slope and are shifted to higher
concentrations. There is also a characteristic change in shape
of the receptor potential of an adapted cell. The rise time to
maximum amplitude increases and the time to return to baseline
decreases. Cross adaptation was used to investigate the interaction of the AL cell and the AC cell in both species. It was found
that 1) self adaptation was always more pronounced than cross a-
daptation 2)conditioning with AL did not adapt the AC cell in
either species and 3) conditioning with AC caused some adaptation
in both species. Local stimulation of the sensillum revealed
that receptor potential adaptation can be confined to discrete
areas of the sensory cell dendrite.

PSYCHOPHYSICS AND APPLIED CHEMOSENSORY PHYSIOLOGY

The role of 'primaries' in taste research

Robert P. Erickson

Departments of Psychology and Physiology, Duke University, Durham, NC 27706, USA

One of the most influential factors in our research is our use of the sweet, sour, salty and bitter taste primaries, which figured largely in each of the papers in this symposium. I believe that our use of this concept has such a strong and basic influence on our research and conclusions, that whether this use is valid or not, it merits serious appraisal. What if this basic premise is even slightly incorrect? It would have a profound effect. I will illustrate what I mean with specific comments on the papers in this symposium, as well as some general comments.

General role of primaries. We all know that there are 4 basic tastes; it is built into our thinking. The historian Boring knew it, describing how "the matter was settled" by Henning's taste tetrahedron. That cement-like settling of the matter could be a basic impediment to our science, turning us to the production of answers in terms of the 4 basic tastes, and away from more basic questions. For example, why did the early researchers - reported by Boring - assume that there should be taste primaries? The intense question of "How many primaries are there?" seems to have obscured more basic questions such as "What does the term primary mean, and does taste employ them at all?" Audition, for example, works quite well without primaries.

Since Boring's statement, the term "primary" has come to be used in at least 5 different ways; from the stimulus level "up," I will refer to primaries as 1) stimulus, 2) receptor, 3) neural organization (e.g., are there primary fiber types?), 4) neural coding (are there primary kinds of neural message?), or 5) psychophysical (do we have only 4 taste sensations, or something more complex?).

In each of the papers of this symposium, inferences about primaries have been made from one of these levels to another. But the fact that the concepts of taste primaries are of dissimilar realms presents a basic problem which must be faced; How may findings at one level influence our thinking at another level? Would a finding of 4 psychophysical sensation types (level 5) have clear implications for stimulus types (level 1)?

Stimulus and Receptor Primaries: A visual researcher around 1835 named Brewster concluded, on the basis of psychophysical studies, that there were 3 kinds of light stimuli - red, yellow and blue. He made, in effect, a seemingly simple inference from level 5 to level 1. He now may be remembered for what might be termed "Brewster's Fallacy" in his conclusion that there are 3 kinds of visual stimuli rather than a continuum. What leads Dr. Birch to search for taste stimulus types? Is it psychophysical primaries, or neural primaries? Just as we do not need 3 unique visual stimuli to evoke the basic sensations of red, yellow and blue, we may not have 4 unique stimuli for sweet and sour etc. In fact, this orientation, in its simple form, may turn out to be no more helpful than would a search for the 3 visual stimuli.

Dr. Bujas has evaluated receptor processes in terms of psychophysical primaries, moving between the psychophysical (5th) and receptor (2nd) levels, giving no comfort to the idea of primaries as far as papilla are concerned. He makes the affirmative point, also made by Dr. Birch and the others, that psychophysical ratings are useful tools. But, as I will point out below, the success of these ratings does not indicate the existence of primaries.

Analysis and Synthesis: In the areas of psychophysics, neural coding and neural organization (levels 3-5) the use of taste primaries has led to what can be termed "analysis" in psychophysics, "labeled-lines" in neural coding, and "fiber types" in neural organization. These are the areas touched on by Drs. Bartoshuk, Nowlis and Frank. I believe Dr. Sato has touched all 5 bases.

A brief example from Dr. Pfaffmann and his coworkers will illustrate this "primary" position. They theorized that activity in individual neuron types is labeled as to its meaning, sucrose predominately activating the neuron type signalling "sweet," and NaCl predominately activating "salty" neurons. Thus, the theory is that there are separate sensations - primaries - that are mediated via separate neural lines. In this way, they analyzed the taste of fructose as being both sweet and salty - 2 sensations - for the monkey.

There are 3 separate ideas here, that deserve separate consideration. The first idea, a psychophysical one, is that taste sensations of any complexity appear as "analyzed" into the 4 primaries. The second idea is that each of these primary sensations has its own private set of neurons mediating a particular sensation, thus called "labeled-lines." The third idea is that each group of labeled-lines have identical response characteristics, forming neural groups or types. These 3 uses of "primaries" are usually taken to-

gether as one, in what might be termed the "analytic" position. I believe
the papers in this symposium generally employ this view. For perspective I
will compare this with a "synthetic" view in which taste primaries are not
used.

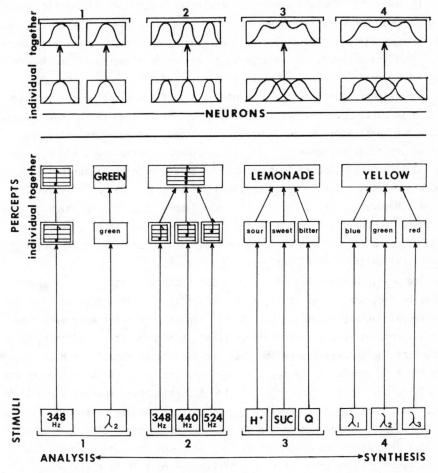

Figure 1

Definitions for analysis and synthesis* in general may be facilitated with
reference to Figure 1. On the far right, panel 4, is the example of color
vision in which each of 3 different wavelengths of light, when taken separately, are experienced as 3 different colors, blue, green and red in this example.
When presented together, the entirely different sensation of yellow arises,
in which the original components are not seen; this is an example of synthesis.
* For a history and discussion of analysis and synthesis (integration) see
C.J. Herrick's "The Evolution of Human Nature."

In panel 1 is an extreme example of analysis. When a visual stimulus and an auditory stimulus are presented separately, they are experienced as green and F. When presented together they are still experienced clearly and separately as green and F, and are not confused by each other in any degree.

In panel 2 is another example of analysis; 3 auditory frequencies each produce their own sensation when presented separately, and when combined each sensation remains distinct. But although the stimuli remain separate, there is an emergent property in addition to those of the elements; there is the important additional property of an F major chord.

In the third panel I have presented a possible description of the situation with taste. In this example there are 3 stimuli which, by themselves, arouse the sensations of sour, sweet, and bitter, and when presented together give us the taste of lemonade. If in the lemonade taste the 3 elements that made it up are not separately distinguishable as in color mixtures (although lemonade or colors can be rated on these 3), then it would be a synthetic system. However, if it is more like the auditory situation in which, within the emergent property (lemonade, or F major chord) individual stimuli are still discernable, then it would be an analytic system. These are brief psychophysical definitions of analysis and synthesis.

The neural definitions of analysis and synthesis might be as follows. Ten years ago, when I was trying to formulate some general principles of sensory neural functioning (Psy. Rev. 1968), and in particular what made some stimulus combinations fuse and others remain separate, it seemed that the mechanisms for synthesis might be that the individual stimuli each would stimulate the same population of neurons (panel 4, top) because these neurons were broadly tuned. On the other hand, in the analytic cases (panels 1 and 2) the stimuli activate separate neural elements, either because these elements are narrowly tuned, or because they belong to different modalities. In brief, the idea is that if the component stimuli activate the same neurons, the system is synthetic; if they activate different neurons it is analytic.

It is well known that in taste the neurons are in general broadly tuned, although there may be some variation in breadth between neurons. Since this is the case, I thought that taste should be a synthetic system. I still don't know if it is, but it seems that the rules at one level (neural in this case) would be more powerful if they could predict events at another level (here, psychophysical).

At any rate, here are provisional definitions of what analysis and synthesis are neurally. I will now relate these definitions to research in taste psychophysics, neural coding, and neural organization.

Psychophysics. The general tactic in taste psychophysics is to categorize or rate taste sensations in terms of sweet, sour, salty and bitter. Two obvious but often overlooked points may be made about this method in addition to its capacity to usefully organize data; first, its success does not demonstrate that the system in analytic with 4 unique sensations, and second that the number 4 is problematical.

Both these points can be illustrated by analogy with a demonstration in color vision, similar to studies by Boynton. We asked subjects to rate 20 evenly spaced Munsell colors, of equal chroma and value, in terms of 2, 3, 4 or 5 standard colors. It turned out that the color naming is successful with 3 or more stimuli, and somewhat with 2 (fig. 2). Color is synthetic, but the naming, like that in taste, is successful. Also, the naming is successful with different numbers of standards. Thus, I feel that psychophysical procedures, as used by the present participants, using 4 basic stimuli, does not demonstrate either that taste is analytic, or that there are 4 basic tastes. Of course, one must be very careful to note when this is, or is not, the goal of any particular experiment, or whether the experiment requires that they be used in this way. Naming tastes in terms of primaries at any level is clearly a useful descriptive tool. For example, Dr. Bujas used the 4 primaries to show that the response characteristics of the individual papilla are not reducible to 4 types, without involving himself in the issue of whether there are 4 primaries.

Neural. On the neural side I earlier defined a synthetic system as one in which the several stimuli activated the same population of neurons. However, in a different definition, the issue of analysis and synthesis has become connected with the issue of whether there are fiber types, and also the separate issue of whether these are "labeled-lines." It would seem intuitively pleasing to have separate fiber types for each sensation type in an analytic system, the meaning of each of these fiber types being unique; that is, "sweet" for the sweet fiber type, etc. These issues may be examined in relation to Fig. 3.

In the top of this figure are 9 neurons tuned along some dimension in which there are clearly not fiber types at all; at the bottom are 9 neurons arranged in 3 very tight groups. In between are 2 intermediate levels of grouping.

Three points may be made about fiber groups, or "neural primaries." The first, as illustrated at the bottom of the figure, is that fiber types do not demand analysis, as is known for color vision. There, fiber types mediate synthesis.

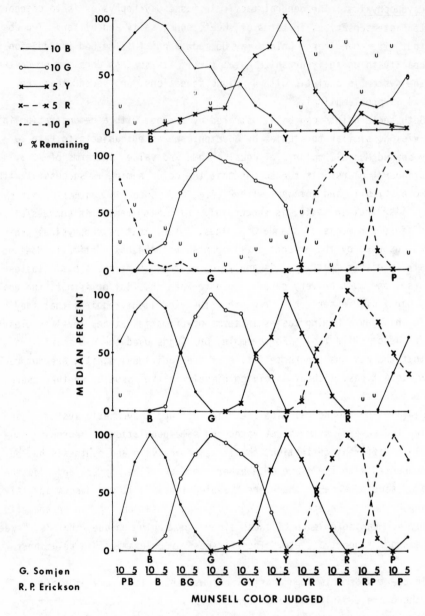

G. Somjen
R. P. Erickson

MUNSELL COLOR JUDGED

Figure 2

Twenty Munsell colors were rated on from 2 to 5 standards from the Munsell series. The "U" symbol indicates the amount of each color unaccounted for by the standards.

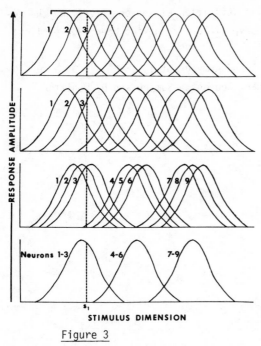

Figure 3

The second point is that the labeled-line position, and therefore analysis, does not require fiber types. The first 3 neurons covered by the bracket on the top line could all signal "salty." That is, each neuron does not have to be centered exactly over its "proper" stimulus, indicated by the "S1" at the bottom and carried across all examples by the dotted line. Mueller understood this clearly, stating in his "doctrine of specific nerve energies" well over 100 years ago that it is not the identity of the stimulus, but the identity of the nerve that is the code. In other words, the "best stimulus" issue, of great concern in modern sensory neurophysiology, is a topic separate from the meaning of the activity of any particular neuron. In brief, the labeled-line or analytic position does not require fiber types.

Concerning whether or not there are fiber types, the third point, I believe that as one progresses from the top to the bottom of this figure there would be differences of opinion as to which cases contain fiber types. And different researchers do not agree on their existence in their data.

There is a mathematical way to decide whether or not there are groups of neurons or stimuli, called hierarchical cluster analysis. We have performed this analysis with a diverse range of stimuli and several samples of up to 50 neurons each. The clear indication, with this particular method, is that there are no neuron or stimulus types, a discouraging as well as illuminating coincidence of data with theoretical position.

Conclusion. Each level of taste research, from stimuli to psychophysics, can be studied in isolation from the others. However, carefully drawn relationships from one level to another, such as between psychophysics and neural coding, or between receptors and stimuli, can serve in a powerful, perhaps essential, way in inspect hypotheses at each level. This relating of levels is sometimes carried out in a very casual, and therefore problematical way, especially with the concept of taste primaries. This concept has been carried across all levels without either its definition at any one level, or the relationships between its usages at several levels, having been made explicit.

Supported by NSF grant BNS 75-22692 and Army grant 14195-L
Assisted by A. Johnson, S. Schiffman, Georgette Somjen and D. Woolston.

Psychophysical studies of taste mixtures

L. M. Bartoshuk

Yale University School of Medicine, 290 Congress Avenue, New Haven, CT 06519, USA

ABSTRACT

When substances are mixed, their taste qualities can usually be recognized but the intensities of those tastes may be decreased (i.e., mixture suppression) or increased (i.e., enhancement or synergism). Previous mixture research was based on the assumption that the taste qualities of the component substances determined these changes. However, recent data suggest that the psychophysical functions relating taste intensity to stimulus concentration of the unmixed components is a better predictor of mixture interactions than are the qualities of the components. Psychophysical functions are said to show compression when successive increments in concentration produce progressively smaller increments in perceived intensity and to show expansion when successive increments in concentration produce progressively larger increments in perceived intensity. Compression appears to predict suppression while expansion appears to predict synergism at least for substances with similar taste qualities.

CLASSIC MIXTURE STUDIES

Taste mixture studies have historically been divided into two categories: Those that deal with substances that have different taste qualities and those that deal with substances that have similar taste qualities.

Mixtures of substances with different taste qualities. Mixtures of substances with different taste qualities were first systematically studied by Kiesow in 1896[1]. He believed that taste qualities were analogous to colors so he constructed mixtures of pairs of the basic tastes to see if he could produce a taste phenomenon similar to the loss of hue resulting from the mixing of complementary colors. Kiesow's results showed that taste mixtures were quite different from color mixtures. Two colors can fuse in a mixture to form a new color that is qualitatively distinct from the components. For example, red and green fuse to produce yellow. However, two tastes remain recognizable in a mixture but their perceived intensities are usually less than when unmixed. Kiesow found only one case of apparent cancellation of taste quality; weak sucrose and weak NaCl produced a flat taste. Surprisingly enough, this one phenomenon received more attention from Kiesow's contemporaries than the mixture suppression that he observed.

Kiesow's work was followed by a series of studies using a variety of techniques but all of those studies tested pairs of basic tastes. That is, the studies were based on Kiesow's implicit assumption that taste interactions would depend on the nature of the taste qualities of the components in the mixture. These studies produced a variety of results. In general, the studies supported Kiesow's overall conclusion, that a mixture tastes less intense than the sum of its parts[2-4] but some studies reported cases of enhancement[5-9] and there was general disagreement over the degree to which suppression occurred for particular pairs.

Mixtures of substances with similar qualities. Research on mixtures of substances with similar tastes comes from a different tradition. Much though not all[10] of this research has dealt with sweeteners[11-15] perhaps because of the important economic implications of sweetener substitutions in food products. One of the major issues in this area has been whether such mixtures result from the summation of concentrations or the summation of the perceived intensities of the components. That is, whether a mixture of two sweeteners simply provides a higher concentration of the sweet stimulus or whether the mixture is the simple sum of the perceived sweetness of each component. Since the exact mechanism for the production of sweetness is unknown, there was no direct way to add the concentrations of two different sweeteners so the "addition" was accomplished indirectly by expressing each sweetener in terms of the concentration of a standard sweetener that was equally sweet.

"Synergism" has been mentioned frequently in connection with studies on mixtures of substances with similar tastes. Although the term is not always used in the same way, it generally refers to a mixture that is more intense than the simple sum of the component tastes.

Moskowitz[10, 14-16] has provided an excellent summary of the studies on mixtures of substances with similar taste qualities and those of substances with different taste qualities. He suggested that suppression results when substances with different tastes are mixed such that the more different the tastes the greater the suppression, while simple addition of perceived intensities or synergism is the rule when substances with similar tastes are mixed.

AN ALTERNATE VIEW OF TASTE MIXTURES

The generalizations above correctly summarized the existing literature but contradict some insights about taste mixtures that come from electrophysiological studies. Pfaffmann[17] and Beidler[18] both noted that the shape of the function relating magnitude of neural response to concentration determines the magnitude of the neural response produced by a mixture of substances both of which stimulate the same receptor mechanisms. We can apply this logic to psychophysical data in the following way. Figure 1 shows three hypothetical psychophysical functions for taste substances. These are power functions but the following argument is not restricted to this class of functions. Consider the simplest case of adding substances with similar tastes: adding a substance to itself. The perceived intensity of concentration 1.0 of A added to concentration 1.0 of A, that is, of concentration 2.0 of A, is 1.4. The same operation on B and C would produce perceived intensities of 2.0 and 2.8, respectively. Function A is said to show compression while C shows expansion[20]. "Mixtures" of A with A would show "suppression" and those of C with C would show "synergism." Simple additivity would occur only for "mixtures" of B with B. Note that the functions in Figure 1 are plotted in linear coordinates. Plotted in log-log coordinates, compression is shown by slopes less than one and expansion is shown by slopes greater than one.

Mixtures of substances with similar tastes: Results that contradict the classic view. If the logic above is extended to substances with similar tastes, then certain predictions must follow. When substances with similar tastes produce compressed psychophysical functions, mixtures of these substances should produce suppression. In addition, if the shapes of the psychophysical functions are changed, then the mixture interactions should change as well. These predictions were tested for mixtures of sugars, mixtures of acids, and mixtures of substances with bitter tastes[21].

This challenge to the classic view of mixtures of substances with simi-

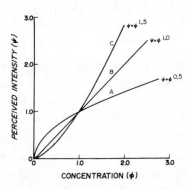

Figure 1. Linear plots of hypothetical psychophysical functions showing compression (A) and expansion (C). (From 19. Reprinted by permission)

lar tastes was possible because of the body of literature that has accumulated using magnitude estimation to produce psychophysical functions in taste. In particular, Meiselman[22] has shown that the shape of these psychophysical functions can vary from compression to expansion by changing the way in which a stimulus is tasted. In the first three experiments to be discussed below, solutions near body temperature were flowed across the subject's tongue[23] because this procedure tends to produce compressed functions.

These experiments were designed to permit direct comparisons between the psychophysical functions of the unmixed components and a mixture function constructed in the following way. In each of the experiments, concentrations of four substances with similar tastes were chosen so that they were of approximately equal perceived intensity. These four stimuli were then used to construct the six possible two-component mixtures, the four possible three-component mixtures and the one possible four-component mixture. The average responses to the mixtures of one, two, three, and four components could then be compared to responses to the unmixed components and to two, three, and four times these original concentrations. For example, Figure 2 shows such a comparison for four acids. Note that the data are plotted in log-log

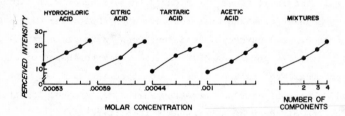

Figure 2. Log-log plots of psychophysical functions for four acids and for mixtures of acids. The slopes of the best-fitting straight lines are: hydrochloric acid, 0.49; citric acid, 0.57; tartaric acid, 0.54; acetic acid, 0.54, and mixtures, 0.55. (From 21. Reprinted by permission of Academic Press, Inc.)

coordinates. The four functions on the left, the psychophysical functions for the unmixed components, show compression, that is, their slopes are less than 1.0. The mixture function on the right shows suppression, that is, the mixtures were less intense than the simple sum of the components. This is shown most dramatically by looking at the four-component mixture. The average intensity of each unmixed component was 10. Thus the simple sum of all 4 is 40 but the mixture of all four was much less intense than that. Figures 3 and 4 show the results for four bitter substances and four sugars, respectively. For all three experiments, the mixture functions look much like the

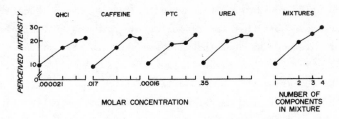

Figure 3. Similar to Figure 2 but for bitter substances. The slopes are: QHC1, 0.60; caffeine, 0.62; PTC, 0.56; urea, 0.60; and mixtures, 0.77. (From 21. Reprinted by permission of Academic Press, Inc.)

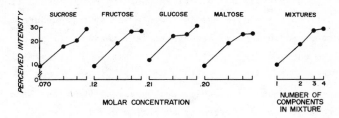

Figure 4. Similar to Figure 2 but for sugars. The slopes are: sucrose, 0.75; fructose, 0.78; glucose, 0.69; maltose, 0.70; and mixtures, 0.80. (From 21. Reprinted by permission of Academic Press, Inc.)

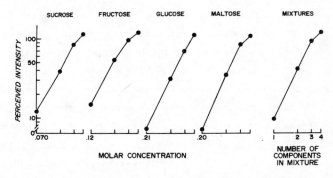

Figure 5. The stimuli were the same as for Figure 4 but the method of tasting was varied. The slopes are: sucrose, 1.67; fructose, 1.54; glucose, 1.97; maltose, 2.01; and mixtures, 1.87. (From 21. Reprinted by permission of Academic Press, Inc.)

psychophysical functions for the unmixed components. The mixture suppression evident in these results contradicts the conclusion that substances that taste similar show simple additivity or synergism.

Figure 5 represents an even more impressive demonstration of the relation between the shapes of the psychophysical functions and mixture interactions. The same stimuli as those in Figure 4 were tasted at room temperature with the sip and spit procedure. This method of tasting can produce expanded functions for sugars. Note that the slopes of the four psychophysical functions on the left are much greater than 1.0 and note that the mixtures show strong synergism. The contrast between Figures 4 and 5 is illustrated particularly well by comparing the perceived intensity of the mixture of all four sugars with the simple sum of the perceived intensities of the four unmixed sugars. The simple sum of the four unmixed sugars was set at 40 in both experiments. The perceived intensity of the mixture of all four sugars tasted with the flow procedure was 29 and that for the sip and spit procedure was 123. That is, the mixture was 0.7 times the simple sum in the flow procedure but was 3 times the simple sum in the sip and spit procedure.

It is important to note that there is no real contradiction between these data and the earlier data on mixtures of substances with similar tastes. It appears that the substances and methods of tasting used in the earlier studies were those that tend to produce psychophysical functions like B or C in Figure 1 so that simple additivity or synergism would be expected on the basis of the logic described here.

Is there a relation between the shape of the psychophysical function and mixture interactions in substances with different tastes? There is no obvious reason why mixture interactions among substances with similar tastes should be related to the presence of compression or expansion in the psychophysical functions of the unmixed components; however, the results of a recent mixture experiment[19] suggest the possibility of such a relation, nonetheless. This experiment used the magnitude estimation-profile method developed by Smith and McBurney[24] to evaluate the tastes of two, three, and four component mixtures constructed from NaCl, sucrose, HCl and quinine hydrochloride (QHCl). That is, subjects broke the total magnitude of the sensation into component magnitudes for the recognizable qualities. Judgments were written on sheets labeled Sweet, Salty, Sour, Bitter, and Other Responses. The last category was rarely used. The stimuli were flowed across the subjects' tongues.

The left part of Figure 6 shows what happened to each quality as the number of components in the mixture increased. For example, the points on the bitterness curve (the curve on the right) reflect, respectively, the bitterness of QHCl alone, the average bitterness of the three two-component mixtures containing QHCl, the average bitterness of the three three-component mixtures containing QHCl and the bitterness of the four-component mixture.

Note that bitterness was severely suppressed by the addition of other

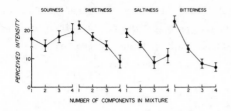 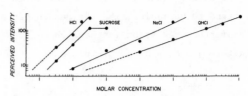

Figure 6. The left part shows the average perceived intensity ± 1 S.E. of each of the four basic taste qualities in mixtures. The right part shows log-log plots of psychophysical functions. The slopes are: HCl, 0.89; sucrose, 0.67 (lower portion, 0.94); NaCl, 0.43; and QHCl, 0.32 (From 19. Reprinted by permission.)

taste substances, sourness was not suppressed at all and sweetness and saltiness fell between these two. The right part of Figure 6 shows the psychophysical functions produced by scaling these four substances with the flow procedure. QHCl showed considerable compression, HCl showed almost none and sucrose and NaCl fell between these two. These results suggest that a substance that shows compression when added to itself will show suppression when something else is added to it.

If lower concentrations of these stimuli are tasted at room temperature with the sip procedure, the psychophysical function for HCl shows compression and those for NaCl and sucrose do not. The mixture interactions change as expected. Sourness decreases as the number of components increases and saltiness and sweetness remain about constant.[25]

The possibility of synergism among substances with different tastes is unresolved. The apparent enhancement of certain components in earlier mixture studies is not unequivocal evidence for such synergism. For example, the sweetness of sucrose has been reported to increase when weak NaCl is added[5]; however, weak NaCl tastes sweet so the apparent increase may be simply addition of common qualities.

CONCLUSIONS

We do not know whether or not all operations that change the shapes of psychophysical functions will change mixture interactions as well. However, the results of these studies show that mixture laws cannot be stated simply in terms of the qualities of the substances to be mixed. Additive properties of taste substances as reflected by psychophysical functions are important.

The view of mixtures discussed here may help explain some of the apparent contradictions in the mixture literature. Since the early studies were based on the implicit assumption that mixture interactions were determined by the taste qualities of the component substances, there was no reason to attend to variables like the method of tasting, temperature of solutions and so forth. Variation in these conditions would, in the light of the present data, have caused the mixture interactions to vary across studies.

REFERENCES

1. Kiesow, F. (1896) Phil. Stud. 12, 255-278
2. Moskowitz, H. R. (1972) Percept. Psychophys. 11, 257-262
3. Pangborn, R. M. (1960) Food Res. 25, 245-256
4. Pangborn, R. M. (1961) J. Food Sci. 26, 648-655
5. Beebe-Center, J. G., Rogers, M. S., Atkinson, W. H., and O'Connell, D. N. (1959) J. Exp. Psychol. 57, 231-234
6. Fabian, F. W. and Blum, H. B. (1943) Food Res. 8, 179-193
7. Kamen, J. M., Pilgrim, F. L., Gutman, N. J., and Kroll, B. J. (1961) J. Exp. Psychol. 62, 348-356
8. Pangborn, R. M. (1962) J. Food Sci. 27, 495-500
9. Pangborn, R. M. and Trabue, I. M. (1967) Percept. Psychophys. 2, 503-509
10. Moskowitz, H. R. (1974) J. Exp. Psychol. 4, 640-647
11. Cameron, A. T. (1947) The Taste Sense and the Relative Sweetness of Sugars and Other Sweet Substances, Scientific Reports of the Sugar Research Foundation, No. 9, New York
12. Stone, H. and Oliver, S. M. (1969) J. Food Sci. 34, 215-222
13. Yamaguchi, S., Yoshikawa, T., Ikeda, S., and Ninomiya, T. (1970) Agri. Biol. Chem. 34, 187-197
14. Moskowitz, H. R. (1973) J. Exp. Psychol. 99, 88-98
15. Moskowitz, H. R. (1974) in Sensation and Measurement, pp. 379-388, Reidel, The Netherlands
16. Moskowitz, H. R. (1972) Percept. Psychophys. 11, 257-262
17. Pfaffmann, C. (1959) in Handbook of Physiology, Vol. I, Sect. I, pp. 507-533, American Physiological Society, Washington D.C.
18. Beidler, L. M. (1961) Prog. Biophys. Biophys. Chem. 12, 107-151
19. Bartoshuk, L. M. (1975) Phys. Behav. 14, 643-649
20. Stevens, S. S. (1958) Science 127, 383-389
21. Bartoshuk, L. M. and Cleveland, C. T. (1977) Sen. Proc. 1, 177-186
22. Meiselman, H. (1971) Percept. Psychophys. 10, 15-18
23. McBurney, D. H. and Pfaffmann, C. (1963) J. Exp. Psychol. 65, 523-529
24. Smith, D. V. and McBurney, D. H. (1969) J. Exp. Psychol. 80, 101-105
25. Bartoshuk, L. M. Unpublished data.

Psychophysical approaches to food and flavor: bridging the gap between the laboratory and the real world of foods

Howard R. Moskowitz

MPI Sensory Testing, Inc., 770 Lexington Avenue, New York, NY 10021, USA

ABSTRACT

With the advent of new methods of psychophysical scaling, mathematical techniques, and a better understanding of perception, it may be time to attempt a new integrative approach to sensory evaluation. This paper offers one approach, which can be called "pragmatic psychophysics." The premises are: (1) One should use the most powerful sensory scaling tools available, to relate physical and subjective variables. (2) It may be impossible to ever discern the true, underlying laws relating variables and sensory responses. (3) If a reproducible model (even an ad hoc model) can be developed to describe the data, then that model may be a more than adequate first step. (4) The appropriate test of the model, independent of its invariant biological truth, is whether the experimenter, by using the model, can produce desired and measured sensory changes by known variations in the physical system. If one knows how physical variations predict sensory responses, then one should be able to aim towards a desired sensory response, and by manipulating the physical variables in a quantitative and predictable way through the model, be able to achieve that response.

INTRODUCTION

This paper concerns approaches to "Bridging the Gap Between the Laboratory and the Real World of Foods." Its thrust is both philosophical and substantive. Philosophically, it argues for a pragmatic psychophysics, with the aim to develop actionable equations relating 'objective' measures of food to sensory or perceptual responses. Substantively, it shows how ad hoc psychophysical functions can be constructed to describe foods and how the functions are used to develop new foods.

PRAGMATIC PSYCHOPHYSICS - PHILOSOPHICAL FOUNDATIONS

In 1953, S.S. Stevens[1] reported on provocative study, which was later to develop into a major stream of psychophysical research. He presented observers with stimuli (e.g., lights of varying luminance) and instructed them to assign numbers to match intensity (viz. brightness). The numbers (called magnitude estimates), reflecting perceived brightness could be plotted against physical luminance to yield a psychophysical curve. Twenty-five years of research using this paradigm produced numerous psychophysical functions. The consensus function relating sensory intensity (S) and physical intensity (P) turned out to be a power function, written as: $S = KP^N$

In evaluation of foods, where one can vary one ingredient alone (e.g., sucrose level in a cherry beverage), experimenters have recovered power functions. Power functions describe how sensory intensity increases with physical magnitude for hardness[2], for cherry flavored beverages, [with varying flavoring and sucrose levels][3] and for simple food aromas[4].

The laws of food perception uncovered in this way illustrate some, and only some, of the nuances of the psychophysics of food. They fail to account for (a) the inhomogeneity of foods, which is the rule, rather than the exception (b) the failure of nature to provide us with uni-dimensional changes in ingredients, (c) the existence of interactions not apparent in simple systems.

In order to bridge the gap between basic research approaches possessing highly refined methodology and empirical requirements for adequate evaluation of real-world foods, we must be able to apply psychophysical measurement in non-laboratory settings. We must maintain the rigor and quantitative usefulness of those measures, but at the same time be sufficiently flexible to realize what pragmatic modifications in the philosophical basis and experimental design are needed to obtain the best data under non-ideal conditions. Furthermore, we must be able to develop a system of measurement and data analysis that produces answers efficiently; for if it takes several years to understand and develop a detailed model of perception for a given food, then in the long run the sciences involved in food perception will be relegated to academic curiosities.

Pragmatic psychophysics offers a possible solution to this problem of real-food evaluations. An application and implications are discussed in the experimental section. The bases of pragmatic psychophysics are discussed below.

(1) The experimenter must be able to use the most powerful, reproducible, and scientifically valid methods for sensory assessment. The method of magnitude estimation[5] has become increasingly popular as a method for relating instrumental measures to sensory responses. It is sensitive to large and small differences, and the numbers have ratio-scale properties.

(2) The experimenter must develop a data-base for a representative set of product variations. Often, the variations will not be uni-dimensional. The experimenter may wish to vary ingredients in known ways (i.e., by

investigating smaller subsets of all possible changes to yield a fractional factorial design). With variations in a half a dozen or more ingredients, and with a proper experimental design, the experimenter should discern relations between ingredient changes and sensory responses. In order to discern these relations, the experimenter must (a) choose those ingredients he wishes to vary, (b) decide the range of variations and the number of levels in that range for each ingredient, (c) develop a statistical design, which covers the range of variation, but does not have to cover all possible interactions. For instance, if the experimenter wishes to evaluate the variations of 6 ingredients, each of which can be present at 4 levels, he may need to choose a set of 12, 16, 20, etc., products to investigate, rather than the total 4^6 combinations.

(3) The experimenter must be prepared to abandon the hope that he will find through experimentation a simple well behaved, invariant function to relate sensory and physical magnitudes. Power functions for sweetness may not be recovered when half a dozen ingredients, including sucrose, are varied in a beverage or pudding. Power functions may describe simple systems, but they would probably fail when a complex, interactive food system is evaluated, in which only a partial set of the potential hundreds of combinations are evaluated. Rather, simple linear functions probably would do just as well to describe the data, in an ad hoc way. The equations would appear as Sensory Intensity = k_1 (Ingr 1) + k_2 (Ingr 2)....K_n (Ingr N) + C [nonlinear equations may be used if there is ample reason, a priori, to expect the data to follow such equations].

(4) The linear or non-linear equation must allow the experimenter to predict sensory changes, given physical modifications (pure data description), but must also allow the experimenter to induce a desired perceptual change by an ingredient modification. If the experimenter knows, for instance, that Sweetness = 2.0 (Ingr A) + 1.5 (Ingr B) + 3 (from empirical evaluations), and wishes to make a 2.0 unit change in sweetness, then the model should allow him to do that. That is, the model must be actionable and not just a device for describing data.

EXPERIMENT - DEVELOPMENT OF A SPICY MEAT SAUCE

Not all experiments can be designed in such a manner as to vary all ingredients across all levels. The experimenter must decide whether psychophysical scaling and design will dictate the experiment (and, thus, allow for investigation of sensory perceptions), or whether psychophysical scaling will be used for ordering physical stimuli into a practical configuration for foods. This experiment concerns the latter half of psychophysics, with the aim to develop a real food product, with the following requirements:

(1) More than one or two ingredients must be varied (here there were 4).

(2) There are certain practical limits to the levels of the ingredients (from a technological point of view).

(3) The combination of food ingredients must produce a product that will be consumed, and which will be purchased by consumers exhibiting specific expectations (cognitive inputs), and realistic likes and dislikes.

In the study, the product was a sauce, comprising 4 ingredients. With 4 ingredients, and 3 levels for each of the ingredients, it is logistically difficult to investigate adequately the total range of variation, or even a representative large range. A full evaluation would require 3^4 = 81 different formulations. That number is impractical in a real-world setting.

In order to develop the product, using psychophysical methodology, the following approach was designed, using the ECLIPSE* method.

(1) An experimental design was developed, comprising 18 of the possible 81 formulations, [which evaluated on the 3 levels of each of the 4 ingredients, plus a representative, but by no means complete set of interactions. See Table I].

(2) Panelists, who were meat sauce users, each evaluated 4 of the 18 product formulations, and for each sample, they scaled 9 specific sensory characteristics + overall liking/disliking by magnitude estimation.

(3) Since the physical composition of each test product was known, it was possible to develop an ad hoc equation, relating a linear combination of ingredients to the sensory intensity. Table I shows the ad hoc descriptor equations, for 3 attributes. Each of the attributes requires a different combination of the same ingredients. Each regression equation represents a different combination rule of the same set of 4 ingredients.

(4) In addition, the same panelists generated a hypothetical profile of a sauce that they would like to have (viz. ideal sauce), using the same magnitude estimation scales and the same attributes as they used to profile the test products.

(5) The equation system was reversed, through the use of goal programming. Originally, the data matrix provided a series of equations which would yield, for a given set of ingredients, the estimated sensory profile. The reversal of the system allows the experimenter to (a) designate a desired

*TRADEMARK

TABLE I

(A) Ingredient and Sensory Profiles for Four of the Formulations

Product	Ingredient				Liking	Attributes		
	A	B	C	D		Aroma	Sweetness ...	Spiciness
01	0.8	0.85	0.3	0.2	-12.8	58.5	78.9	79.0
02	0.8	0.65	0.3	0.3	5.8	72.2	82.3	83.1
03	0.9	0.85	0.4	0.3	- 5.4	75.0	75.8	101.6
......								
18	0.9	0.85	0.1	0.3	18.1	77.7	84.0	93.0
99	?	?	?	?	85.5	-84.9	74.4	97.4

Concept to be matched by product (Ideal)
Product 99 = Concept, presented after the test formulations were evaluated.
.Consumers profiled the ideal on aroma, sweetness ... spiciness and liking
as if it were another test product.

(B) A Sample of the Regression Equations Relating Ingredients (A,B,C,D) to Perceptions.

Aroma Strength = 50.8 + 13.3(A) + 2.8(B) + 7.8(C) + 14.0(D)   (R = .41)
Sweetness = 109.4 - 29.2(A) + 4.0(B) - 5.9(C) - 16.1(D)   (R = .55)
Spiciness = 41.8 + 9.6(A) + 35.6(B) + 4.7(C) + 37.9(D)   (R = .70)
Sharpness = 25.9 + 25.6(A) + 40.5(B) + 17.4(C) + 31.2(D)   (R = .78)

(C) Solution of ECLIPSE Approach and Expected Sensory Profiles

    (a)   The recipe corresponding to the desired sensory profile...
         Level (%) of ingredient A = 0.90
         Level (%) of ingredient B = 0.65
         Level (%) of ingredient C = 0.11
         Level (%) of ingredient D = 0.30

    (b)   A comparison of the desired and expected sensory profiles...

Attribute	Desired Level (See A)	Optimal (ECLIPSE) Recipe Should Provide (Based on Equations)
Aroma	100.9	69.9
Sweetness	74.4	80.6
Spiciness	97.4	85.4
E	104.4	67.2
F	70.8	80.4
G	82.8	82.8
H	103.4	71.6
I	116.6	70.0
J	92.2	82.3
K	1.02	1.32

sensory profile, (b) establish limits of ingredients and (c)   determine the
levels of ingredients which in concert produce a sensory profile as close as
possible (in a statistical sense) to the desired profile.   (See Table I for
the results.)

DISCUSSION AND CONCLUSIONS

Is there a relation between psychophysics and food evaluation?

    One of the most oft-heard pleas and raisons-d'être for research in
psychophysical methodology, especially as it concerns the chemical senses

of taste and smell, is that only by such research can we really apply the power of formal, psychophysical designs to an understanding of how we perceive food. The unstated continuation of that hypothesis is that by understanding food product perception through psychophysical research, we may be able to engineer sensory responses to foods by knowing what specific aspects of foods to vary in order to produce a set of desired sensory percepts.

Unfortunately, the cross-fertilization between basic psychophysics, food science and sensory evaluation has not yielded the general fund of knowledge which is necessary. Consequently, we lack adequate information to engineer foods precisely so as to produce, in an exact fashion, desired textural, taste and aroma perceptions. What we possess today, rather, is information that provides only very general correlations.

Despite the lack of direct transference of knowledge from psychophysical scaling to food product evaluation, there is a bright light at the end of the research tunnel. What may be needed is a re-evaluation of sensory psycho-physics, to more adequately define which of its aspects can be tied to real-food analysis. It may be that the methods of measurement and the use of functional relations are the critical aspects. At the same time, it may prove impractical to continue the search for invariant laws of product per-ception, and to prolong the attempt to uncover for complex foods, psycho-physical functions which parallel the simple sensory laws governing model systems.

One approach may be to consider a new and pragmatic direction. As the ECLIPSE approach showed, actionable, albeit ad hoc, psychophysical relations can be constructed, even for a complex food. Those relations can be used to modify a food by altering its ingredients. The premise of pragmatic psy-chophysics is that a model which describes relations among ingredients and perceptions is the critical thing to develop in food psychophysics. The contributions of traditional psychophysics are scaling method and functional relations. Concomitant with those methods and equations must be the reali-zation that the translation and analogy from model systems to real foods at that point must cease. A separate set of new analytical methods (e.g., goal programming) must be then developed to deal with the complex set of stimuli inherent in the food, and the complex perceptions which the food provokes. At that point, the logic of experimentation must yield to other, more relevant and practical methods of analysis, outside the realm of sensory psychophysics.

SPECULATIONS ON PRAGMATIC PSYCHOPHYSICS AND THE MIXTURE QUALITY OF ODORS

An interesting extension of the foregoing methods can be made to develop odor mixture from constituent chemicals. We can assume that an odor mixture comprises (a) a desired sensory quality, given by a quality profile (b) chemical components at varying concentrations. The same logic used by the ECLIPSE method to develop foods from ingredients (so that the foods produce a desired sensory impression) may well be applicable to odor. It would be very exciting from the point of view of quality mechanisms in olfaction to have a procedure which could produce similar-smelling odors from a variety of different chemical mixtures. The realization of such a demonstration with odor stimuli awaits the hand of an adept sensory scientist.

REFERENCES

1. Stevens,S.S.(1971)Science,118,573
2. Moskowitz,H.R.,Segars,R.A.,Kapsalis,J.G.,& Kluter,R.A.(1974)J.Food Sci., 39,200-202
3. Moskowitz,H.R.,Kluter,R.A.,Westerling,J.,& Jacobs,H.L.(1974)Science,184 583-585
4. Moskowitz,H.R.(1977)in Chemical Senses and Nutrition II,Academic Press, N.Y., (in Press)
5. Stevens,S.S.(1975) Psychophysics: An Introduction to Its Perceptual Neural and Social Prospects,John Wiley,N.Y.

Flavour characterization and its development

Roland Harper

Department of Food Science, University of Reading, London Road, Reading, Berks, UK

ABSTRACT

A comprehensive list of flavour qualities is presented and discussed. These constitute a representative sample of all possible terms. The chemical stimuli responsible for flavour are examined in a similar manner, contrasting the chemical involved in the flavour of actual products with the stimuli selected for research in taste and olfaction. An agreed set of reference standards should be developed. Knowledge gained from odour characterization studies going back over more than ten years is summarized in a series of dogmatic propositions. Finally, a few examples of the application of descriptive analysis confirm its effectiveness.

ON FLAVOUR QUALITIES

Just as a comprehensive vocabulary exists and forms an essential tool, so a special set of terms is necessary to describe flavours. Many different sources are involved in compiling such a list including:-

Previous systems of odour classification as far back as Linnaeus[1] - All relevant words in the Concise Oxford Dictionary[2] - Many existing glossaries - The technical literature dealing with flavours and off-flavours in many different commodities[3].

A distinction between flavour and off-flavours, or foreign flavours is important. The flavour of a product is a complex pattern involving many separate constituents, both chemical and sensory. Off-flavours are normally additional 'notes' which can often be named in terms of their likely origin.

The first comprehensive list of terms was developed c. 1965 in a project on odour characterization and odour classification[4]. An up-to-date version of this list is given in Table 1.

The original list contained 44 terms each of which was scored on a 5-point scale (0-5) thus indicating the degree or extent to which each of the qualities was present in the sample or stimulus assessed. These terms

TABLE 1

1. ODOURS		
Acid	Hay-like	Like-Urine
Ammonia-like	Honey-like	
Animal		Vegetable-like (raw)
Aromatic	Malty	Vegetable-like (cooked)
	Medicinal	
Beery	Metallic	Warm
Broth-like	Meaty (raw)	(Watery)
Burnt	Meaty (cooked)	Waxy
Butyric	Minty/Peppermint	Woody
	Musky	
Camphor-like	Musty	Yeasty
Cheesy		
	Oily	
Diacetyl		2. TASTES
(Dry/Powdery)	Petrol/Solvent	
	Putrid	Sweet
Earthy		Acid
Estery	Rancid	Salt
Etherish	Resinous	Bitter
	Rubbery	
Faecal		
Fatty	Sharp	3. TACTILE
Fishy	Smoky	
Floral	Soapy	Astringent
Fragrant	Sour	Cool, Cooling
Fruity (citrus)	Spicy	Warm
Fruity (other)	Sulphurous	(Metallic)
Fresh	Sweaty	Puckery
	Sweet	Pungent
Garlic/Onion		
Greasy	Tallowy	
Green	Toasted	

formed a representative sample of all possible terms and covered a broad range
of odour qualities sufficient to provide a general system. The complete range
of terms in the English language numbers over 800 items[5].

THE CHEMICAL STIMULI

The chemical stimuli used in any particular study is governed by many
different factors. In product or process-orientated studies the choice is
fixed by the actual constituents of the particular flavour complex. Micro-
chemical analysis provides basic information about the identity and concentration of these constituents, each of which requires its own sensory
weighting factor. The threshold values for each component has been used, but
characterization data and an assessment of the actual perceived intensity of
the separate components is important. In creating a perfume which 'copies
nature' (or another manufacturer's product) the dominant components are first
identified by chemical _and_ sensory methods, which may include sniffing the
outlet of the Gas-chromatographic system. A crude version of the final
product is then made and is 'topped up' by further components to round out the
flavour and so that it approximates better to what is intended. This action
is based entirely on experience and involves testing with the trained nose.

In contrast, experimental studies of tastes and odours requires the
conscious selection of stimuli. Too little attention is given to the underlying logic of selection. A representative sample of all possible odours
should be available. A number of proposals have been made with a view to
establishing a set of chemicals suitable for research in olfaction and taste.
The matter remains open to discussion and action. The Norwich project
included between 45 and 50 odorous chemicals, mostly selected from a composite
list of all those used by previous investigators, well distributed over odour
qualities, molecular size and functional groups. This balanced sample meant
that a number of unpleasant odours which usually have to be avoided in human
studies were included. Detailed Odour Profiles were prepared of each of these
chemicals[6,7,8]. Subsequently, 14 of the stimuli proposed as suitable for
research in olfaction at the 1966 Gordon Research Conference were included.
Only half of these were found to correspond with the qualities they were intended to represent[9]. The various 'character-impact compounds' provide another
interesting group of odour/flavour stimuli[10].

CHARACTERIZATION IN PRACTICE

Limitations of space prevents the use of many relevant examples and

makes it necessary to exclude the analysis of data using Multidimensional
Statistical Methods. A number of general conclusions which can be supported
by experimental data are presented as a series of dogmatic propositions:

a. According to particular interests it is possible to emphasize
    consistency or variability (individual differences) in
    characterizing the same stimulus.

b. In spite of both facts, effective discrimination and prediction
    can be made from descriptive information.

c. Individual differences may take different forms. Some individuals
    use many more terms than others. Many individuals show personal
    idiosyncrasies not shown by others (e.g. the use of Sweet and
    Sickly characterizing Hexyl Butyrate).

d. In Information Theory terms odour and flavour characterization
    is a 'noisy activity'. For example, if the data for a group of
    individuals is tabulated in full for a particular stimulus over
    all 44 qualities many gaps will be apparent in the general
    pattern. These gaps may represent genuine individual differences
    or purely accidental events (omissions or commissions). For
    example, the term Almond was recently omitted in the characterization
    of Benzaldehyde in spite of the fact that this term had already
    been entered on the form of a spontaneous comment.

e. A very similar pattern is obtained if all the existing systems
    of odour classification are tabulated together. No single
    quality runs through all the systems. No single system includes
    all the qualities. The differences may represent idiosyncrasies
    in the perception of the individual who proposed each particular
    system.

f. In order to be certain that all relevant qualities have been
    identified, the results of at least 10 assessors should be
    combined.

g. Considerable differences exist between spontaneous and directed
    characterization, using a prepared list. Fewer terms are used
    in spontaneous characterization.

h. Beginners use fewer terms than experienced assessors. Beginners
    also seem to use higher characterization values. Studies should
    be extended to professional perfumers and flavourists as opposed to

people who are simply experienced in smelling chemicals.

i. The difference between beginners and an experienced assessor
    has recently been confirmed in an extensive study involving 10
    replicate assessments. As the study progressed the two beginners
    used progressively more terms, the experienced assessor progressively
    less. The ratio of the number of terms used by the two beginners
    (N_1 and N_2) and the experienced assessor in the first and the tenth
    replications were as follows: N_1 = 91:140; N_2 = 32:68; and
    E = 78:37 respectively. The experienced assessor might be described
    as 'zoning in' to a previous degree of skill, gradually becoming
    more precisely aware of what qualities were relevant and what were
    not. In this instance corresponding data are available for 1965.
    Lower characterization values and lower sensitivity to some of
    the odour stimuli are apparent in the recent study[11].

j. Many odours seem to become more complex with experience and to
    become unique. Characterizing them in terms of a set of general
    qualities fails to give a complete picture and many odours are
    best described in terms of themselves. For example, Eugenol may
    be more Clove-like than any other quality including Spicy.

k. A single figure rarely does justice to the characterization
    data. Three figures are required. The frequency of actual use,
    the maximum possible frequency of use (i.e. the total number of
    assessors) and the average rating for each of these conditions.
    The average overall assessors may underestimate the degree to
    which a particular quality is present for those who perceive it.
    In reporting the data the common core will be noted together
    with those terms used more than 7 times out of ten.

SOME APPLICATIONS

    A number of different applications are noted. Some of these contributed
to the method which has been outlined, others applied this method. In the
1930's the staling of coffee and loss of freshness was investigated using
a matching technique with samples stored for different periods either in the
bean or when ground. The data clearly indicated about one month's advantage
for coffee in the bean[12]. About the same time Crocker and Henderson proposed
a system of odour classification based on the four qualities Fragrant, Acid,
Burnt and Capryllic. A set of reference standards was developed and could be

purchased and an unknown odour could be matched with the appropriate member
of each series, thus providing a four-figure number for F, A, B, and C [13,14].
Crocker was a member of the Arthur D. Little Inc. organization which
developed and popularized the Flavour Profile in the 1950's[15]. This involved
an expert panel who developed their own vocabulary for each product covering
aroma, taste, flavour and after-taste, each quality being assigned an appropriate number on a scale from 0-3. The limitations of the flavour profile
lie in its use of a single consensus figure which precludes statistical
treatment and therefore provides no information about variability including
individual differences.

The first major application of the characterization system which has
been outlined earlier was due to von Sydow and his colleagues. In this
instance the panel was also trained specially and the original five-point
scale was extended to ten points. The first study dealt with the flavour
of bilberry juice, although the specific term 'Bilberry' was not included
in the terms used[16]. More recently the same approach was used to examine
the effects of cooking time on the flavour of canned meat products. Sensory,
chemical and statistical techniques were combined and the particular chemical
responsible for an off-flavour known as Retort Flavour was identified. By
changing the recipe this chemical and its associated off-flavour could be
eliminated. Optimal recipes and processes were established. It was also
possible to distinguish between accidental, predictive and causal relationships (correlations). Causal relationships normally require experimental
manipulation of the variables to identify them[17,18].

Two investigations relating to beer will be mentioned. Wren developed
a method of quality specification based upon desirable values for qualities
which are wanted and tolerance limits both for these and for undesirable
qualities or off-flavours[19]. Clapperton developed a detailed vocabulary
covering the whole range of qualities required and a series of reference
standards to define these qualities. These are used to train beginners.
One simple example is the term 'Hoppy' which can be defined in terms of hop
oil, or dried hops. The data obtained have been examined in many different
ways which indicate the reliability of average data. The correlation between
different panels ranged from 0.9 for experts to 0.62 for others. The use
of Principal Components Analysis separated different types of beer in terms
of the sensory data very effectively, and only trivial misclassifications
were made in predicting the type of beer. In two studies 80/92 and 86/92
classifications were correct. Both the sensory qualities and the chemical

constituents most effectively discriminating between the beers were also identified[20,21].

It would be possible to add to this list the investigations carried out by Williams but these will be described by him later[22]. Many other examples could be added. A number of individuals and groups now offer a service which includes these descriptive methods of analysis. Finally, Sensory Analysis in all its aspects has become a matter of international application and standardization[23,24]. At the same time, the characterization of taste, odours and flavours has an important part to play in future research, both fundamental and applied.

REFERENCES (selected)

1   Linnaeus, K., (1756) Amoenitates Academicae, 3, 183.
     Lars Sylvius, Stockholm.

2   Harper, R. (1956) Abstract. Bull. Brit. Psych. Soc.
     Harper, R. (1972) Proc. Inst. Food Sci. and Technol., 5, 211-216.

3   Land, D.G. (1977) ARC Research Rev., 3 (1), 5-8.

4   Harper, R., Bate-Smith, E.C. and Land, D.G. (1968) Odour Description
     and Odour Classification. Churchill; London.

5   Dravnieks, A. (1973) Report to Task Group 04.05 (Sensory Evaluation)
     American Soc. Testing and Materials, Philadelphia.

6   Harper, R., Bate-Smith, E.C., Land, D.G. and Griffiths, N.M. (1968)
     Perfum. and Essent. Oil Rec., 59, 22-37.

7   Harper, R., Land D.G., Griffiths, N.M. and Bate-Smith, E.C. (1968)
     Brit. J. Psychol., 3, 231-252.

8   Harper, R. (1975) Chem. Senses and Flav., 1, 353-357.

9   Land, D.G., Harper, R. and Griffiths, N.M. (1970)
     Flavour Ind., 1, 842-846.

10   Nursten, H. (in press) Proc. Int. Symp. on Sensory Properties of Food.
     National College of Food Technol., Univ. Reading.

11   Data collected by Dr. Miles Sawyer on leave of absence from the
     Department of Food Science and Nutrition, University of Massachusetts
     at Amherst, May-July 1977.

12   Punnett, P.W. and Eddy, W.R. (1930), Food Ind. 2, 401-404.

13   Crocker, E.C. and Henderson, L.F. (1927), Amer. Perfumer essent. Oil
     Rev., 22, 325-327, 356.

14   Crocker, E.C. (1945) Flavour. McGraw-Hill, New York.

15   Caul, J.F. (1957),   Advanc. in Food Res., 7, 1–40.

16   von Sydow, E., Anderson, J., Anjou, K., Karlsson, G., Land, D.G. and
     Griffiths, N.M. (1970).   Lebensm. Wiss. u Technol., 3, 11–17.

17   Persson, T., von Sydow, E. and Akesson, C. (1973)
     J. Food Sci., 38, 386.

18   von Sydow, E. (1975) Proc. Roy. Soc., 191B, 145–153.

19   Wren, J.J. (1972) J. Inst. Brewing, 78, 69–75.

20   Clapperton, J.F., (1973) J.Inst. Brewing, 79, 495–508.

21   Clapperton, J.F., Dalgliesh, C.E. and Meilgaard, M.C. (1975)
     MBBA Quarterly, 12, 273–280.

22   Williams, A.A., (1975) J. Sci. Food Agric., 26, 567–582.

23   British Standards Institution Committee on Sensory Analysis was
     established in 1968 and has published a glossary on terminology,
     and is about to publish one on methodology in sensory analysis.

24   The International Standards Organization (ISO) has a sub-Committee
     on the Sensory Analysis of Agricultural Products and periodically
     issues documents on recommended practices derived from discussions
     between the representatives from different countries.

Flavour research - a return to sensory evaluation

Anthony A. Williams

University of Bristol, Cider and Fruit Juices Section, Research Station, Long Ashton, Bristol, UK

ABSTRACT

In the field of flavour chemistry a great deal of emphasis over recent years has been placed on evaluating the flavour significance of compounds found in foods and beverages. This paper briefly reviews the methods which are being used and discusses some of the more complex sensory procedures which are developing and the problems of relating such information to preference assessments and, eventually, consumer acceptance.

INTRODUCTION

The development and refinements of sophisticated instrumental techniques over the last twenty years opened up a complete new dimension in the scientist's ability to identify and quantify components potentially responsible for flavour. The result of this is that large compilations of compounds present in individual foods and beverages now exist. These are, however, of little value to the flavourist or industry in general, unless they can be related to some aspect of flavour and quality enabling the information to be used in quality control and product improvement. It is to try and satisfy this need that many flavour chemists are directing an increasing proportion of their effort to sensory techniques. In our own research, whereas ten years ago obtaining such information was mainly intuitive, it now forms an integral part of a three directional research programme on quality evaluation[1,2]. Objective profile assessment is used to define the flavour characteristics of a product and to obtain information on the variation of these characteristics due to external factors such as variety, storage and processing. By relating such objective information to the physico-chemical data and to hedonic evaluation from either small laboratory or consumer panels, the cause of the various descriptive terms being used can be discovered and their importance to acceptance and overall quality established.

METHOD OF ASSESSING THE ORGANOLEPTIC IMPORTANCE OF COMPONENTS

Three general procedures have been used to interpret some of the information obtained from the analysis of potential flavour components in foods. Broadly speaking they cover all approaches from assessing the components in isolation, building up the information to interpret the complex aroma and flavour patterns to assessing the aroma and flavour in their entirety and comparing the information with the analytical data.

Sensory assessment of separated components

The sensory assessment of components as they are being separated by gas or liquid chromatographic techniques is a valuable means of obtaining an indication of the flavour characteristics of components[3,4,5,6]. In most flavour laboratories such techniques are now fairly common practice, participants being asked to describe components in their own terms or using predetermined adjectives. In work on apples this rather simple approach has led to flavour significance being attached to such compounds as ethyl 2-methylbutyrate, hexanal, 2-hexenal[7], 4-methoxyallylbenzene[8] and damascenone[4], hexyl acetate and hexyl 2-methylbutyrate (Williams and Lewis, unpublished results). Trapping, followed by examination of fractions in solution, enables this concept to be extended and various combinations of components to be evaluated together rather than individually, a technique which has been put to admirable use recently by Parliment and Scarpellino[9] enabling them to identify linalool and trans 2-hexenal as being important to the characteristic flavour of American blueberry.

Threshold values

The use of threshold values of compounds as a means of estimating their relative flavour potential was first used in 1957[10], the logic being that the smaller the amount of a compound that one can detect the more likely it is to contribute to the flavour of any product in which it is found. By indicating the degree by which the concentration of a compound in a food or beverage exceeds its threshold value it is possible to get an indication of the contribution it makes to the overall flavour. This idea has been used by many authors, the quotient $\dfrac{\text{concentration of compound in product}}{\text{threshold concentration}}$ being given various names from odour values to flavour units[11,12,13].

Typical of the information which the use of such quotients can give is shown by their application to the volatiles isolated from ciders[14] (Table 1). From such information one can get an indication of the relative flavour-contributing potential of the various compounds present. In foods and beverages, however, compounds are perceived not as individual components but

TABLE 1. A selection of compounds of potential organoleptic significance in cider

Compound	Approximate concentration in cider (ppm)	Selected threshold value (ppm)	Odour value concentration threshold	Description
3-Methylbutanol	80	40	2.0	Choking, alcoholic, winey
2-Phenylethanol	50	58	1.0	Roses, honeylike
4-Ethylphenol	2	1.0	2	Woody, medicinal, cidery
4-Ethylguaiacol	1	0.1	10	Phenolic, spicy
Acetic acid	150	80	1.9	Sour, pungent
Ethyl 3-methyl-butyrate	4	0.1	40	Fruity, apple, banana
3-Methylbutyl acetate	10	2	5.0	Fruity, sweet, pear drops
Ethyl hexanoate	0.2	0.19	1.0	Fruity, winey
2-Phenylethyl acetate	4	4	1.0	Sweet, fruity, roses, cidery

as complex mixtures. Limited information can be obtained on how compounds interact by comparing threshold values and flavour characters of mixtures with odour values of the constituent components, information of this nature having been used to predict flavour differences in beers[15]. To extrapolate information obtained at threshold levels to the higher concentrations and the completely different situation existing in foods and beverages, however, the concept of odour values assumes an analogous increase in perceived intensity for all compounds and mixtures, an assumption which is not altogether justified[16,17,18,19,20].

Correlations between analytical and sensory data

The third broad approach to elucidating the flavour significance of compounds in foods hinges on discovering mathematical relationships which exist between sensory descriptions of the product and the analytical data as a whole. The techniques which have been used range from purely visual comparison such as was used in the early work reported by McCarthy et al on bananas[21] to the much more sophisticated computer based methods of the last ten years, as expounded by workers in the USA[22] and Sweden[23]. Stepwise discriminant, multiple discriminant and various ranking techniques have been used to indicate the analytical parameters which enable a series of products to be distinguished or categorised from the point of view of some sensory attribute or variable such as blend composition, price or source. It has been used successfully on many products ranging from Pepsi and Coca Cola[24] to orange oils[25], but apart from the recent publication by Qvist et al[23] its use has been restricted to general characteristics such as flavour scores and overall acceptance.

Regression techniques have also been used to discover relationships between sensory attributes and the analytical data. All the available information may be used deriving a general regression equation[26], or alternatively one may restrict the data to various combinations and functions of the analytical results using psychophysical concepts, as has been done by the workers at the Swedish Institute of Food Preservation and Research[27,28,29].

Normal discriminant and regression techniques at their best are limited to the relationship of one variable in one set of data (e.g. one sensory attribute) with a set of variables in the other set (the analytical data). In real life, however, one perceives an overall sensation from a food rather than separate sensations from individual stimuli. In an attempt to simulate this overall relationship, canonical correlation and multiple regression between the principle variables or groups of variables obtained by factor or principal component analysis or multidimensional scaling techniques can be used[30,31,32].

With all the methods discussed for relating sensory and analytical data it must be remembered that any relationships established are in the first instance purely statistical and only hold within the context of the experimental data examined. Ability to extend a relationship beyond this point so that it can be used to predict responses from new sets of data makes the relationship of value in a quality control situation, but even so, it is only a mathematical relationship and need not necessarily involve causative stimuli. The repeated occurrence of similar compounds in predictive models, however, makes it highly probable that causative stimuli are involved. The only true way to check whether established relationships are causative, however, is to alter the amounts of postulated important compounds and submit the product to further sensory evaluation.

SENSORY EVALUATION (OBJECTIVE)

To enable sensory data to be related meaningfully to analytical data and to act as the link between consumer acceptance and the analytical results, the sensory information obtained must be as detailed and precise as the analytical data.

The development of defined vocabularies based on the terminology described by Harper et al[33], rather than the relatively simple approach of the original profile procedures[34], has therefore been the trend over the last few years. In our work on cider and whole apples[1,35] once a vocabulary was agreed upon, the various descriptions were defined by reference to standards or by association with other foods, terms and standards being checked to ensure that they were meaningful to panelists by performing blind assessments and by studying correlation coefficients and principal component vectors after the language had been in use for a period of time.

Definition of a vocabulary is only one of the problems associated with sensory evaluation. Estimation of the level of an attribute can be equally as problematical. When using scaling techniques, difficulties arise due to the skew nature of the raw sensory data and due to the fact that different people score at different levels. From work of Powers and co-workers[36] it also appears that people tend to operate different intervals between different scores.

SENSORY EVALUATION (SUBJECTIVE)

Objective sensory assessment provides a valuable tool for evaluating differences and changes in foods and for relating such changes to analytical data. To be of real value to a producer, however, such information must be capable of being related to preference, quality and consumer acceptance. Although there are a number of successful reports in the literature[22,37] relating hedonic assessments directly to instrumental data, we have felt it unwise to do this because different people may have different reasons for preference. We believe it wiser to use the trained objective panel as an intermediary.

Considering overall acceptance and quality not all attributes play an equal role. Examination of the relationship between overall quality of Cox apples and the ratings given to such general attributes as external and internal appearance, colour, external and internal aroma, taste, texture and feel of the apple from a number of assessors (Table 2) illustrates this point. It also indicates that different attributes are not of equal importance to all panelists. Whilst taking means, therefore, is justifiable when interpreting objective assessments, when handling hedonic data it is more appropriate to divide the population into sub-sets according to similarity of reasons for preference.

The problem of interpreting quality is further complicated by the fact that attributes, whether of a specific or general nature as described above, may not have the same relative importance throughout the hedonic range. It

TABLE 2. Correlation coefficients for attribute ratings with overall rating
from a selection of individual assessors

			Tasters				
	A	B	C	D	E	F	G
External appearance	0.84	0.71*	0.38	0.40	0.50	0.65	-0.23
External colour	0.82	0.58	0.06	0.44	0.42	0.30	0.52
Internal appearance	0.88	0.29	0.23	0.32	0.52	0.40	0.012
Internal colour	0.85	0.42	-0.10	0.08	0.49	0.57	0.31
External aroma	0.80	0.39	0.42	0.31	0.17	0.55	0.61
Internal aroma	0.88	0.29	0.61	0.36	0.60	0.56	0.71
Taste	0.91	0.56	0.78	0.70	0.77	0.62	0.80
Texture	0.92	0.67	0.50	0.53	0.88	0.70	0.19

* Underlined figures = correlation coefficients > 0.70

is highly probable that certain attributes, such as texture and taste, exert
their maximum effect only up to a particular level of quality. Above this
point previously less significant characteristics start to play a dominant
role.

CONCLUSION

Flavour and quality are sensory responses and although much information
can be gleaned about a product by modern analytical techniques, the two must
be related if results are to be of any value to industry. To satisfy this
end, flavour research must of necessity involve effort from three directions,
objective sensory assessment to discover what characteristics are present in
a food or beverage, analysis to discover their cause and the consumer to
pronounce on desirability. Many problems, in particular the psychophysics
of odour mixtures above threshold levels and the interpretation of consumer
response, still need to be solved if we are to understand fully the interrelationships of these three aspects. It is only by solving these problems,
however, that the flavour chemist will produce criteria which will enable a
manufacturer to produce products with the sensory qualities his customers
want.

ACKNOWLEDGMENTS

The co-operation of C.R. Baines, M.J. Lewis and Caroline S. Carter is
gratefully acknowledged in respect of work taken from current projects in
this publication.

REFERENCES

1. Williams, A.A. (1975) J. Sci. Food Agric. 26, 567-582
2. Williams, A.A. and Knee, M. Ann. Appl. Biol. (in press)
3. Von Sydow, E., Andersson, J., Anjou, K., Karlsson, G., Land, D.G. and Griffiths, N. (1970) Lebensm.-Wiss. Technol. 3, 11-17
4. Nursten, H.E. and Woolfe, M.L. (1972) J. Sci. Food Agric. 23, 803-822
5. Stern, D.J., Guadagni, D.G. and Stevens, K.L. (1975) Am. J. Enol. Vitic. 26, 208-213
6. Noble, A.C. (1976) J. Agric. Food Chem. 24, 321-323
7. Flath, R.A. Black, D.R., Guadagni, D.G., McFadden, W.H. and Schultz, T.H. (1967) J. Agric. Food Chem. 15, 29-35
8. Williams, A.A., Tucknott, O.G. and Lewis, M.J. (1977) J. Sci. Food Agric. 28, 185-190
9. Parliment, T.H. and Scarpellino, R. (1977) J. Agric. Food Chem. 25, 97-99
10. Patton, S. and Josephson, D.V. (1957) Food Res. 22, 316-318
11. Guadagni, D.G. (1968) in Correlation of Subjective-Objective Methods in the Study of Odour and Taste, American Society for Tasting and Materials Special Publication No.440, pp. 36-47, American Society for Testing and Materials, Philadelphia
12. Salo, P., Nykanen, L. and Suomalainen, H. (1972) J. Food Sci. 37, 394-398
13. Meilgaard, M.C. (1975) Tech. Q. Master Brew. Assoc. Am. 12, 151-163
14. Williams, A.A. (1974) J. Inst. Brew. 80, 455-470
15. Stenroos, L.E., Siebert, K.J. and Meilgaard, M.C. (1976) J. Am. Soc. Brew. Chem. 34, 4-13
16. Reese, T.S. and Steven, S.S. (1960) Am. J. Psychol. 73, 424-428
17. Cain, W.S. (1969) Percept. Psychophys. 6, 349-354
18. Patte, F., Etcheto, M. and Laffont, P. (1975) Chem. Senses and Flavour, 1, 283-305
19. Koster, E.P. (1968) Olfactologia 1, 29.41
20. Cain, W.S. (1975) Chem. Senses and Flavour 1, 339-352
21. McCarthy, A.L., Palmer, J.K., Shaw, C.P. and Anderson, E.E. (1963) J. Food Sci. 28, 379-384
22. Powers, J.J. and Quinlan, M.C. (1974) J. Agric. Food Chem. 22, 744-749
23. Qvist, I.H., Von Sydow, E. and Akesson, C.A. (1976) Lebensm.-Wiss. Technol. 9, 311-320
24. Young, L.L., Bergmann, R.E. and Powers, J.J. (1970) J. Food Sci. 35, 219-223
25. Gostecnik, G.F. and Zlatkis, H. (1975) J. Chromatogr. 106, 73-81
26. Aishima, T. and Nobuhara, A. (1977) Food Chem. 2, 81-93
27. Persson, T., Von Sydow, E., Akesson, C. (1973) J. Food Sci. 38, 682-689
28. Karlsson-Ekstrom, G. and Von Sydow, E. (1973) Lebensm.-Wiss. Technol. 6, 86-89
29. Akesson, C., Persson, T. and Von Sydow, E. (1975) Proceedings of the IVth International Congress of Food Science and Technology, Madrid 1974, Vol. II, pp. 187-189, Instituto Nacional de Ciencia y Tecnología d'Alimentos Consejo Superior de Investigaciones Cientisicas, Valencia, Spain
30. Tanaka, T. and Saito, N. (1969) J. Ferment. Technol. 47, 780-789
31. Vuataz, L., Sotek, J. and Rahim, H.M. (in press) Proceedings of the IVth International Congress of Food Science and Technology, Madrid 1974, Vol. I (abridged version only consulted)
32. Powers, J.J. and Bergmann, R.E. in Flavour Quality: Objective Measurement, Am. Chem. Soc. Symposium, Series No. 51, Am. Chem. Soc. (in press)
33. Harper, R., Bate-Smith, E.C., Land, D.G. and Griffiths, N.M. (1968) Perf. Essent. Oil Rec. 55, 22-37

34. Caul, J.F. (1957) Adv. Food Res. 7, 1-39
35. Williams, A A. and Carter, C.S. submitted to J. Sci. Food Agric.
36. Powers, J.J. (1975) Proceedings of the IVth International Congress of Food Science & Technology, Madrid 1974, Vol. II, pp. 173-182, Instituto Nacional de Ciencia y Tecnología d'Alimentos Consejo Superior de Investigaciones Cientisicas, Valencia, Spain
37. Von Sydow, E. and Akesson, C.A. (1977) Paper presented at the Symposium on Sensory Properties of Food, Weybridge, England

Sensory aspects of flavour in alcoholic beverages - the strength and quality of whisky aroma

Paula Jounela-Eriksson[x]

Research Laboratories of the State Alcohol Monopoly (Alko), Box 350, SF-00101 Helsinki 10, Finland

ABSTRACT

The factors affecting the flavour experience in a beverage are smell and taste, but also appearance and the mouth-feel, which is mainly dependent on touch. The compounds identified in the flavour of alcoholic beverages include higher alcohols, fatty acids, fatty acid esters, lactones, and carbonyl, phenolic, sulphur and nitrogen compounds. Nevertheless, it is not yet possible to determine the aroma of even the volatile fraction in terms of the aroma compounds, even though these continuously grow in number. A method was developed for estimating statistically checked odour thresholds. A whisky imitation with 67 ingredient substances and rectified grain spirit was used as a model. The odour thresholds were used with quantitative gas chromatography to describe the role played by aroma components in producing the aroma of the whisky imitation. These relative odour intensities revealed several possible kinds of interaction in the aroma complex. Additionally, a study was made of how added aroma components, which were observed to compose the core of the aroma in the whisky imitation, affected the aroma of some genuine whiskies.

INTRODUCTION

The use of alcoholic beverages arises from both the intoxicating effect and the pleasant sensory experience obtained from them. When drinking alcoholic beverages our senses tell the colour, aroma nuances, taste characteristics and even the suppleness of the beverage. In addition to the characteristics of the beverage, many factors, such as mood, company, environment, food accompanying the beverage and so on have an influence on the experience. A person drinking the beverage perceives the sensations and associates them with the environmental factors already mentioned, the result being a pleasant or unpleasant overall impression at different levels. The flavour of an alcoholic beverage has, however, an intrinsic meaning within the sensation. Flavour has traditionally been one of the most important quality factors of alcoholic beverages. Unfortunately it is nearly impossible to obtain an unambiguous picture of the flavour of a beverage without tasting it.

THE SENSES AND THE FLAVOUR OF ALCOHOLIC BEVERAGES

When drinking alcoholic beverages our senses provide us with an overall impression generally called the aroma of the beverage. This in fact means the flavour of the beverage describing primarily the overall impression of odour and taste but also involving the other senses. In addition to odour and taste, sight as well as feelings transmitted by tactile and pressure senses in the regions of the mouth, nose and larynx and by sense cells reacting to temperature come into play.[1]

Sight creates the first impression of the beverage, revealing its colour and clarity or turbidity. Most alcoholic beverages have their own characteristic colour if the beverage is not completely colourless. On the other hand clarity is a desired qualitative positive feature. A human being acts under the control of his sense of sight to such an extent that a certain flavour is recognized for a product of a particular colour on the basis of visual memory and conceptual impressions.[2] The colours of food and beverages in particular are associated with previous qualitative experience, and thus act as immediate indicators of the fitness of a product.

The sense of smell follows in forming an impression of the beverage consumed. A person can more easily distinguish between different odours than various levels of intensity. Although the quality and intensity of odour are perceived at the same time, the sensation of pleasantness or disagreeableness is more dominant than intensity. The intensity of odour produced by a volatile substance can be most conveniently analysed at the threshold level, whereas phenomena occurring above or below this level are explained by means of mathematical models requiring certain hypotheses. These hypotheses cannot be verified until the origin of the odour sensation has been determined. The volatile aroma fraction of alcoholic beverages is always made up of many smells mixed together. The quantities of most components can vary within certain limits while the total aroma still remains acceptable. Since the odour of the mixture can either be stronger, weaker or the same than the strength of individual odours in the mixture, it is a pity that the phenomena cannot today be satisfactorily explained mathematically in mixtures consisting of more than two or three components.[3] On the other hand, the conception of pleasantness greatly varies from one individual to another as does human sensitivity to various odours. Thus statistical methods are necessary when charting aroma preferences and likewise cannot be neglected when analysing the intensity of the aroma.

Although the flavour nuances of distilled beverages especially are mainly based on different odours, the importance of taste should not be under-estimated. The quality of water used in a beverage does not often emerge until later in the taste of the beverage. Even though the sensation of odour is prevalent in the flavour of a distilled beverage, its taste must charac-terise it and, in the first place, be flawless. The combined effects of taste and odour in undistilled beverages are inseparable to the extent that the flavour of wine or beer cannot be discussed without taste sensations. The mutual interactions of taste sensations are better known than those of odour sensations, and in addition ethyl alcohol has its own effects. An experienced wine producer attempts to control the relationships between alcohol content, sweetness and acidity in order to attain the most harmonious flavour in the product or the typical taste characteristic for a particular wine.

In addition to the senses of smell and taste ethyl alcohol provokes a third sense reacting to chemical stimulants, called the general chemical sense. The burning or hot sensation in the mucous membranes of the mouth and throat produced by diffuse nerve endings can be perceived most clearly when consuming alcoholic beverages in which the concentration of extracts is low but alcohol content high, as it is for instance in vodka. A slight stimulative pheno-menon is sought after thorough flavouring in order to accentuate aroma. There are also diffuse and specialized nerve cells functioning as the tactile sense in the mucous membranes of the mouth. During drinking or thereafter, a so-called mouth-feel is recorded on the mucous membranes. This is primarily determined by the viscosity of the beverage but also by its density, surface tension and other chemical or physical properties. As a result of the stimu-lation of the tactile sense we feel the suppleness of the beverage as well as its smoothness or hardness. The beverage's mouth-feel is at its best when its various components form a harmonious whole. The mellowness of wine resulting from an appropriate degree of maturity of the grapes is a typical feature perceived with the tactile sense. In the same manner, the effect of carbon dioxide rests not only on its more rapid transfer of substances pro-ducing scents to the reach of the sense of smell but also on its capability to stimulate the tactile sense. The so-called astringent sensation caused by tannic substances appearing as a "puckerish and dry" feeling in the jaws especially deserves mentioning as well. This phenomenon arises from the combined effect of several senses on the mucous membranes of the mouth. Additionally a great number of sense cells react to temperature in the mouth. Temperature also affects the action of the other senses and the physical characteristics of the beverages, especially the volatility of aroma components.

Every sensory experience results in a pleasant or unpleasant feeling on various levels. A person does not assess different sensations so much according to intensity as to pleasantness. The scale of preferences varies with each individual. It has been noticed in wine tasting tests performed at the Slovakian Technical University[4] for instance that preferences arising from chemical, visual and tactile sensations are determined individually. Tests have also indicated that in experiencing flavour the brain does not sum up individual sensations but instead multiplies them. In the equation developed to describe a wine's sensorial total value the degree of preference therefore appears as an exponent.

$$R = V_1^{0.1} \cdot V_2^{0.3} \cdot V_3^{0.5} \cdot V_4^{0.1}$$

where R = Sensorial total value of wine (with the exponents of experts)

V_1 = Value for visual observation V_3 = Value for taste observation

V_2 = Value for odour observation V_4 = Value for tactile observation

Experimentally specified exponents of various sensations are so divided that the taste sensations of experts were clearly weighted more heavily, whereas sight and tactile sensations turned out to be of minor significance. On the contrary, students representing typical consumers preferred visual sensations to those of smell and taste. Thus a human's sensory world resting firmly on visual sensations is apparent in evaluating wines as well, though they are traditionally appreciated according to taste and aroma.

THE CHEMICAL COMPOSITION OF ALCOHOLIC BEVERAGES

The flavour sensed in alcoholic beverages is created by compounds called the aroma components either originating in raw materials or produced during fermentation. The less volatile components primarily influence the taste of the beverage. They abound in undistilled beverages such as wines and beers. Research on the flavour of alcoholic beverages chiefly concentrates on volatile aroma substances appearing in all alcoholic beverages.[5-6]

Different raw materials for beverages seem to produce only minor effects on the aroma composition of the beverages.[7] Both in wines and beers as well as in distilled beverages the same volatile aroma components comprise the bulk of the aroma (Fig. 1). Yeast apparently produces the quantitatively important aroma substances in the fermentation solution, so the aroma of beverages produced by fermentation is dependent on the type of yeast used and the fermentation conditions. When producing distilled beverages distillation methods

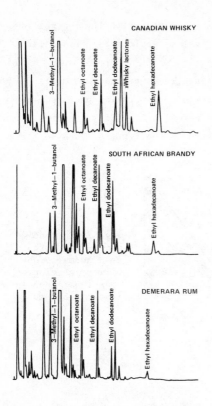

Fig. 1. Gas chromatograms of some of the major aroma components isolated from different alcoholic beverages.[5]

play a decisive role in the composition of aroma. Because the aroma of fresh distillates is generally raw and pungent, many of the beverages are matured for years before consumption.[8] It must also be remembered that the brand names of distilled beverages as well as many wines are blends containing many dozens of distillates or production batches.

Along with the growth in the number of known aroma components it becomes increasingly difficult to conclude what components chiefly produce the characteristic aroma of a beverage. In spite of the similarity in the chemical aroma composition of different beverages, they can be easily differentiated with the senses. Sensory physiology and chemical analytics operate in different ways. A human being senses flavour as a totality, whereas the chemical analysis only reveals individual aroma components and their concentrations.

For this reason merging sensory evaluations and chemical analysis has not always fulfilled the hopes set for it, at least in aroma research. It is possible, however, to analyse dependencies between various types of data with today's statistical methods. The aim of the combined research is to describe the sensed impression by means of known taste and aroma components and to analyse how components create flavours.

THRESHOLD VALUES

Aroma is the sensory response evoked by volatiles. Aroma components and their concentrations are known but also it is evident that concentration does not alone determine the intensity of the aroma produced by a component. Threshold value is one useful basic unit of measuring sensation intensity. Since individual differences are great in threshold values the definitions of threshold values must be based on iterative and statistically controlled methods. A method to define odour threshold values employing a triangular test has been developed at the Research Laboratories of the Finnish State Alcohol Monopoly.[9] The threshold levels were determined by using the percentage-above-chance scores as a function of logarithmic concentration and assuming the distribution of the scores to follow the normal probability function (Fig. 2). The threshold values were determined at the level of 50 % positive responses.

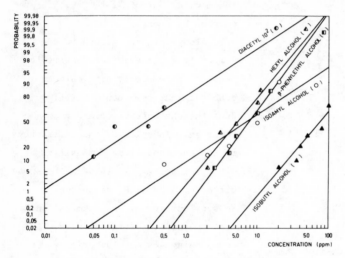

Fig. 2. Percentage-above-chance scores as a normal probability function of logarithmic concentration of some alcohols and diacetyl.[9]

WHISKY IMITATION AND INTERACTIONS OF AROMA COMPONENTS

Those compounds influencing the intensity of total aroma can be isolated from numerous aroma components by comparing the relationships of threshold values and concentrations of aroma substances. Nevertheless, the mutual interactions of the components can create the flavour impression to be sensed. Attempts to analyse these interactions were made using an artificial Scotch whisky imitation. The whisky imitation consisted of nine carbonyls, 13 alcohols, 21 acids, 24 esters and highly rectified grain spirits. Phenol and sulphur compounds as well as heavy compounds were excluded from the imitation, which contained only one lactone, β-methyl-γ-octalactone.[10] In addition to the threshold values for individual compounds, the threshold values for some compound mixtures and the aroma fractions of alcohols, esters, acids and carbonyls were also determined. The relative contribution of each component, mixture or fraction to the odour was estimated by dividing the concentration by the respective threshold. This quotient was called the "odour unit".

As it proved difficult to express the relative intensity of aroma fractions and mixtures as a sum of the odour units of the separate components, an attempt was made to develop a method to reveal the prevailing interactions. At the threshold level of a mixture, its odour was just perceptible, and the sum of the odour unit values of the components should be equal to the odour units of the mixture, assuming components did not interact.[11]

$$O_B + O_C + O_D \cdots = O_1$$

were O_B, O_C, O_D.... = odour unit values of the components B, C, D....
O_1 = odour unit value of a mixture 1.

In other words, by measuring the odour unit value of an individual component with the odour unit value of the mixture a proportion value was constructed which should sum to 1 for a mixture - or to 100 to simplify calculations - if the components were additive. If the components sum to less than 100, they are synergistic, and if the sum exceeds 100, they interact suppressively. Uncertainties in the threshold values were considered when deciding whether the calculated sum of proportion values significantly deviated from the expected value of 100.

The effect of some alcohols in the whisky imitation on the aroma intensity of the alcohol fraction is presented in Table 1. All alcohols seemed additive. The proportion value for 3-methyl-1-butanol did not, however, deviate significantly from the proportion value for the whole fraction.

Table 1.

	'Odour unit'		'Proportion value'	
	in Mixture	in alcohol fraction	in Mixture	in alcohol fraction
Alcohol Mixture 1 (9 alcohols with odour units less than 0.5)		2.1		4.7
Alcohol Mixture 2		5.0	103.0^{ns}	11.0
iso-Butyl alcohol	2.3		46.0	
2-Methylbutan-1-ol	2.9		57.0	
3-Methylbutan-1-ol		36.0		78.6
β-Phenethyl alcohol		0.6		1.3
Total alcohols		45.4		95.6^{ns}

ns = Total value does not deviate significantly from the expected value of 100 (P > 0.10).

Table 2.

	'Odour unit'		'Proportion value'	
	in Mixture	in acid fraction	in Mixture	in acid fraction
Acid Mixture 1 (13 acids with odour units less than 0.1)		0.8		1.9
Acid Mixture 2		3.3	24.6^{xxx}	8.4
iso-Butyric acid	0.3		9.6	
Butyric acid	0.2		7.2	
Hexanoic acid	0.3		7.8	
Acid Mixture 3		57.4	16.6^{xxx}	144.0
Acetic acid	1.4		2.3	
iso-Valeric acid	4.3		7.4	
Octanoic acid	0.9		1.6	
Decanoic acid	1.8		3.2	
Dodecanoic acid	1.2		2.1	
Total acids		39.8		154.0^{xx}

xx = Total deviates significantly from the expected value of 100 (P < 0.01).
xxx = Total deviates highly significantly from the expected value of 100 (P < 0.001).

Table 1 and Table 2. Contributions of alcohols and acids to strength of aroma in whisky imitation.[11]

Thus 3-methyl-1-butanol would dominate the aroma intensity of the alcohol fraction. Correspondingly in the acid fraction of the whisky imitation (Table 2), acid mixture 3 seems to form the majority of the aroma, but suppressive interactions appear in the fraction. In the ester fraction on the other hand synergistic effects apparently dominate. Nevertheless, it has generally been found that most odours are usually weaker in mixtures than when sensed individually.[3] By means of these relative values mentioned above, the achieved results need not be interpreted to mean that these types of interactions would necessarily dominate among the compounds analysed in every case. This research seeks to analyse those compounds in the composition of whisky aroma important from the standpoint of aroma intensity as well as those fluctuating in concentration apparently affecting the intensity or quality of aroma.

THE EFFECT OF ADDED CONCENTRATIONS OF COMPONENTS ON AROMA

The methods depicted above have sought after compounds in the jungle of aroma components in whisky which are assumed to be of prime significance in whisky aroma. The following was considered a prerequisite in examining what kind of concentration changes would apparently be detectable organoleptically. Since the test was also meant to be performed with genuine whiskies, only an increase in concentrations by means of chemical augmentations was considered satisfactory. Removing aroma components or fractions from whisky is unsuccessful, resulting in a product which has no longer anything to do with whisky.

When various aroma fractions were added to the whisky imitation, it was noticed that a 3-4 times higher concentration caused a perceptible change in aroma intensity (Fig. 3). Deviation was largest in the alcohol fraction, apparently caused by 3-methyl-1-butanol where deviation was greater than that in the entire alcohol fraction. The threshold value of 3-methyl-1-butanol has also been observed to vary individually to a large degree. The ester addition seemed to have the most rapid influence on the aroma of the whisky imitation not withstanding the fact that the aroma composition obviously included in this case a disproportionate number of esters when compared with genuine Scotch whiskies.

With genuine whiskies it was impossible to make a corresponding addition of the total fraction, but adding single components or their mixtures had to suffice. In this case the subject of study was a Scotch whisky bottled in Finland as well as a Sotch whisky blended in Finland in which Finnish grain

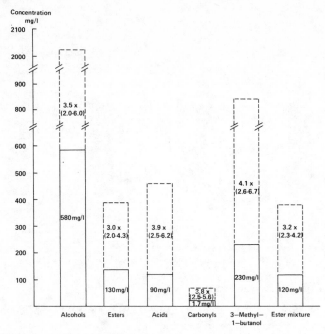

Fig. 3. Additions of various fractions to whisky imitation producing perceptible changes in aroma. Ester mixture consisted of ethyl acetate, octanoate, decanoate, dodecanoate and 3-methylbutyl acetate.

spirits had been substituted in place of grain whisky. Differences in the concentrations of fusel alcohols in these are smaller than in the whiskies generally. The results reveal that it was possible to add a mixture of iso-butanol and 2-methyl-1-butanol to both of them with a 3 times higher concentration before the panel could differentiate with statistical significance between the augmented whisky and the original (Fig. 4). Phenethyl alcohol clearly differs from the fusel alcohols; it was necessary to add more than 40 times as much before a distinction could be made in the whisky aroma. In general phenethyl alcohol parallels esters as an aroma component but in this context it did not behave as esters do.

In the same way, ester and acid mixtures were added to whiskies. The composition was the same as that of the ester and acid mixtures referred to above, with a heavy influence on the aroma of the whisky imitation. Acetic acid and ethyl acetate were omitted, however. An addition of one-quarter or one-half concentration to the esters is sufficient to make a statistical difference, but with the acids a 2.5 concentration is required before the panel can differentiate with statistical significance (Fig. 4). Thus a relatively small change in the concentration of esters affects the intensity of the whisky aroma. On the contrary, a really conclusive divergence in the concentration of acids and especially fusel alcohols must occur before a

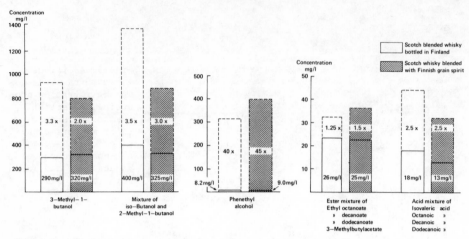

Fig. 4. Additions of some fusel alcohols, esters and acids producing a perceptible change in aromas of two Scotch whiskies.

perceptible change takes place in the whisky aroma.

What is presented above indicates that at least the aroma of whisky – or other alcoholic beverages – cannot be determined by means of analysed compounds. Also specific components essential to aroma cannot be listed as generally accepted. Instead, development of different applications has succeeded to meet the practical needs of aroma quality control and product development.

^{x}former Salo

REFERENCES

1. Le Magnen, J. (1976) Proceedings of 4th Nordic Symposium Sensory Properties of Foods, March 18-20, 1976, Skövde, Sweden, pp. 5-22

2. Harper, R. (1972) Human Senses in Action, pp. 154-159, Churchill Livingstone, Edinburgh and London

3. Moskowitz, H.R. (1975) Lebensm. Wiss. + Technol. 8, 237-242

4. Malik, F. (1975) Vinohrah, 13, (1) 14-15

5. Suomalainen, H., Nykänen, L. and Eriksson, K. (1974) Amer. J. Enol. Viticult. 25, 179-187

6. Suomalainen, H. (1975) Ann. Technol. Agr. 24, 453-467

7. Suomalainen, H. and Lehtonen, M. (1976) Kemia-Kemi, 3, 69-77

8. Salo, P., Lehtonen, M. and Suomalainen, H. (1976) Proceedings of 4th Nordic Symposium, Sensory Properties of Foods, March 18-20, 1976, Skövde, Sweden, pp. 87-108

9. Salo, P. (1970)
   J. Food Sci. 35, 95-99

10. Salo, P., Nykänen, L. and Suomalainen, H. (1972)
    J. Food Sci., 37, 394-398

11. Salo, P. (1975) in Aroma Research, Proceedings of the International
    Symposium on Aroma Research, Central Institute for Nutrition and Food
    Research TNO, Zeist, Netherlands, May 26-29, 1975, pp. 121-130,
    Centre for Agricultural Publishing and Documentation, Wageningen

Taste and chemical composition of drinking water

B. C. J. Zoeteman, G. J. Piet, C. F. H. Morra and F. E. de Grunt

National Institute for Water Supply, P. O. Box 150, 2260 AD Leidschendam, Netherlands

ABSTRACT

15% of the population of The Netherlands qualified the taste of tapwater, derived from surface water, as objectionable or worse. Water from 8 groundwater supplies tasted significantly better than water from 12 surface water supplies. Suboptimal levels of the hydrocarbonate-ion (less than 300 mg/l) were related with a slight adverse effect on the taste of water derived from groundwater. The present levels of saltions in tapwater could not be related to impaired taste of water prepared from surface water. Sensorily perceptible organic compounds in those tapwaters were e.g. geosmin, nonanal and octene, which were possibly introduced due to growth of organisms in reservoirs, as well as some insufficiently removed contaminants of water of the river Rhine, such as chlorinated benzenes and 1,3,5 trimethylbenzene. Consumption of water as such was 50% lower for individuals qualifying the taste as objectionable or worse compaired to those assessing water taste as good.

INTRODUCTION

Although drinking water should be tasteless and odourless for all consumers practical circumstances can often result in a water quality deviating largely from this requirement. A questionnaire held in The Netherlands in June 1976, among 3073 individuals of 18 years or older, by the Central Bureau of Statistics (Voorburg) and the National Institute for Water Supply (Leidschendam) showed that 91.7% of the population assessed water odour as good or not perceptible, while 82.7% qualified the taste of their tapwater in these categories. It was further found that impaired taste quality mainly occurred when tapwater was derived from surface water in stead of groundwater. Table 1 shows that 91.4% of the individuals assessed the taste as good or not perceptible in the case of groundwater supplies which figure is only 66.9% for surface water supplies.

Among the groundwater supplies those supplies with a low water hardness (2 meq/l or less) generally obtained a better taste rating, for the water as well as for tea derived from this water, than supplies with hard waters (4 meq/l or more).

Table 1.: Type of water source and taste assessment of tapwater in The
Netherlands

Water source	% of persons scoring in a taste category				
	good	not perceptible	weak, not objectionable	objectionable	very bad
Groundwater	38.69	52.73	5.83	1.78	0.76
Surface water	14.90	52.03	18.51	10.05	4.52

Inorganic ions as well as organic micropollutants have been related to
water taste [1-6]. Some ions have to be present in drinking water in a minimum
quantity, comparable to the concentration of ions in saliva, to give the
water a neutral taste. Impaired water taste seems to be particularly related
to organic substances of biological or industrial origin, which can cause e.g.
an earthy smell or a chlorine like smell of the water.

In order to identify the chemical compounds responsible for the impaired
taste of tapwater derived from surface water in The Netherlands 20 types of
drinking water were sampled in 1976 and presented to a selected panel for sensory evaluation and analysed for inorganic as well as organic components. The
next chapters describe the panel, the selected water supplies and the results
of the sensory assessment and chemical analysis of the tapwaters. The possible
effect of a number of identified individual chemicals on water taste will be
discussed and finally the impact of water taste on water consumption habits
is evaluated.

THE PANEL

A panel of about 50 subjects was selected which was as representative as
possible for the national population as far as age, sex and domicile distribution is concerned. Only subjects of 18 years and older were selected. Subjects showing a low odour sensitivity for aqueous solutions of isoborneol and
o-dichlorobenzene were excluded [4]. Besides the main test results it was found
that for the panel members smoking in combination with increased age resulted
in a significantly reduced odour sensitivity for o-dichlorobenzene (t=-2.77
for odour thresholds of subjects of 18 - 35 years versus subjects of 50 years
and older). However for isoborneol it was found that smoking increased the
odour sensitivity for all ages (t=2.35 for non-smokers versus smokers). All
panel members smoking more than 1 cigarette/day were considered to be smokers.
The sex of panel members was not found to influence significantly the odour
sensitivity for o-dichlorobenzene and isoborneol.

For the sensory evaluation of the 20 tapwaters 3 panel sessions were held. During each session 8 tapwaters were presented to the panel 20 times. The subjects were instructed to smell and taste the sample, without swallowing it, and to note on a punch card the item on a taste (odour) scale which resembled most closely the perceived sensations. The descriptive terms at the scale and the 1-dimensional solution for the scale values, constructed by the method of triads[7] after treatment by multidimensional analyses[8], are given in table 2.

Table 2.: Items and scale values for taste and odour description

Item number	Descriptive terms	Scale value
1	It tastes (smells) good	0.00
2	It has no perceptible taste (smell)	0.74
3	It has a weak, hardly objectionable taste (smell)	1.41
4	It has an objectionable taste (smell)	2.07
5	It tastes (smells) bad	2.87

Also the character of the water taste and odour had to be noted by indicating items like: chlorine like, earthy, putric, metallic and faint-unqualifiable. The sensory experiments were prepared and carried out in co-operation with Prof. Dr. E.P. Köster c.s.[4] of the Laboratory of Psychology, University of Utrecht, The Netherlands.

THE TYPES OF DRINKING WATER

A total number of 8 groundwater supplies and 12 surface water supplies were selected in such a way that during each panel session tapwaters belonging to both types and tapwaters with large differences in salt content were available. Furthermore two types of tapwater were represented during all 3 sessions to provide a basis for comparison and an indication of seasonal changes.

Among the 12 surface water supplies 7 applied chlorination and 3 ozonization. 10 of these supplies used water directly or indirectly originating from the river Rhine.

The water samples were collected in glass bottles of 25-50 liter for the sensory evaluation by the panel and in stainless steel vessels of 200 liter for most of the chemical determinations, which will be described in detail elsewhere.

SENSORY ASSESSMENT OF TAPWATER AND CHEMICAL SUBSTANCES

Generally smell of water samples was detected much less easily than water taste. Samples with mean taste ratings varying from 1.03-1.95 obtained mean odour ratings varying only from 0.83-0.98. Table 3 gives a survey of the mean taste scale values and the detected levels of the major cations.

Table 3.: Classification of 20 tapwaters according to the taste rating by a panel and presence of saltions

Tapwater type number	Main type of raw water		Type of storage	Mean taste scale value	Cations			Anions		
	ground water	surface water			Na^+ mg/l	Ca^{2+} mg/l	Mg^{2+} mg/l	HCO_3^- mg/l	Cl^- mg/l	SO_4^{2-} mg/l
1	+			1.12	33	95	14	308	64	8
2	+			1.16	40	72	10	246	51	13
3	+			1.16	7	38	4	112	11	6
4	+			1.16	21	62	10	177	39	25
5	+			1.19	8	29	4	84	13	6
6	+			1.19	9	36	5	115	15	11
7		+	Dune inf	1.20	27	97	10	262	51	58
8	+			1.21	82	173	31	634	134	1
9	+			1.23	12	24	4	66	17	13
10		+	Dune inf	1.30	79	114	16	270	135	78
11		+	Dune inf	1.48	101	104	14	182	187	98
12		+	Dune inf	1.55	74	100	9	195	147	72
13		+	Dune inf	1.59	61	85	5	182	118	86
14		+	Reservoir	1.68	79	54	12	104	82	108
15		+	Bankfiltr	1.70	86	104	16	274	156	30
16		+	Reservoir	1.81	124	98	20	70	242	144
17		+	Bankfiltr	1.91	46	75	13	180	92	41
18		+	Bankfiltr	2.01	75	88	17	193	154	71
19		+	Reservoir	2.06	120	53	16	91	175	88
20		+	Bankfiltr	2.06	80	104	17	230	158	55

The detected levels of cations were not high enough to affect seriously water taste, as shown in similar experiments with individual salt in water solutions[4]. Furthermore the highest levels found in tapwater derived from groundwater compared to surface water were not significantly different. It has also been shown that particularly $NaHCO_3$ contributes to the pleasant neutral taste of tapwater[4]. Such a tendancy was also present among the groundwater derived tapwaters, where the optimum quantity corresponds with a HCO_3^- content of 300 mg/l, which is normally present in saliva.

The data of table 3 further indicate that dune infiltration results in a product with a better taste than water treatment by means of storage of surface water in open reservoirs or by means of bankfiltration.

It is of great interest to identify those organic chemical compounds which are the causes of impaired taste of water derived from surface water. Such determinations have been carried out by means of gaschromatography and mass-spectrometry. A first indication of compounds of potential interest are those organic compounds which are particularly found in water supplies using open reservoirs as a mean of water storage.

During storage,growth of algae and bacteria can cause the formation of earthy and musty smelling compounds into the water. A survey of compounds, particularly present in tapwaters derived from reservoirwater and of possible importance to water taste is given in table 4. Known earthy tasting compounds among these substances are 2-methylisoborneol and geosmin, metabolites of certain blue-green algae and streptomycetes.

Another category of compounds are those water contaminants which are insufficiently removed during riverwater treatment. Interesting in this respect is the fact that the taste of a number of waters,derived by means of bankfiltration of water of the river Rhine,was qualified as "chlorine like" while no chlorination was applied during treatment. Chlorinated chemicals, already present in the river water, must have been responsible for this effect.

Table 4.: Taste impairing organic substances, possibly introduced by growth of organisms in storage reservoirs of surface water supplies

Compound	Highest concentration found in tapwater ($\mu g/l$)	Odour Threshold Concentration in water ($\mu g/l$) [10]	Ratio C/OTC
Octene-1	0.03	0.5	0.06
2-Ethylhexanol-1	3.0	300	0.01
2-Methylisoborneol	0.003	0.02	1.5
Geosmin	0.03	0.015	2.0
Heptanal	0.1	3.0	0.03
Octanal	0.03	0.7	0.04
Nonanal	0.1	1.0	0.1
Decanal	0.1	2.0	0.05
Heptan-3-one	0.1	7.5	0.01

Such compounds have to be incorporated in the so called "grey list" of compounds of which the concentration should be lowered in relation to the recently accepted convention against the chemical pollution of the river Rhine[11].

Some of the relevant chemical compounds in this context are presented in table 5. Other chemicals, which could not yet be identified or for which odour threshold concentrations in water have not yet been determined will be added to this list.

Table's 4 and 5 contain compounds for which the C/OTC ratio is 0.01 or higher. Low value's of 0.01 or more have been included as the Taste Threshold Concentrations of chemicals in water will generally be substantially lower than the Odour Threshold Concentrations, but insufficient taste thresholds are reported up till now in literature to provide a suitable basis for comparison.

Table 5.: Some potential taste impairing organic compounds in drinking water, originating from the river Rhine

Compound	Highest concentration found in tap-water ($\mu g/1$)	Odour Threshold Concentration in water ($\mu g/1$)[10]	Ratio C/OTC
1,3,5 Trimethylbenzene	0.7	3	0.2
Hexachlorobutadiene	0.1	6	0.02
o-Dichlorobenzene	0.1	10	0.01
p-Dichlorobenzene	0.3	0.3	1.0
1,2,4 Trichlorobenzene	0.3	5	0.06
bis(2-Chloroisopropyl) ether	3.0	300	0.01

TASTE AND TAPWATER CONSUMPTION HABITS

As a part of the questionnaire, mentioned in the introduction, individuals have been asked to indicate the daily consumed quantity of tapwater for drinking as such and for drinking as tea. It was found that particularly water consumption is considerably affected by the taste assessment by the individual consumer, as shown in table 6.

Table 6.: Effect of tapwater taste assessment on water consumption habits in The Netherlands (n=3073, 18 years and older)

Tapwater taste category	Daily consumed water volume (ml/person)	
	water as such	water as tea
good	316	320
not perceptible	202	310
weak, not objectionable	203	302
objectionable	145	305
very bad	163	303

These data clearly indicate the need to create such environmental conditions and such water treatment systems that the sensorily perceptible quality of drinking water, derived from surface water, meets the requirements for drinking water of tastelessness. As long as considerable parts of national populations are deprived of such a quality of their tapwater much work in the laboratory as well as in the field of enforcement and water treatment remains to be done.

REFERENCES

1. Bruvold, W.H., Ongerth, H.J., Dillehay, R.C. (1969)
   Journ. Am. Water Works Assoc., 61, 575-580
2. Pangborn, R.M., Trabue, J.M., Little, A.C. (1971)
   J. Food Sci., 36, 355
3. Bartoshuk, L.M. (1974)
   J. Comparative and Physiol. Psychol., 87, 2, 310-325
4. Zoeteman, B.C.J., de Grunt, F.E., Köster, E.P., Smit, K.G.J.,
   Punter, P.H. (1977)
   Chem. Senses and Flavor (in press)
5. Kölle, W., Koppe, P., Sontheimer, H. (1970)
   Water Treatm. Exam., 2, 120
6. Zoeteman, B.C.J., Piet, G.J., (1974)
   Science Tot. Env., 3, 103-115
7. Torgerson, W.S. (1967) in
   Theory and Methods of Scaling, 7th ed., Wiley, New York
8. Roskam, E. (1970),
   Nonmetric multidimensional scaling "Minissa-1", version for triadic
   data, University of Nijmegen, Psychological Department, The Netherlands
9. Zoeteman, B.C.J., (1977)
   On sensorily perceptible contamination of drinking water, thesis in
   preparation, University of Amsterdam, The Netherlands
10. van Gemert, L.J., Nettenbreijer, A.H. (1977)
    Compilation of odour threshold values in air and water.
    (RID/CIVO publication, obtainable at the National Institute for Water
    Supply, P.O.Box 150, 2260 AD Leidschendam, The Netherlands)
11. Tractatenblad, (1977), nr. 31-34
    (Staatsuitgeverij, 's-Gravenhage)

Fundamental considerations and methods for measuring air pollution odors

Andrew Dravnieks

Odor Sciences Center, IIT Research Institute, Chicago, IL 60616, USA

ABSTRACT

Characterization of odors associated with pollution requires use of methods that would yield communicable values: data obtained on the same stimulus by different laboratories should agree within reasonable statistical significance limits. Cooperative experiments organized by the Sensory Evaluation Committee of American Society for Testing and Materials and other work elsewhere demonstrated a potential utility of some methods. An odor intensity reference scale based on 1-butanol gave more coherent results than a 0 to 5 category scale. Odor character comparison by χ^2 analysis of individual response profiles based on a redundant (136) descriptor list yielded a sensory distance measure ($-\ln$ of the association coefficient) which correlated between laboratories at $p < 0.001$: as well as the direct similarity comparisons based on a 0-7 scale. Forced-choice methods for odor threshold measurements may become the preferred practice, but some agreement on the parameters of stimulus/subject interface is needed. Hedonic evaluations of odors in the laboratory may assist in gross estimates of their pollution impact.

INTRODUCTION

Responses to odorous air pollution generally involve the following chain of processes, Figure 1.

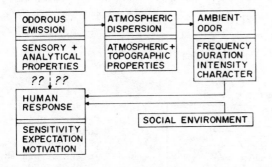

Fig. 1 Processes in Odorous Air Pollution

An odorous emission, with certain sensory and analytical properties, undergoes weakening and distortion by atmospheric dispersion determined by atmospheric conditions and topography, and is converted to an ambient odor stimulus of varying frequency, duration, and sensory properties. The response of the ultimate panel--the population in its daily life--is determined by the sensory properties of the ambient odor, as well as by the sensitivities, expectations, and motivations of the individuals.

A direct path that would relate the characteristics of the odorous emission to the population response is uncertain; all indicated factors need to be considered. This discussion will be limited to the properties of emission and ambient odors. In their characterization, the need is to find procedures which will measure pollution-relevant properties and yield comparable values when practiced by different groups. Much of the material in this paper resulted from cooperative studies by task groups within Sensory Evaluation Committee, E18, of the American Society for Testing and Materials (ASTM), on model odorants.

SENSORY PROPERTIES

The principal sensory properties are perceived odor intensity, hedonic tone, and quality (character). Odor dilution threshold and detectability are subsidiary properties, not imminently evident when smelling an odor. Their significance is for estimates of the needed degree of odor control since they indicate how much non-odorous atmospheric air will be needed to eliminate the odor by dispersion.

ODOR INTENSITY

Suprathreshold intensities can be characterized by category scales, magnitude estimates, or reference scales. In communicating data to other groups, the first two approaches invite the use of calibration samples. Hence a direct comparison to a set of intensity-graded reference samples is an almost inevitable development. Turk[1] used a mixture scale for diesel exhaust odors. For general use, a scale based on some pure and stable odorant is preferred. ASTM E18 committee compared, in a cooperative exercise of several laboratories, category and 1-butanol odor reference scales, Figure 2. Constant concentrations of 1-butanol and anethole were evaluated using a 0 to 5 category scale

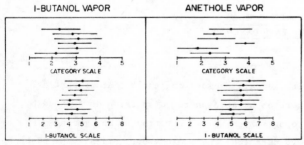

I-BUTANOL VAPOR   ANETHOLE VAPOR

CATEGORY SCALE   CATEGORY SCALE

I-BUTANOL SCALE   I-BUTANOL SCALE

SCALE VALUES

Fig. 2 Performance of Category and 1-Butanol Reference Odor Intensity Scales

and a 1-butanol vapor scale of 8 levels, from approximately 10 to 2000 ppm v/v in binary steps. Each segment represents a different laboratory, indicating its mean and standard deviation. The reference scale produced better agreement than the category scale. The mean values for anethole dispersed only slightly more than for 1-butanol when matched against its own scale.

Subsequently, ASTM issued a Standard Recommended Practice E544, which proposes reporting intensities in terms of 1-butanol concentration that exhibits an odor intensity which matches that of the sample. Other experience indicated that despite differences in the sensitivities of individuals to different odors, groups of 8 or more yield values comparable usually within less than one binary scale step to the results by other groups.

The 1-butanol scale has not yet been extensively studied for evaluations of low-intensity odors, such as odors in ambient air.

The odor intensity equivalents in ppm 1-butanol are not proportional to the perceived intensities. Moskowitz et al[2] proposed that

$$S = 0.261 \text{ (ppm vol/vol 1-butanol in air)}^{0.66}$$

The resulting S scale gives values in simplified proportion to the perceived intensity magnitudes; at $S = 10$, the odor is twice as strong than at $S = 5$, and equals the odor intensity of 1-butanol at 250 ppm and a 160 ml/min flow rate; and is of substantial intensity. Thresholds are below $S = 1$. This equation is based on magnitude responses pooled from many groups of panelists. The individual functions may exhibit quite different coefficients[3].

Flow rate of the stimulus to the nose is significant. We found that an increase in the 1-butanol test stimulus rate from 160 to 5000 ml/min increased its S value by a factor of 12[4].

DILUTION vs. ODOR INTENSITY

Atmospheric dilution models for the prediction of ambient odors require knowing how odor intensity changes with dilution. It has been usually assumed that a simple power function relates both:

$$S = k \text{ (SAMPLE CONCENTRATION IN AIR)}^{n}$$

By measuring the intensities at several dilutions vs. 1-butanol scale, k and n can be calculated for different emissions. Relative significance of several odor sources in local environment can then be estimated.

Some odors do not behave so simply. Figure 3 shows some exceptional functions. A simplistic explanation is that two types of chemoreceptors may operate, one at the lower, another at a higher level, and inbetween they somewhat counteract.

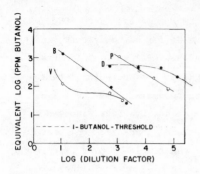

Fig. 3 Some Dose-Response Functions
P, pyridine; D, diacetyl
B, benzaldehyde; V, vanillin

ODOR THRESHOLD

The signal detection theory as applied to the perception of weak odors postulates that individual judgements on the presence of a "signal" (odor, in this case) in a stimulus containing "noise" (other sensory inputs and extraneous odors) depend on two factors: sensitivity and judgement criterion (when to decide if signal is present). This theory, applied to odorous pollution by Lindval[5], produces a detectability index, d', isolated from the criteria. Its use requires a very substantial number of responses at marginally low odor intensities. At present, this approach is not yet well understood by personnel dealing with pollution odors.

In many methods presently practiced in the pollution odor measurements, one sample at a time is presented, and the judgement criterion is important. In the forced-choice multiple sample methods, in which subjects must select from several samples that which is odorous, the criteria effect is suppressed[6]. The multiple choice methods are common in food science[7,9]; also, used in some odorous pollution work[10,11]. One of the most common is the triangle method: two blanks and one test sample. According to Frijtens[12], it yields threshold values not influenced by positional bias (selection of sample in a certain preferred position) or timing in sniffing. The forced-choice method solves the most pressing practical problem of "controls": it provides obvious evidence that the subject did not detect odor if he made an incorrect choice.

An olfactometer that utilizes the triangle forced-choice procedure on odorous gaseous samples was introduced in 1975[11,13]. Subsequently, TRC[14] compared odor dilution thresholds of 5 malodorant-containing stimuli at 3 concentration levels using 4 different measurement systems but the same panelists. Figure 4 shows plots of the results of three dynamic olfactometric procedures (left-dynamic olfactometer; center-high flow rates from sniffing ports; right, a mask device) vs. ASTM D1391 syringe dilution method data; correlation co-

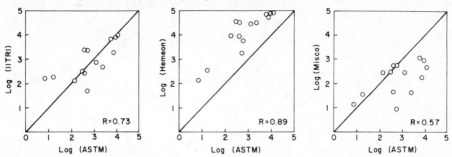

Fig. 4   Correlations between Odor Thresholds for 3 Olfactometric Systems vs. ASTM Syringe Method.

efficients are indicated.   The correlations are reasonable, but the fast flow results in a higher sensitivity, and, paradoxically, the mask results in a lesser sensitivity, although the rationale for the mask is to eliminate any loss of stimulus between the olfactometer and the nose.

An obvious problem is the selection of the most suitable stimulus flow rate to the nose.   Repeated measurements on the same odorous sample by the same 9 subjects yield group thresholds which differ with a standard deviation of 0.1 logarithmic units.   However, the rate of flow from ports influences the threshold, Figure 5.

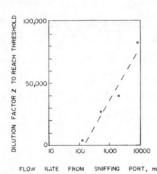

Fig. 5   Dependence of 1-Butanol Odor Threshold on Stimulus Flow Rate.

HEDONIC TONE

A measurement of hedonic tone (pleasantness/unpleasantness) on air pollution samples in the laboratory gives results only remotely related to the hedonic impact of the same odor when it is a component of a pollution emission. An otherwise pleasant odor may not be tolerated out of context of a perfume, and unpleasant odors will be even more so in the form of a pollution emission.

The hedonic tone of an odor changes with the perceived intensity.   A compilation of hedonic data obtained by magnitude estimation on many industrial air pollution odors and plotted vs. odor intensities is shown in Figure 6.

"Moderately unpleasant" corresponds to a value of 100. A mean value line is indicated. A new sample can be rated with respect to this line to estimate its relative potential for annoyance, as compared with other industrial odors.

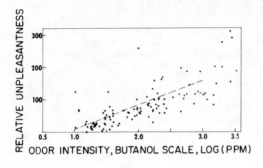

Fig. 6 Distribution of Hedonic Values of Industrial Air Pollution Odors.

ODOR QUALITY (CHARACTER)

In odorous pollution measurements, qualitative characterization of odors may serve several purposes. An ambient odor may need to be compared to odors of several possible emission sources. This can be done by comparing the odors, or else the sample may be analyzed in a gas chromatograph equipped with a sniffing port to characterize odors of GC-separated components. The latter method yields much more information. An emission odor can be handled similarily, to establish which processes are the main odor determinants. If an emission is treated, e.g. by scrubbing or additives, odor character changes may be of interest.

Odor quality is evaluated in terms of similarities to other odors, either real (presented as reference samples) or characterized by descriptors. The ASTM E18 committee conducted cooperative studies with some of the techniques.

In one study, 12 laboratories (8 within the U.S.A.) described, by freely selected terms, odors of 9 substances (1-butanol, pyridine, cyclohexanol, p-cresyl methyl-ether, ℓ-carvone, acetophenone, anethole, phenylethanol, low-odor propylene glycol) when smelled from a bottle and at 3 different concentrations in a GC effluent. Statistically highly significant agreement was found between the clustered odor profiles of same odorant in 4 presentation modes, except for weak odors. Statistically significant agreement existed also between the composite profile and profiles by the separate laboratories. Thus, despite the diversity of subjects and terms, the GC effluent sniffing method is a useful comparison technique for characterizing the odor quality of GC effluent components.

In another study, 4 laboratories characterized iso-intense odors of dilute solutions of 10 odorants (8 as above, plus 1-hexanol and 1-heptanol) using two methods. In one, each odor was compared to each odor, including cases of same vs. same, rating their dissimilarity from 0 (= no difference) to 7. The correlation between different laboratories, for dissimilar pairs, were at $p < 0.001$ level (R = 0.80). In the other method, each odor was rated twice, many days apart, for the applicability of each of 136 descriptors[15]; (an expanded Harper's list[16]). For comparison of the descriptor profiles, logarithms of the coefficients of association (via χ^2) were calculated for each pair of odors comparing each subject's ratings separately. This procedure eliminates the effect of differences in odor perception and descriptor use and was adapted from Döving's[17] treatment of electrophysiological data. Correlations of the values of this similarity index between laboratories was at $p < 0.001$ level (R = 0.81).

Recently, we added 10 descriptors (alcohol-like, important since 4 odorants were alcohols; dill-like; chemical; cresote; green pepper; nail polish remover; fermented fruit; cherry; varnish; sour milk) and repeated the above exercise. Figure 7 is a plot of resultant -ℓn (coefficient of association) vs. direct sensory distance category rating. The relation is curvilinear, but becomes linear with the square root of the ordinate.

Thus, it is feasible to communicate odor similarity/dissimilarity data using measures derived from the multidimensional semantic scaling.

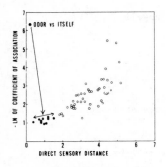

Fig. 7 Correlation between Descriptor-Derived and Categorized Sensory Distance Measures.

TOTAL ANNOYANCE POTENTIAL

A tridimensional representation may be needed to reflect the annoyance potential of an emission. Odor dilution threshold is clearly insufficient: two emissions may have the same threshold but different slopes in Fig. 3, and since the odor will be detectable, but less frequently, also at the dilutions below "threshold", the emission with a lesser slope will have a higher probability to be detected below its 50 percent threshold. Furthermore, if two emissions have identical threshold and slope, that which is more unpleasant or, if pleasant, more distinct in quality, would have a higher annoyance potential. Developing an annoyance "space" is another problem in odorous air pollution.

REFERENCES

1. Turk, A.(1967) Selection and Training of Judges for Sensory Evaluation of Diesel Exhaust Odors
    U.S. Public Health Service Publ. No. 999-AP-32

2. Moskowitz, H.R., Dravnieks, A., Cain, W.S. and Turk, A.(1974)
    Chem. Senses and Flavor 1,235-237

3. Cain, W.S.(1971)
    Perception and Psychophysics 9,478-479

4. Dravnieks, A.(1977) in Flavor Quality: Objective Measurement
    pp.11-28, ACS Symp. Ser. 51 Washington, D.C., Scanlan, R.E. Editor

5. Lindvall, T.(1970) On Sensory Evaluation of Odorous Air Pollution Intensities
    Nord. Hygienisk Tidskrift Suppl. 2, Stockholm

6. Swets, J.A.(1964) Signal Detection and Recognition by Human Observers
    p.142, Wiley & Sons, New York

7. Guadagni, D.G., Buttery, R.G. and Okano, S.(1963)
    J. Sci. Food Agr. 14,761

8. Takken, P., van der Linde, L.M., Boelens, M., and Takken, J.J.(1975)
    J. Agr. Food Chem. 23,638

9. Meilgaard, M.C.(1975)
    MBHA Technical Quarterly 12, 151-168

10. Cederlöf, R., Edfors, M.L., Friberg, L. and Lindvall, T.(1965)
    Tappi 48, 405-411

11. Dravnieks, A. and Prokop, W.H.(1975)
    J. Air Poll. Control Assoc. 25, 28-35

12. Frijters, J.E.R.(1977)
    Chem. Senses and Flavor 2, 301-311

13. Dravnieks, A.(1975) in Industrial Odor Technology Assessment
    pp.27-44, Ann Arbor Sci. Publ. Inc., Ann Arbor, Mich.,
    Cheremisinoff and Young Editor

14. TRC, The Research Corporation of New England (1975) Evaluation of Four Odor Measurement Systems
    Illinois Env. Prot. Agency, Springfield, Illinois

15. Dravnieks, A.(1975)
    J. Soc. Cosm. Chem. 26, 551-571

16. Harper, R., Land, D.G., Griffiths, N.M., and Bate-Smith, E.C.(1968)
    Brit. J. Psychol. 59, 231-252

17. Döving, K.B.(1966)
    Acta Physiol. Scand. 68, 404-419

Quality, intensity, and time in olfactory perception[21]

Birgitta Berglund

Department of Psychology, University of Stockholm, Box 6706, S-113 85 Stockholm, Sweden

ABSTRACT

Experiments on odor perception are classified in terms of number of odorous substances and temporal patterns of stimulation used in the designs. This classification leads to four well-known sensory functions: the psychophysical, the interactive, the self-adaptive, and the cross-adaptive. These functions were analysed in experiments with hydrogen sulfide and dimethyl disulfide as odorous stimuli. It is concluded that the olfactory system attenuates the input so that the perceived intensity grows more slowly than the stimulus concentration. Attenuation is also characteristic for the chemical compounds that stimulate the system simultaneously, as reflected by the vector model of odor interaction. When self-adapted, the system responds with attenuation as is true for the cross-adapted system except for near-threshold concentrations where perceived intensity is facilitated. The four sensory functions of the human olfactory system are also discussed in relation to the odor quality coding mechanism.

INTRODUCTION

Knowledge of the perceptual processes constitutes the foundation for meaningful correlations of psychophysical data to physiological data. This report presents some basic functional principles of olfactory perception and discusses them within a common empirical framework.

In a number of experiments, perceived odor intensity (ψ) was measured as a function of various concentrations (φ) of one or two odorous substances (i & j) presented simultaneously ($t_i = t_j$) or successively. Classification of experimental designs in terms of number of odorous substances and temporal patterns of stimulation leads us to four well-known sensory functions: the psychophysical, the interactive, the self-adaptive, and the cross-adaptive, see Table 1. The four functions have here been determined using the same substances (H_2S - hydrogen sulfide; DMDS - dimethyl disulfide), the same type of scaling method (equal-intensity matching; magnitude estimation), and the same equipment for olfactory stimulation (olfactometer; air-conditioned test chamber with two odor-exposure hoods; gas chromatographic analyses of odorants).

Table 1. Perceptual functions of the olfactory system.

Number of odorous substances	Simultaneous stimulation $(t_i = t_j = k)$	Successive stimulation $(t_i = t_j \text{ or } t_i \neq t_j)$	
One (i)	Psychophysical functions $\psi_i = f\,(\varphi_i, t_i),$	Self-adaptation functions $\psi_i = f\,(\varphi_i, t_i),$	$(t_i = k$ or $\varphi_i = k)$
Two (i,j)	Interaction functions $\psi_{i,j} = f\,(\varphi_i, \varphi_j, t_i, t_j)$ or $\psi_{i,j} = f\,(\psi_i, \psi_j, t_i, t_j),$ alternatively, $\psi_i' = f\,(\varphi_i, \varphi_j, t_i, t_j)$ or $\psi_i' = f\,(\psi_i, \psi_j, t_i, t_j)$	Cross-adaptation functions $\psi_i = f\,(\varphi_i, t_j)$ or $\psi_i = f\,(\psi_j, t_j),$	$(t_i = k$ or $\varphi_j = k$ and $\psi_j = k)$

The technical equipment and scaling procedures have been described elsewhere.[17]

If possible, all the relationships in Table 1 should be investigated throughout the full dynamic range[19] from the weakest detectable to the strongest concentration the observer can tolerate, provided, as a matter of ethics, that it is below the maximum allowable concentration (MAC) for inhalation during an 8-hour exposure in the working environment. For both H_2S and DMDS the MAC-values are at present 10 ppm. For the olfactometer and exposure conditions used in the present research, the absolute thresholds for the two substances are close to 1 ppb, thus leaving us with a dynamic range of about 4 log units for both odors.

PSYCHOPHYSICAL FUNCTIONS

The most basic problem for psychophysicists has been to determine the mathematical form of the psychophysical function relating perceived intensity to stimulus intensity.[3] Psychophysical functions for H_2S and DMDS are shown in Fig. 1. The functions[18] were obtained by matching various concentrations of the one substance to a set of concentrations of the other so that they

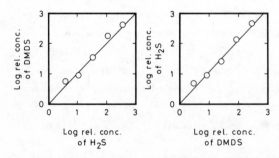

Fig. 1 (from Svensson & Lindvall[18]). Equal-intensity matching functions for H_2S and DMDS. The left-hand diagram shows the results when DMDS was matched against five concentrations of H_2S and the right-hand diagram when H_2S was matched against five concentrations of DMDS.

were perceived as equally intense. The matching functions show linear trends in log-log coordinates indicating that power functions govern the relationship. The slopes of these functions are close to one, meaning that the exponents of the power functions for DMDS and H_2S are approximately equal.[20]

For all odorous substances investigated so far, perceived intensity has virtually always been possibly described as a power function of concentration,[3]

$$\psi_i = c \, \varphi_i^n \, , \tag{1}$$

where c and n are constants. The use of the exponent n for odor classification has been attempted for a set of 21 substances.[1,3] The exponents were correlated and submitted to factor analysis. From the same group of observers and for the same substances, matched in perceived intensity, similarity estimates of odor quality were collected and analysed with a multidimensional scaling (MDS) procedure.[1,4] The configuration obtained from MDS did not show any obvious relationship to the exponent variation. Since the inter-observer concordance for both estimates of perceived intensity and exponents of the power functions was much higher than for the similarity estimates,[1] it may be concluded that the exponents carry more basic information about the odorous substances than do similarity estimates of odor quality.

INTERACTION FUNCTIONS

The second sensory function presented in Table 1 is odor interaction, studied by having observers inhale the vapors of two substances at once. The perceived odor intensity of the mixture is studied as a function of either concentrations or perceived intensities of the constituents.

While the odor interaction process has not yet been described mathematically in psychophysical terms, it has been described in perceptual terms.[2,5] The intensity of the mixture seems always to be less than the sum of the subjective intensities of the constituents but more than a simple average of the two, a finding substantiated in a number of experiments. The perception of a total of 10 two-odor mixtures has also been demonstrated to conform to a vector sum[5,12], first derived by Berglund et al.,[8]

$$\psi_{ij} = \sqrt{\psi_i^2 + \psi_j^2 + 2 \, \psi_i \, \psi_j \, \cos \alpha_{ij}} \tag{2}$$

where the vector ij refers to the mixture and the parameter (α) can be conceived as an angle between two vectors i and j, which represent the constituents smelled separately.

Fig. 2 illustrates the fit of the vector model for mixtures of H_2S and DMDS. The data were obtained by mixing all combinations of 5 concentrations of each substance and then scaling these, as well as the 2 x 5 constituents, by magnitude estimation.[8] The findings to date show that the change in odor intensity caused by the term of interaction is characteristic for the pair of odors. α has been found to range from 100-120°. This opens the prospect of using α for classification of odor substances: If a set of odor substances is studied, it would be possible to factor analyse a full matrix of cos α-values[2].

In the experiments on odor interaction where the effect has been scaled in terms of perceived intensity, it has often been studied for the mixture perceived as a single quality (the component odors blend). Table 1 shows that there is another possibility, namely to ask observers to estimate the perceived odor intensity of the one or the other component inside the mixture (ψ_i') and study its relationship to the perceived intensity outside the mixture. However, no such experiment has yet been reported.[5]

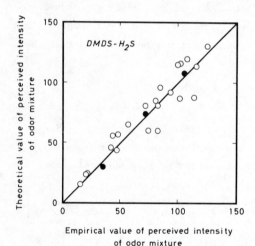

Fig. 2 (from Berglund et al.[4]). The odor interaction function for mixtures of H_2S and DMDS. Empirical scale values of perceived odor intensity of the mixtures are plotted against the theoretical values computed according to the vector model in Eq. 2. (The filled symbols refer to equally intense component odors).

SELF-ADAPTATION FUNCTIONS

The third function presented in Table 1 is self-adaptation. By self-adaptation is here meant that the adaptation substance and the test stimulus are identical. Olfactory sensitivity is known to decrease rapidly when observers are exposed to a constant stimulus. The perceived odor intensity of a set of concentrations may be studied as a function either of the duration of the preceding stimulus or of its intensity. In the first case, the effects of adaptation are studied in terms of a time-course function while in the latter, of a psychophysical function.

Time-course functions of self-adaptation

The time-course of self-adaptation was first determined by Ekman et al.[14] and later verified in several studies.[9,11] For various concentrations of H_2S, it was found to be well described by an exponential function

$$\psi_i = a + b\, c^{t_i}, \qquad (c < 1) \qquad (3)$$

where a is the asymptote, $a+b$ the initial perceived intensity value, and c a constant related to the rate of adaptation. The exponential function may be derived by assumptions about the role of breathing in olfactory perception.[9]

Fig. 3 shows the time-course of adaptation for H_2S and DMDS for a low versus a high concentration.[6] The general trend here agrees well with earlier findings. Perceived intensity does not reach zero nor does it appear that it would do so at any concentration. The constant c, reflecting the rate of adaptation, seems to be invariant with odorous substance and concentration, but published data are still too sketchy to allow a final conclusion.

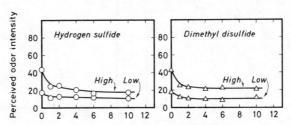

Fig. 3 (from Berglund et al.[6]). Time-course functions of self-adaptation for H_2S and DMDS at a high and a low concentration representing two levels of equal perceived odor intensity. The curves fitted to the data are exponential functions according to Eq. 3.

Psychophysical functions of self-adaptation

Cain[10] was the first to determine the psychophysical function after adapting the olfactory system to various concentrations for various periods of time. The mathematical form of the psychophysical function for an adapted system has not been finally established.

Fig. 4 illustrates typical functions resulting from the self-adaptation of the system to a low and a high concentration of H_2S and DMDS.[7] In these plots the concentration values on the abscissa have been replaced by the perceptual scale values for the unadapted system. Quite simply, any deviation from the principle diagonal reflects the effect of adaptation. Sensitivity is reduced in a systematic manner by adaptation. This effect may be described by Ekman´s reformulated power function,[13] suggested to apply by Engen[15]

$$\psi_i = k \, (\varphi_i - \varphi_o)^n \qquad (4)$$

where φ_o is a constant speculated to have a relation to the momentary threshold under conditions of adaptation. The psychophysical data for H_2S can be described well by this function but the DMDS-data would require a negative value of φ_o. Although a good fit of the reformulated function is possible to obtain, it is somewhat unclear what the meaning of a negative φ_o would be. Perhaps it reflects the sensory noise in the system. The results obtained for H_2S and DMDS agree with earlier ones: A general decrease in perceived intensity accompanies a steepening or flattening of the function in the low stimulus range.

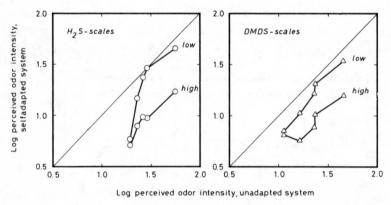

Fig. 4 (from Berglund et al.[7]). Perceived intensity scales obtained for unadapted and self-adapted olfactory systems plotted against each other. The adaptation stimulus was either a low or a high concentration of H_2S or DMDS. The concentrations were matched in perceived odor intensity.

CROSS-ADAPTATION FUNCTIONS

Lastly, Table 1 presents a cross-adaptation function. The olfactory system is now adapted to one odorous substance and its sensitivity to another is tested. As for those of self-adaptation, the effects of cross-adaptation may be studied either in the form of time-course or psychophysical functions. Experiments may be designed on the assumption that odors of equal concentration or of equal perceived intensity cross-adapt symmetrically.

Time-course functions of cross-adaptation

While the time-course function of self-adaptation has been determined for many odorous substances, Berglund et al.[6] seem to be alone in dealing thus with cross-adaptation. Fig. 5 shows the results of cross- and self-adapting

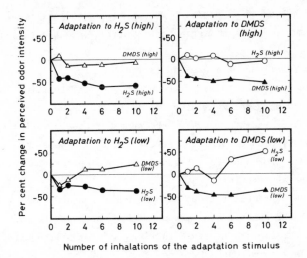

Fig. 5 (from Berglund et al.[6]). Time-course functions of self- and cross-adaptation for H_2S and DMDS. The effects are expressed in per cent change in perceived intensity relative to the unadapted state of the system. The two upper diagrams show the effects at a high and the two lower diagrams the effects at a low concentration.

the olfactory system to H_2S and DMDS. The odorous substances were matched to be equal in perceived intensity for two low and two high concentrations. The results are expressed as per cent change in perceived intensity when the system is adapted as compared to unadapted.

A larger effect on perceived intensity is found for self- than for cross-adaptation, the latter showing inconsistent results. The cross-adaptation effect is nearly nonexistent for high concentrations, whereas for low concentrations, perceived intensity increases with number of inhalations, i.e., facilitation occurs. The self-adaptive and cross-adaptive powers are about the same regardless of substance. The data are based on few observations and it may be too early to determine the mathematical form of the time-course function of cross-adaptation (i.e., cross-facilitation).

We found that facilitation of perceived intensity increases with number of inhalations. Engen and associates,[15,16] studying odor detection, found that facilitation increased with the length of the interval between the offset of the adaptation stimulus and the onset of the test stimulus. Both findings may reflect the same mechanisms, namely, a post-responsive system with a build-up in sensitivity with number of inhalations. We are here dealing with a facilitation effect that is bound to the temporal order of stimulation because the simultaneous presentation of H_2S and DMDS (and many other two-odor mixtures) results in inhibition of response. However, the cross-facilitation may also result from simultaneously mixing a test stimulus with the residuals of the adaptation stimulus.

Psychophysical functions of cross-adaptation

Cain[11] was the first to study the psychophysical function for cross-adaptation under varying conditions of stimulation and showed that, in principle, the effects of cross-adaptation were the same as those of self-adaptation. As the adaptation stimulus grows stronger the function becomes steeper, especially near threshold. For odorous substances of equal perceived intensity the effect seems to be asymmetric.

Fig. 6 shows effects of cross-adaptation to H_2S and DMDS at various concentrations.[7] The results are not shown in the usual psychophysical plot (since these data exhibit a picture very much like that for self-adaptation, cf. Fig. 4, Eq. 4) but in a form that makes them easily comparable to the results of the time-course functions (Fig. 5). Fig. 6 shows the per cent change of perceived intensity due to both cross- and self-adaptation as a function of concentration of the adaptation stimulus. Two levels of concentration (a high and a low) were investigated and within each pair, the odors were equally intense.

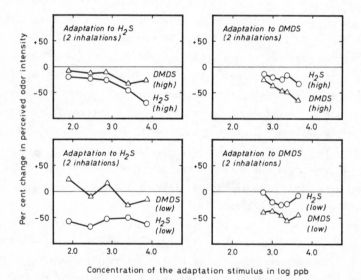

Fig. 6 (from Berglund et al.[7]). Psychophysical functions of self- and cross-adaptation for H_2S and DMDS. The effects are expressed in per cent change in perceived intensity relative to the unadapted state of the system. The two upper diagrams show the effects at a high and the two lower diagrams the effects at a low concentration.

Cross-adapting the system, then, seems to bring a decrease in sensitivity as the concentration of the adaptation stimulus increases. For the two high concentrations the effects are very much like those of self-adaptation but weaker. For the low concentrations, self-adaptation to an ever stronger concentration brings a constant, proportional decrease in perceived intensity while cross-adapting the system gives an accelerated effect. Again (cf. Fig. 5), facilitation seems to exist for cross-adaptation at near-threshold concentrations.

CONCLUSIONS

The processing of intensity as a function of quality

The olfactory system processes the information from one odorous substance according to a power function with an exponent less than one. It attenuates the input so that perceived intensity grows more slowly than the concentration. A second attenuation, linked to the nature of the chemical compound which stimulates the system simultaneously, is reflected in the vector model of odor interaction. A third attenuation is found when cross-adapting the olfactory system to different concentrations at equal duration. At low concentrations, the decrease in perceived intensity is a constant proportion of the increase in the concentration of the adaptation stimulus, whereas at high concentrations, that decrease is an ever-growing proportion. The attenuation of perceived intensity found for single compounds, mixtures of compounds, and compounds presented successively has not yet been explained in terms of the particular compound combination or of different mathematical formulations.

The processing of intensity as a function of time

The olfactory system is fatigued under ongoing constant stimulation by an odorous substance so that the perceived intensity of the adapting stimulus decreases according to an exponential function. This process of self-adaptation gives a decrease of perceived intensity in a constant proportion per unit time of adaptation. Again, the olfactory system responds by attenuating the input. However, when the system is cross-adapted by ongoing constant stimulation, it responds with facilitation of perceived intensity at near-threshold concentrations. For strong concentrations, it is unclear whether cross-adaptation or cross-facilitation takes place.

The processing of odor quality

A classical approach to studying odor quality is to group chemical compounds according to their similarities and dissimilarities in function when perceived in mixtures or after cross-adaptation. In other words, the constants of the hypothetical functions in Table 1 are possible to use for the grouping

of odors. Obviously the philosophy behind this approach is that functional
properties of the olfactory system reveal an odor quality coding mechanism.
To investigate whether this approach is fruitful, a first step must be to prove
that the same groupings of odors can be obtained from the different sensory
functions presented in Table 1.

The power function is known to have an exponent that is characteristic
for the odorous substance involved. This would lead to one type of grouping.
A second type could be created from the constant α of the vector model of odor
interaction. The exponential function and the reformulated power function of
self-adaptation might also reflect some constants specific to odorous substances. The cross-adaptation functions are of course important candidates for the
odor classification although the empirical data on this process are incomplete.

So far, the classical approach has not been applied systematically to the
problem of odor qualities. In my opinion, it seems more likely to provide valid
correlations to physiological findings than the alternative approach of multidimensional scaling of odor quality. The latter gives a cognitive representation of odor qualities in an odor space, and may thus be more open to influence
by cognitive and emotional factors than by basic physiological properties of
the olfactory system.

REFERENCES AND NOTES

1. Berglund, B. (1971) Rep. Lab. Psychol., Univer. Stockholm, Suppl. 6.

2. Berglund, B. (1974) Ann. N.Y. Acad. Sci. 237, 35-51.

3. Berglund, B., Berglund, U., Ekman, G., and Engen, T. (1971) Percept. &
    Psychophysics 9, 379-384.

4. Berglund, B., Berglund, U., Engen, T., and Ekman, G. (1973) Scand. J.
    Psychol. 14, 131-137.

5. Berglund, B., Berglund, U., and Lindvall, T. (1976) Psych. Rev. 83,
    432-441.

6. Berglund, B., Berglund, U., and Lindvall, T. (1977) In preparation (a).

7. Berglund, B., Berglund, U., and Lindvall, T. (1977) In preparation (b).

8. Berglund, B., Berglund, U., Lindvall, T., and Svensson, L.T. (1973)
    J. Exp. Psychol. 100, 29-38.

9. Berglund, U.(1974) Ann. N.Y. Acad. Sci. 237, 17-27.

10. Cain, W.S. (1970) Percept. & Psychophysics 7, 271-275.

11. Cain, W.S. (1974) ASHRAE Trans. 80, 53-75.

12. Cain, W.S. (1975) Chemical Senses and Flavor 1, 339-352.

13. Ekman, G. (1958) J. Psychol. 45, 287-295.

14. Ekman, G., Berglund, B., Berglund, U., and Lindvall, T. (1967) Scand.
    J. Psychol. 8, 177-180.

15. Engen, T. (1971) in Handbook of Sensory Physiology, Vol IV (Part I), pp. 216-244, Springer Verlag, Berlin.

16. Engen, T. (1973) Ann. Rev. Psychol. 24, 187-206.

17. Lindvall, T. (1970) Nord. Hyg. Tidskr. Suppl. 2.

18. Svensson, L.T., and Lindvall, T. (1974) Percept. & Psychophysics 16, 264-270.

19. Teghtsoonian, R. (1973) Amer. J. Psychol. 86, 3-28.

20. In other experiments, H_2S and DMDS have been shown to have different exponents (.45 and .20, respectively) when scaled by magnitude estimation. However, in those experiments different groups of observers as well as different stimulus ranges were used, both known to affect the exponent of the power function pronouncedly.[2,19]

21. Supported by grants from the Swedish Council for Social Science Research. Dr. Ulf Berglund and Dr. Martha Teghtsoonian have given valuable comments on the manuscript.

Perception of composite odorous air pollutants

Thomas Lindvall

Department of Environmental Hygiene, The National Swedish Environment Protection Board, S-104 01 Stockholm, Sweden

ABSTRACT

The value of H_2S for the prognosis of odor from pulp mills is surprisingly inconsistent. Perceptual interaction explains part of the inconsistency. Subliminal levels of NO enhances the odor strength of H_2S and carbonyl sulfide. Acid fumes seemingly increase the sensitivity of observers to H_2S, probably because of a shift in the H_2S protolysis equilibrium.

INTRODUCTION

There is a close link between problems of odor control in the environment on the one hand and chemosensory physiology and psychophysics on the other. This is illustrated by a series of studies carried out to elucidate inconsistencies in applied odor data from the kraft pulp mill industry.

Kraft pulp mills emit strongly odorous gases, i.a. from soda recovery furnaces and lime kilns. The dominating odorous substance in these gases is hydrogen sulfide. Because of the seemingly simple composition of these gases from an odor point of view, emission limit values for hydrogen sulfide have been established. In Sweden the content of hydrogen sulfide in soda recovery furnace effluents may not exceed 10 mg/m^3 more than 5-10% of the time monthly [1]. It is thus assumed that a change in hydrogen sulfide concentration will lead to a corresponding change in odor strength.

Laboratory investigations show that hydrogen sulfide varies in odor threshold concentration (in recent studies roughly between 10^{-5} and $10^{-6.5}$ mg/l [2]). In flue gases from recovery furnaces and lime kilns this variation is even more pronounced [3].

Between 1965 and 1973 two pulp mills with comparable processing techniques were checked twice with basically the same sensory technique. Fairly good correlations were found between the concentration of hydrogen sulfide and the dilution needed to reach the odor threshold (log units, r=0.74-0.96)

as far as the recovery furnaces were concerned [3]. Figure 1 presents in log coordinates the regression lines of odor strength expressed as ED-50 thresholds and hydrogen sulfide concentrations in ppm. For the one mill, A, hydrogen sulfide is a suitable odor indicator but for the other, B, its prognosis value is doubtful. In pulp mill B a high concentration of H_2S in the recovery furnace effluents corresponds to a high odor strength, but a lowering of the concentration gives a marginal reduction in odor strength.

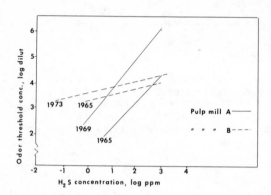

Figure 1 (from [3]) Relationships between odor threshold and H_2S concentrations in recovery furnace flue gases.

In pulpmill B the prognosis value of hydrogen sulfide for the perceived odor strength of effluent gases has been studied in further detail [4], Figure 2. The perceived odor strength of the effluents of the main stack (mainly emitting gases from a recovery furnace) and of a lime kiln was estimated by an equal-intensity matching procedure [5] in a mobile sensory laboratory at the stack base. H_2S equivalents were obtained from observers who adjusted the odor strength of H_2S by varying its concentration until it was equal to the odor strength of the effluents. The effluents were studied at different dilutions with air.

In Figure 2 the dotted line is the relationship between H_2S in the effluents and the matched H_2S, that would be expected if H_2S were the single determinant of the perceived odor strength of the effluent. It is clear from the figure that this is not the case. Other properties of the effluents must contribute to the odor.

The practical conclusion from these findings is that the prognosis value of hydrogen sulfide must be determined for each recovery furnace individually. This is possible but costly and this unsatisfactory situation demands further

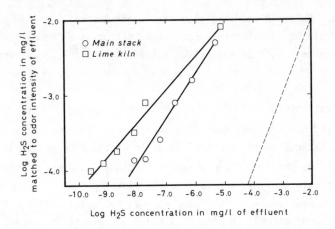

Figure 2 (from [4]) The H_2S concentrations matched to be equally intense to the effluent odors plotted against the H_2S concentration of the effluents.

research.

The inconsistencies in the results of the H_2S studies may be explained by interactions between odorous and non-odorous factors in the effluents and in the exposed humans. We are presently undertaking systematic studies in order to reveal possible mechanisms of interaction, both response interactions and stimulus interactions. After a brief mention of response interactions, the emphasis in this paper will turn to possible interactions between odorous and non-odorous gases present in the pulp mill effluents and to the influence of acid or alkaline fumes on the detectability of hydrogen sulfide, i.e. mainly stimulus interactions.

RESPONSE INTERACTION

Our studies on response interaction have focused on mixing odor perceptions [6] and odor adaptation [7]. These matters together with cross-adaptation phenomena are discussed by another member of the research group at this conference [8].

By using a vector model of odor interaction for the pulp mill odors [4] it was shown that the proportion of unexplained odor strength was large. Factors other than the odorous constituents known to exist in the effluents were therefore assumed to be responsible for the total odor perceptions. Not surprisingly, a careful chemical-physical study of gases from a soda recovery furnace have revealed the presence of another odorous sulfide, carbonyl sulfide, that previously has been disguised in the gas chromatograms by hydrogen sulfide peaks. Sulfur dioxide is also present in the effluents in concentrations that should be perceivable. Further laboratory studies will elucidate the role of carbonyl sulfide and sulfur dioxide in the perceptual interaction process.

STIMULUS INTERACTIONS

Odorous and non-odorous gases - In addition to the odorous gases mentioned above, ozone from the electrofiltration of the flue gases and nitrogen oxides produced by the combustion of waste cooking liquid are present in non-odorous amounts (at ground level) in the recovery furnace effluent gases. The question now arises: Do these non-odorous gases affect the perception of the odorous gases? In Figures 3 and 4 are plotted perceived odor strength of H_2S (8-1600 ppb) and carbonyl sulfide (160-10 000 ppb) with and without simultaneous presentation of realistic amounts of ozone (73±3 ppb) and nitrogen monoxide (677 ± 41 ppb) resp. Perceived odor strength was measured by cross-modal magnitude matching and magnitude estimation (12 observers).

In Figures 3 and 4 the diagonal represents no effect on perceived odor strength. At this concentration ozone does not affect the perception of the two sulfides. This is in agreement with studies on masking for ozone [9]. On the contrary, NO enhances the perceived odor strength of the two sulfides.

What is the mechanism behind the reinforcing effect of NO? In control studies conducted on all the observers, the NO and O_3 concentrations used

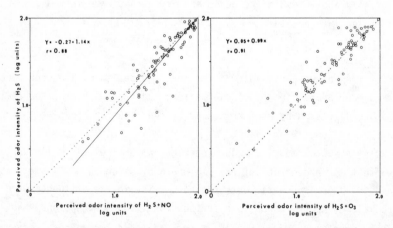

Figure 3 Perceived odor strength of H_2S plotted against H_2S + NO and H_2S + O_3 respectively.

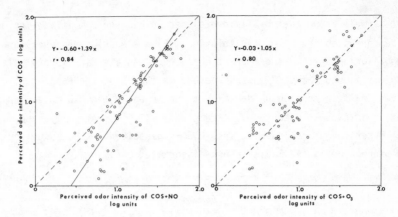

Figure 4 Perceived odor strength of carbonyl sulfide (COS) plotted against
COS + NO and COS + O$_3$ respectively.

could not be distinguished from air alone. Thus perceptual interaction is not
likely to be taken place. NO may stimulate Nervus trigeminus, but if so, not
enough to create a sensation in itself. Undoubtedly trigeminal stimulation
accounts for parts of most odor sensations [10, 11], but subliminal interaction
is unknown to the author. NO may affect the nasal mucosa or the mucus, hence
rendering the two sulfides more powerful in stimulating the odor receptors.
For instance, NO may oxidize to NO$_2$ and further to nitric acid which may affect the pH of the mucus. A change in pH may affect not only the solubility
of the odorants in the mucus but also the chemical dissociation of the sulfide
molecules. For hydrogen sulfide the latter is probable, as will be elaborated
upon later. It has also been shown that the electrical responses of the olfactory cells may be affected by the ionic content of the mucus [12].

The reinforcing effect of NO on the sulfide odors is most evident at the
lower intensity levels. This is easily explained by the attenuating effect
of the olfactory system with increasing stimulation.

H$_2$S and the pH of nasal mucus - Perhaps the most intriguing explanation
of the difference between pulp mills with regard to H$_2$S as an odor indicator
would be that the pH of the mucus of the nose is influenced by the composition
of inhaled flue gases. Soda recovery furnaces often produce acid gases and
lime kilns alkaline gases. Already in the 1940´s Manci [13] claimed that the
odor sensitivity to ketone musk and quaiacol was affected by the ionic equilibrium of the mucosa. Manci´s study, however, aimed at revealing the role of
thiocyanic acid as an oxidative catalyzer in the nasal mucus. The starting
point may be somewhat different when H$_2$S is discussed.

It is well known that H_2S is protolysed in HS^- and S^{2-} in varying proportions depending on the pH of the solution. Figure 5 shows the hydrogen sulfide equilibrium system at different pH's. H_2S has its first protolysis
constant at a pH of about 7 which is close to the pH of the nasal mucus[14].
Thus even small changes in pH may affect the number of the H_2S-molecules present at the olfactory receptors. A pH change will theoretically have a dual
effect. When the pH is lowered, less H_2S is dissolved in the mucus, but a
larger proportion is available as non-dissociated H_2S.

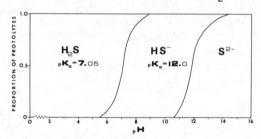

Figure 5   The protolysis equilibrium system of H_2S.

Assuming that the most effective part in the H_2S protolysis system for
stimulating the odor receptors is the H_2S molecule, a moderate lowering of
the pH of the nasal mucus would result in an increased sensitivity to the
hydrogen sulfide odor. A series of studies have been undertaken recently to
test this hypothesis[15]. In the first experiment an attempt was made to affect
the pH of the nasal mucus by exposing 8 observers during 5 min. to buffer
aerosols of sodium citrate at pH 5.3, 6.6 and 9.3 resp. Before and after the
buffer aerosol exposure the individual odor thresholds for H_2S were determined. The test order between sessions and subjects was balanced. In Figure
6 the relative change in H_2S odor threshold concentration (log ppb) is shown
for different pH's of the buffer aerosol inhaled and for a control condition
with no aerosol.

The trend is that the sensitivity to H_2S is elevated by lowering the
pH. It should be noted that the threshold determinations were made with a
forced choice technique[2] to avoid expectancy effects. In a parallel study
on an organic sulfide, dimethyl monosulfide, no effect of the acid aerosol
was found compared to the control condition.

In a second experiment the same buffer aerosols were presented to the observers but now simultaneously with the hydrogen sulfide presentations, Figure
7. The trend is the same as in Figure 6.

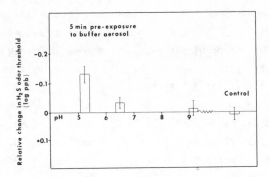

Figure 6 Relative change in H$_2$S odor threshold concentration as a function of pH of pre-exposure to buffer aerosol ($\bar{x}$, SE).

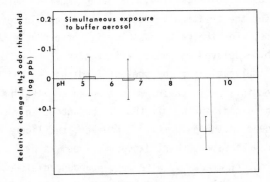

Figure 7 Relative change in H$_2$S odor threshold concentration as a function of pH of buffer aerosol presented simultaneously ($\bar{x}$, SE).

Although the changes achieved by using the buffer aerosols point in the direction of the hypothesis, they are fairly small. As we do not know the buffer capacity of the olfactory mucus itself and have no practical means of measuring the pH change achieved by the buffer aerosol, an attempt was made to "acidify" the noses by exposure to realistic amounts of sulfur dioxide, after which the same two experiments as before were conducted. The SO$_2$ level (114 $\pm$ 3 ppb) was well below the detection threshold but about the same as the level of the flue gas dilutions presented in the field sensory analyses.

Although the dispersion in data is large and the differences small, the trend is as before; the sensitivity of the observers towards the H$_2$S odor is seemingly increased by the SO$_2$ inhalation. The relative change in H$_2$S odor threshold concentration brought about by 5 min. pre-exposure to SO$_2$ was 0.14 $\pm$ 0.10 log ppb and the change by simultaneous presentation of H$_2$S and

SO$_2$ was 0.03 $\pm$ 0.10 log ppb. All comparisons are made with experiments conducted without using SO$_2$. Together with the aerosol experiments the data
support the view that the pH of the nasal mucus does influence the sensitivity of the olfactory system towards H$_2$S, most probably by a shift of the
protolysis equilibrium in the H$_2$S system.

Other factors may be of importance. Nasal mucus can be brought into
alternating gel and sol by shifting the pH [16], namely, the mucus becomes a
gel below about pH 7.5. This may affect the solubility and dissociation of
the odorous molecule. Further, a shift of mucus pH may alter the interface
potentials at the receptor cells [17] which may affect the receptor sensitivity
to H$_2$S.

It is not likely that the pH effect is caused by trigeminus stimulation
from the buffer aerosol because, if so, the effect must be persistent for
several minutes after the treatment. Such an effect should be evident for
dimethyl monosulfide. For the same reason it is not probable that the pH
effect is caused by a delayed response-facilitation [18].

The practical implication of the present findings is that H$_2$S is probably
more easily detected in an acid environment than in an alkaline. The effect
is not large enough to explain in full the discrepancies in the odor prognosis value of H$_2$S found in the pulp mills. However, the laboratory studies
have been conducted with fairly short exposure times. A prolonged exposure
to the air of the factory areas may give more pronounced effects. In the
real-life situation, psychological, chemical and physiological interactions
may unite to provide a satisfactory explanation of the perceived odor strength
of the pulp mill effluents. This is a basic research problem of great applied
importance.

CONCLUSIONS

1. Odor threshold concentrations of hydrogen sulfide vary much between
laboratories.

2. For some recovery furnaces in kraft pulp mills hydrogen sulfide can
be a suitable odor indicator, but in other cases its prognosis value is
doubtful.

3. Perceptual interaction between odorous constituents may account for
part of the unexplained pulp mill odors, but is not the full answer.

4. Nitrogen monoxide in nonperceptual but realistic amounts has been
shown to enhance the odor strength of hydrogen sulfide and carbonyl sulfide
at the lower intensity levels. Ozone did not display such an effect. The

cause of the NO response facilitation remains unclear.

5. The detectability of hydrogen sulfide is seemingly influenced by the pH of the fumes inhaled. At a lower pH, observers sensitivity to H_2S is slightly increased. The reason for this probably is a shift in the pH-dependent dissociation equilibrium of the sulfide. A delayed trigeminal effect or a delayed response facilitation is not likely. The results point to still more difficulties in determining the effective stimulus at the olfactory receptor sites.

This work was supported by grants from the Swedish Environment Protection Board.

REFERENCES

1. Swedish Environment Protection Board (1973)Guidelines for air protection
    Publication No. 8 p. 1, Stockholm (in Swedish)

2. Lindvall, T. (1970)
    Nord. Hyg. Tidskr. Suppl 2, 1-181

3. Grennfelt, P. and Lindvall, T. (1976)
    Svensk Papperstidn. 79, 389-393

4. Berglund, B., Berglund, U. and Lindvall, T. (1973) in Proceedings of the
    Third International Clean Air Congress
    pp A 40-A 43, VDI-Verlag, Düsseldorf

5. Lindvall, T. and Svensson, L.T. (1974)
    J. Appl. Psychol. 59, 264-269

6. Berglund, B., Berglund, U., Lindvall, T. and Svensson, L.T. (1973)
    J. Exp. Psychol. 100, 29-38

7. Ekman, G., Berglund, B., Berglund, U. and Lindvall, T. (1967)
    Scand. J. Psychol. 8, 177-186

8. Berglund, B. (1977) in Proceedings of the 6th International Symposium on
    Olfaction and Taste

9. Cain, W.S. (1974)
    ASHRAE Transactions No. 2295, 53-75

10. Cain, W.S. (1974)
    Ann. New York Acad. Sci. 237, 28-34

11. Tucker, D. (1971) in Handbook of Sensory Physiology (Beidler, L.M. Ed.)
    Vol. 4, pp. 151-181, Springer Verlag, Berlin

12. Tucker, D. and Shibuya, T. (1965)
    Cold Spring Harbour Symposium 30, 207-215

13. Manci, F. (1946)
    Riv. Clin. Med. 46, 367-378
    cited from
    Jones, F.N. and Jones, M.H. (1953)
    J. Psychol. 36, 207-241

14. Negus, V.E. (1958) Comparative Anatomy and Physiology of the Nose and Paranasal Sinuses, Livingstone, London

15. Grennfelt, P. and Lindvall, T. (1977)
    Manuscript in preparation

16. Breuninger, H. (1964)
    Arch. Ohr. Nas. Kehlk. Heilk. 184, 133

17. Niccolini, O. (1942)
    Arch. Psicol. Neurol. Psichiat. Psicoterapia 3, 31-78
    cited from
    Jones, F.N. and Jones, M.H. (1953)
    J. Psychol. 36, 207-241

18. Engen, T. and Bosack, T.N. (1969)
    J. Comp. Physiol. Psychol. 68, 320-326

Sensory behaviour of a nose panel towards bad odours: application to diesel exhaust odours

Paul Degobert

Institut Français du Pétrole, F 92506 Rueil Malmaison, France

ABSTRACT

Diesel odour measurement began in 1956 in the U. S. A. specially to reduce odour from Diesel city buses.   This paper presents first the mechanisms leading to odorant formation and surveys the investigations carried out in the USA which resulted in the development in 1974 of the Arthur D. Little odormeter, based on liquid chromatographic analysis of the exhaust and correlations with sensory data collected in particular conditions.
Energy saving in European cities pushes towards an increase of Diesel vehicles, which may afford an odorous level unbearable for welfare.   Thus IFP presently studies Diesel odours in order to develop reliable measurements methods, starting from ADL liquid chromatography and sensory evaluation.   Present results show that until new developments in chemical analysis appear, sensory evaluation remains the most reliable method.   Future prospects, based on the MAC LEOD's differential olfactometer are presented.

INTRODUCTION

Diesel cars, delivery vans, urban buses are due to increase in city traffic, as they present versus spark-ignition engines a better efficiency, very interesting for energy saving. In that case, annoyance from Diesel exhaust malodors may reach levels unbearable for population welfare and official authorities and manufacturers push to study generation mechanisms and measurement of exhaust odours and means to reduce them.

This paper reports the status of the exhaust odours development with a peculiar emphasis on the investigations now in progress at the INSTITUT FRANCAIS DU PETROLE.

GENERATION OF EXHAUST ODOURS FROM INTERNAL COMBUSTION ENGINES

Incomplete combustion occuring in the engine combustion chamber generates partially oxidized products of medium molecular weight which are strong odorants. It is a matter of common knowlegde that the smell of compressing-ignition (Diesel) engines is both stronger and more disagreeable than that of spark-ignition (gasoline) engines.

Diesel and spark-ignition engines differ essentially in the type of air-fuel mixture. The fuel-oxidizer charge in a spark-ignition is a relatively homogeneous mixture, in contrast to the heterogeneous mixture found in a Diesel combustion chamber ; that heteregeneous combustion is primarily responsible for the noxious character of Diesel exhaust (1).

In spark-ignition engines, unburned hydrocarbons are mainly attributed to the wall quench phenomenon in rich mixtures, when oxygen quantities are not sufficiently available to convert hydrocarbons to odorant oxygenates (2). In Diesel engines where lean mixtures are the rule, oxygenates are generated at the outskirts of the fuel spray, where oxygen may rapidly attack hydrocarbons cracked in the flame core (3). If such a flame is quenched, or if the main temperature is too low (part load), the residence time too short (high speed), oxygenates cannot burn completely and go directly to exhaust (4). Near full load conditions, incomplete combustion may also happen in the fuel rich core of the Diesel flame (3).

Therefore, although the overall quantity of unburned compounds is generally higher in gasoline than in Diesel exhaust, generation of odorants is greater with Diesel, because of the general presence of oxygen in the exhaust molecules, and also the more complicated chemical composition of the exhaust and of the starting fuel. In fact the basic mechanisms leading to odorant generation are still unknown and as moreover, addition mechanisms of even binary odorous mixtures are far from being completely understood, precise chemical analysis of exhaust cannot at the present time predict the odorous sensation sent by a given Diesel engine in a specific operating condition. For it is worth to notice that a typical Diesel exhaust may contain more than 1000 identified compounds, about 100 of which are odorants (5), and when fed with pure hexadecane,up to 75 identified compounds (1).

STATUS OF THE AMERICAN PREVIOUS WORK

Research on Diesel odour began in 1956 in the U.S.A. and 10 different projects have been in progress since that time with different approaches to the problem (7). Investigations proceeded in different laboratories from universities, technical centres, and engine manufacturers.

Studies refered to Diesel odour measurement techniques by sensory methods, engine and vehicle odour tests, Diesel exhaust chemical analysis. They were partly supported by the Environmental Protection Agency(EPA),and after 1968 by the Coordinating Research Council(CRC) a cooperative body from the Society of Automotive Engineers (SAE) and the American Petroleum Institute(API)-EPA developed sensory methods in contract with Amos TURK (8), and CRC, looking for a measurement device more convenient for automotive manufacturers than a nose panel, tried to develop exhaust chemical analysis correlated with odour ; that project reached its goal in 1973 with the development of the Arthur D. Little Diesel Odor Analytical System (DOAS) (9.).

Now most laboratories are equipped with ADL DOAS and only Southwest Research Institute uses both DOAS and sensory panel (10).

MAIN AMERICAN RESULTS

Sensory measurement techniques All now conventional olfactory psychophysical techniques have been applied to Diesel odour evaluation, some rating only the overall odour intensity, others estimating both odour quality and intensity. Intensity has been estimated by the threshold dilution technique (11) with randomized presentations, a method which cannot give information concerning either the quality or the relative intensity of the various odour characters.

Other methods estimated odour intensity against a standard. We have here to mention the development of the Amos TURK Kit (8), generally accepted in the USA for measuring odour quality and intensity. It comprises 4 odour scales, measuring 4 odour qualities described as burnt/smoky, oily, pungent/acid and aldehydic/aromatic, and one general intensity scale. All standards in sniff-bottles are complex mixtures of specific chemicals, and the general intensity standard a mixture of the first four standards.

The Arthur D. LITTLE odour profile method has also been used in Diesel Odour research. It basically consists in giving descriptive characters of the Diesel odour following previously agreed verbal descriptive terms ; the intensity of each character, as felt by the panelist is given on a 4 point category scale ; odour characters were similar to Amos TURK'S : burnt, oily, oxidized, nose and eye irritation.

Odour presentation systems to nose panels were of different kinds for Diesel Odour evaluation :

. the ASTM syringe method (11)

. the "camera inodorata ", aluminum-clad gas chamber used by ADL (12)

. the "sniff-box" technique, face-mask opened in a duct in which runs the odorant mixture (13)

. the "funnel-type" presentation system (14) (15), in which the sensory assessors sniff the odorant from funnels set in parallel on the main distribution line

Engine and vehicle odour tests Odorous effect of operating conditions and type of fuel have been investigated. Among the parameters studied : load, speed, injection timing injector-type, shape of combustion chamber, type of fuel,

fuel additives, etc ..., conditions favoring the formation of oxidized unburned compounds were found the most odorant (idling, deceleration, high speed/high load) (14) (10). Fuel additives are unefficient; only replacement of poorly designed injectors by improved ones was felt efficient to reduce odour level (16).

Diesel exhaust chemical analysis and correlation with odour level

Chemical species within easy reach by conventional analytical methods were first determined : unburned HC, NOx, aliphatic aldehydes, acroleïn, formaldehyde (17). Tentative correlations between odour and those pollutants (18) show that no combination of such species may predict the odour level and that the unburned HC level was the main factor in the correlation, but unable alone to represent odour.

More accurate determinations were done on exhaust concentrated in suitable traps, either cold, or polymer powder filled traps (Chromosorb), by gas and liquid chromatography combined with mass spectrometry. Illinois Institute of Technology IITRI isolated and identified about 1000 chemical compounds, of which 100 odorants (19). Concerned chemical classes are : alkyl-alkenylbenzenes, indans, naphtalenes, tetralins, paraffinic, aromatic and furannic aldehydes.

Arthur D. Little separated collected trap samples into two fractions, one corresponding to the smoky-burnt, the other to the oily-kerosene character (9). Typical compounds were phenols and aromatic aldehydes and ketones for the first fraction, and substituted tetralins, indans and naphtalenes for the second. After liquid chromatography group analysis with an UV detector, the two fractions were correlated with odour. This good correlation found between odour and the aromatic oxygenates fraction led to the development of the ADL DOAS "Odormeter". Excepted Southwest Research Institute which still makes sensory evaluation (21), DOAS data are now assimilated to odour in the USA (20).

STATUS OF THE EUROPEAN AND JAPANESE WORK

In England, by sensory analysis, Ricardo (22) evaluated the "nastiness" of Diesel exhaust at different operating conditions, within a "camera inodorata", the standard being an engine running in constant conditions : increasing load, decreasing speed, and adding a noble catalyst exhaust muffler reduce odour level. Ricardo owns now an ADL DOAS and Perkins built a similar liquid chromatograph.

In Germany, main investigation happen at Clausthal Technical High School (23). Threshold dilution technique is used (24) with gas chromatography. Tentative correlation between odour and chemical composition points out the high correlation with furannic compounds. Moreover Daimler-Benz uses an ADL DOAS to evaluate odour from its products.

In Sweden, different cars have been studied at the Karolinska Institute by threshold dilution with sniff-box technique (25). Non-heated sampling tube led to the conclusion that Diesel seemed to be less odorant than gasoline cars.

In Japan, some studies deal with irritation effect from exhaust odours(26).

FRENCH INVESTIGATIONS

They started in 1974 under sponsorship of INSTITUT DE RECHERCHES DES TRANSPORTS (IRT). Except some work on spark-ignition engines at the Commissariat à l'Energie Atomique (CEA), most investigations concern Diesel engine with three purposes :

. To establish sensory evaluation methods to reliably measure odour

. To establish connections between odour figures from sensory panels and analytical data, specially ADL DOAS figures, to verify if ADL correlations are valid with European cars and fuels, with the aim of substituting in the future a physical instrument to the expensive sensory evaluation

. To study engine and fuel improvement to decrease exhaust malodour level

The work is still now in its earlier stage. Experimental installation has been erected at the INSTITUT FRANCAIS DU PETROLE (IFP) and some preliminary results have been gained.

Sensory analysis set-up and sensory methods

IFP semi-mobile laboratory is made of a specially designed odour presentation cabin put on a trailer (Fig.1). That air conditioned room houses up to 12 panelists smelling simultaneously diluted exhaust,coming from an engine on a test bench, or a car tail-pipe on a chassis dynamometer (Fig.2). Dilution ratios vary from 1:25 to 1:1000.Funnel-type presentation system allows to get 12 simultaneous verbal answers at a time, without adding engine operation discrepancies (Fig.3).

Odour-freed, thermostated and moisturized air is used both to condition the cabin and dilute the engine exhaust sucked from the exhaust manifold (Fig.4).

A specially trained panel of 16-18 people make the sensory evaluations. After selection following modified TURK'S instructions (8), they were trained to give two verbal answers when presented with odours to be evaluated : one answer concerning the intensity either by matching against standard sniff-bottles arranged in geometrical progression or by magnitude estimation against a standard sent in the presentation funnel, another answer corresponding to the "repulsivity" felt by the subject on a category scale without standard.

As a matter of fact, the training sessions, with pure standard odorants

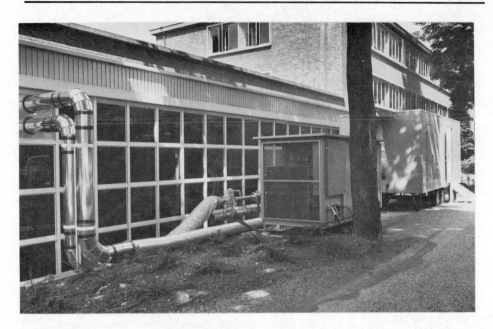

Fig.1 - Sensory Evaluation Set-up. Overall external view

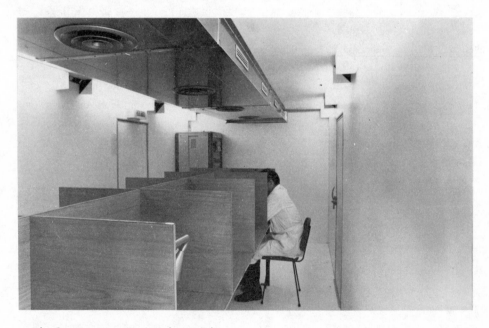

Fig.2 - Sensory Evaluation Cabin

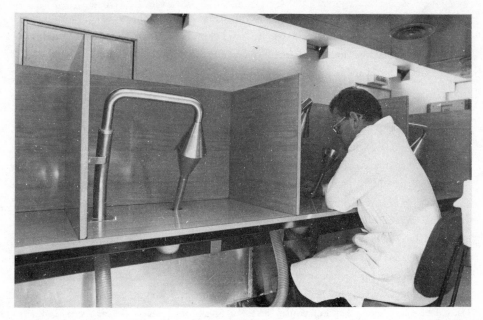

Fig.3 - "Sniff-funnel" odour presentation system

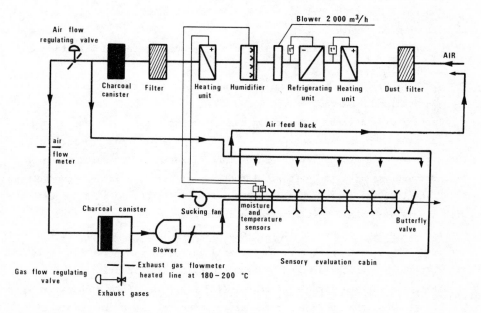

Fig.4 - Air and exhaust gas flow-sheet

taken from the TURK Kit and representing Diesel odour characters, were unable
to bring out a common standard for intensity and repulsivity (27). For intensity, pyridine appeared as the best standard and is used thenceforth, but no common repulsivity standard suits the majority of the panel.

<u>Physico-chemical analysis</u>   The ADL liquid chromatographic odormeter suffers
from at least one basic drawback : solutions from trapped exhaust are, after
injection in the chromatographic loop, split off into 2 fractions : aromatic
hydrocarbons LCA, and aromatic oxygenates LCO. LCA is automatically eluted
from the chromatographic column, but the injection of a polar solvent is necessary to elute LCO. As the main solvent (cyclohexane) is sensitive to oxidation, the oxidation impurities accumulated in the column are freed at once
with the injection of the polar solvent (isopropanol) resulting in an erratic
blank value, of a magnitude similar to the sample value to be measured.

The IFP analysis laboratory overcomes that drawback by using in the loop
since the beginning a mixture of the two solvents with a very low content of
the polar one, which develops successively the two peaks. Besides that special
liquid chromatographic technique, more conventional analyses are carried out:
HC, CO, NOx smoke, aliphatic aldehydes, acroleïn, ...

Prelimary results on French Diesel Engines

Two small French Diesel engines have yet been submitted to olfactory and
physico chemical analysis :
   . a PEUGEOT 504 D engine - 2.11 liter displacement tested with the match-
     ing method (28)
   . a SAVIEM 720 engine - 3.6 liter displacement - tested with the magnitu-
     de estimation method

TABLE 1 presents the 8 operating conditions of the PEUGEOT engine evaluated 12 times each in random order by 16 people at 3 dilution levels. TABLE 2
shows the ranking of the corresponding intensities after transformation on a
linear scale. Ranking is quite similar at any dilution ratio, the gap between
1:100 and 1:200 is greater than between 1:200 and 1:400, in good agreement
with the STEVENS' law. Most intense odours are generated at full load, high
speed (incomplete combustion in rich mixture) and then at part load, low speed
(medium combustion temperature). The overall intensity range is relatively narrow : there is a factor 3 between the most and the less odorant condition.

Nastiness shows a parallel tendancy (TABLE 3). The odorous character does
not change along the operating range tested, and, although trained to make
distinction, people assimilate intensity and nastiness, which remains between
slightly and meanly objectionable.

TABLE 1 -

| CODE | ENGINE OPERATING CONDITIONS | | | | |
	SPEED RPM	LOAD	POWER HP	BEPM kg/cm²	NOTES
①	1,000	0	0	0	∿ IDLE
②	1,500	1 : 4	6	1.7	MIN. SMOKE
③	1,000	4 : 4	12	5.11	MAX. SMOKE
④	3,000	1 : 4	12	1.7	MIN. SMOKE
⑤	3,000	4 : 4	42	5.11	ACCEL. GENTLE SLOPE
⑥	4,500	4 : 4	54	5.11	FULL LOAD MAX. HC
⑦	1,000	1 : 4	6	2.56	MIN. HC
⑧	2,000	1 : 10	3	0.64	RUNNING ON THE FLAT

TABLE 2 - **RANKING OF THE ODOROUS INTENSITIES**

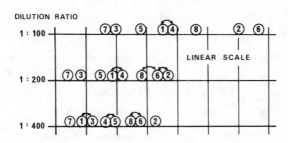

TABLE 3 - **RANKING OF NASTINESS OF THE EIGHT OPERATING CONDITIONS**

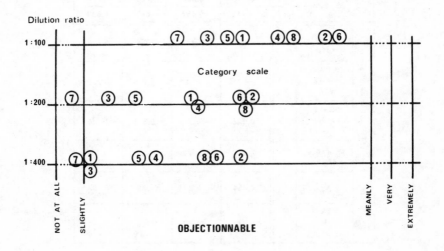

Similar results were obtained with the SAVIEM engine, but with that MAN-type combustion chamber, 1:100 dilution ratio was judged untolerable and idling conditions were the most odorant.

Connections between sensory and analytical data

No relation exists between odour and smoke. TABLE 4 sums up at the top of the table the linear correlation coefficient calculated from our results. No chemical data fits correctly with the odorous intensity, the LCO and LCA figures obtained by the liquid chromatographic analysis akin to ADL odormeter appear worse than unburned HC.That is not specific to our procedure,as we draw the same conclusion from similar calculations starting from American data (10)(21) at the bottom of TABLE 4.

CONCLUSION AND FUTURE PROSPECTS

Although Arthur D. Little has delivered a certain number of "odormeters" on the market , and some companies use exclusively that device to get odour level (20), physicochemical analysis in its present stage of development cannot predict odour. More advanced analytical and correlation work is needed before replacing sensory evaluation.

The application to Diesel odour investigations of the olfactometer inven-

TABLE 4 - CALCULATED CORRELATION COEFFICIENTS BETWEEN SENSORY AND ANALYTICAL DATA

ENGINE INVESTIGATED			ANALYTICAL DATA			
		DILUTION	UNBURNED HC	ALIPH. ALDEHYDES	L CO	L CA
PEUGEOT 504 D IFP DATA		1 : 100	0.679	0.439	0.540	0.516
		1 : 200	0.735	0.536	0.638	0.559
		1 : 400	0.642	0.454	0.667	0.598
DATA SWRi (14) "D" RATINGS	PEUGEOT 504 D	1 :: 100	0.828	0.431	0.276	0.477
	NISSAN DATSUN (Winter)		0.778	− 0.185	− 0.106	0.250
	NISSAN DATSUN (Summer)		0.643	− 0.358	− 0.371	0.314
	MERCEDES 220 D		0.383	− 0.464	0.764	0.701
	OPEL REKORD		0.654	− 0.221	0.568	0.799
	5 CARS ALL TOGETHER		0.941	0.757	0.720	0.814

ted and developed by Dr P. MAC LEOD would afford a solution. That device(29) based on the separated olfactory connections between the brain and the two nostrils, and the inhibition of the less excited connection in favour of the influx coming from the nostril receiving the most intense excitation, will be next tested on Diesel exhaust on the IFP installation, in a cooperative programme between MAC LEOD's laboratory, CEA and IFP under sponsorship of IRT.

If successful, the olfactometer, needing one single sensory assessor, without intense training, and one single presentation would advantageously compete with ADL type odormeter, giving a true odour intensity instead of a chemical analysis.

That work has been partly supported by contract IRT-ATP Pollution n°75060 from INSTITUT DE RECHERCHES DES TRANSPORTS.

REFERENCES
 1. Aaronson, A.E. and Matula, R.A. (1971)
    Combustion Inst. Pittsburgh PA - Symp. Combustion 13th p471-481
 2. Edwards, J.B.(1973) in Engine emissions, Pollutant Formation and Measurement, pp. 33-76, Plenum Press, New York
 3. Henein, N.A. (1973) in Engine emissions, Pollutant Formation and Measurement, pp. 211-266, Plenum Press, New York
 4. Eyzat, P., Lys, X. (1972)
    Rev. Assoc. Franç. Techn. Petrole, 216, pp. 95-105
 5. Spindt, R.S., Barkes, G.J., Somers, J.H. (1971)
    SAE Paper 710 605
 6. Rounds, F.G., Pearsall, H.W. (1957)
    SAE Transactions 65, pp. 608-627
 7. Savery C.W., Matula, R.A. (1974)
    SAE Paper 740213
 8. Turk, A. (1967)
    NTIS report PB 174-707
 9. Levins, P.L. et al. (1974)
    SAE Paper 740216
10. Springer, K.J., Stahmann, R.C.,
    SAE Paper 750 332
11. Barnes, G.J. 1968
    SAE Paper 680 445
12. Kendall D.A., Levins, P.L., Leonardos G. (1974)
    SAE Paper 740 215
13. Reckner, L.R., Squires, R.E. (1968)
    SAE Paper 680 444
14. Stahmann, R.C., Kittredge G.D., Springer, K.J. (1968)
    SAE Paper 680 443
15. Vogh, J.W. (1969)
    J. Air Poll. Control Assoc. 19 (10), pp. 773-777
16. Ford, H.S., Merrion D.F., Hames, R.J. (1970)
    SAE Paper 700 734
17. Linnel, R.H., Scott, W.E. (1962)
    J. Air Poll. Control Assoc. 12 (11) pp. 510-515
18. Dietzmann, H.E., Springer, K.J., Stahmann, R.C. (1972)
    SAE Paper 720 757

19. Dravnieks, A. et al (1970)
    NTIS Report PB 198 072
20. Hills, F.J., Schleyerbach C.G. (1977)
    SAE Paper 770 316
21. Springer K.J., Stahmann R.C. (1977)
    SAE Papers 770 254 - 770 258
22. Lesley S., French C.C.J. (1976)
    SAE Paper 760 554
23. Oelert H.H., Jajontz J., Knuth, H.W. (1977)
    Erdöl und Kohle 30(4) p.183
24. Oelert H.H., Florian, Th. (1972)
    Staub, Reinhalt Luft 32(10) pp. 400-407
25. Lindvall, Th. - Mortstedt S.E. (1970)
    Aktiebolaget Atomenergi (Sweden) Rep. BIL-52
26. Iwai, T., Furui , K., Yoshida, A. Tashiro, M. (1976)
    FISITA Congress - Tokyo Paper NO 2-11
27. Degobert, P. Pasquereau, M. , Nadaud, Y. (1976)
    IFP Report 24202
28. Degobert, P., Pasquereau, M., Nadaud, Y. (1977)
    IFP Report 24 857
29. French Patent 2,210, 298 (1972)

Odor pollution and odor annoyance reactions in industrial areas of the Rhine-Ruhr region[o])

Gerhard Winneke and Joachim Kastka

Medizinisches Institut fuer Lufthygiene und Silikoseforschung an der Universitaet Duesseldorf, Gurlittst. 53, D-4000 Duesseldorf, GFR

ABSTRACT

Odor-annoyance is shown to be a multi-dimensional concept with sensory, social-emotional and somatic aspects as main dimensions. The composite annoyance-scores, derived for these dimensions have been shown to be remarkably reliable over time and have, furthermore, been shown to be related to distance from the source as well as to quantitative odor-exposure data. It is, therefore, concluded that odor-control might eventually improve, if these relationships, some of which are based on preliminary data, are supported by further research.

INTRODUCTION

By extrapolation from representative surveys it has been estimated that about 10% of the american population live in odor problem areas[1]. Similar estimates have been reported for Sweden[2]. Although the necessity of efficient odor control is almost universally accepted, enforcement is lagging considerably behind air pollution control in general, a fact which is illustrated by the diversity of odor control regulations in the U.S.[3,4]. This frustrating state of affairs is fundamentally related to the very nature of odor perception, namely the lack of equipment capable of measuring threshold concentrations of more than a few odorous compounds as well as the lack of methodology for quantifying undesirable odor-effects[4].

Since 1974 we are conducting laboratory and field studies designed to develop concepts and strategies for the development of odor control legislation in the Federal Republic of Germany[5-8]. In making annoyance reactions a key concept of this research we do agree to a large extent with a group of american investigators, stating "...that the only measurable impact associated with a vast majority of odor problems was annoyance and that a proper

means for dealing with such problems must consider the measurement of annoyance as central to success"[4], Before recommen-
ding attitude surveys as a routine tool for gathering basic information for odor control regulation, however, we felt it was
necessary,to study the psychological structure of odor annoyance,
to establish the reliability of annoyance reactions, and to vali-
date annoyance scores in the following stepwise manner: (1) by
comparing a known problem area with a comparable control area,
(2) by relating degree of annoyance to distance from the source,
and (3) by relating annoyance scores to odor concentrations in
ambient air, as measured by the sensory dilution to threshold-
principle[9]. In this paper data will be given, dealing with these
fundamental problems.

THE STRUCTURE OF ODOR ANNOYANCE

The first step of the project was the construction of a struc-
tured questionnaire, the main part of which consisting of 40
rating-scales, dealing with the perception of environmental odors,
and their social, emotional and somatic impact. The first study
was run in the city of Duesseldorf (about 600 000 inhabitants)[5,6].
In collaboration with the local enforcement authorities ("Gewer-
beaufsichts-Amt") an odor-problem area in close vicinity of a de-
tergent and soap plant (about 14000 employees), emitting primarily organic compounds, and two odor-free control areas close to
glass-works (about 500 000 t of glass/year),   and a steel-mill
(about 600 000 t of steel-tubes/year), respectively, were selected
for study. A random sample of about 1000 inhabitants from these
areas was drawn from the census-files, and a final sample of 704
of these was sucessfully interviewed by instructed personnel
(mostly students) in a standardized face-to-face situation. The
complete set of data was subjected to principle-components analysis, which gave rise to six components with eigenvalues larger
than 1.0. A subsequent Varimax-rotation of the component factors
resulted in a clear item-structure, with three main factors accounting for more than 50% of the total variance (table 1).
The first factor (F_1) is primarily characterized by those items,
which stress the sensory aspects of odor perception, its intensity, frequency and quality, reduced possibilities of ventilating
the apartment, as well as formal statements of being annoyed or

ODOR — ANNOYANCE — REACTIONS	F1	F2	F3	F4	F5	F6	C%
Distinct perception of odors in neighborhood	82	9	11	-7	20	-1	75
Intensity of perceived odors	81	21	17	-8	26	-9	82
Frequency of odor perception	80	17	20	-7	8	-7	75
Odor annoyance of people "does exist"	79	15	10	-9	22	-5	74
Degree of annoyance due to malodors	78	22	28	-9	26	-14	85
Degree of disturbance due to malodors	66	19	26	-22	36	-14	75
Windows often shut because of odors	65	32	32	-19	5	-20	73
Discomfort due to environmental odors	61	19	25	-31	30	-9	69
Foul smelling air	60	29	31	-27	36	-7	76
Ventilation of apartment difficult	58	41	36	-12	12	-13	70
"Stinking" air in neighborhood	56	31	31	-28	34	-11	73
Sleeping with windows shut	56	26	48	-14	9	-13	68
Environmental odors unbearable	53	21	28	-4	14	-20	49
Reduced pleasure of taking a walk	53	49	17	-16	13	-9	63
Strange smell in apartment	51	41	24	-16	4	-18	56
Reduced social contacts	-14	75	19	0	18	0	67
No pleasure coming home	-18	71	18	-6	19	-9	62
Odor leads to tensions within family	-9	69	21	-1	11	-11	56
Odor disturbes communication	-27	69	26	-4	1	-14	65
Odor spoils the appetite	-23	63	41	-6	13	-14	67
Odor interferes with the comfort of living	-40	56	34	-11	17	-14	68
Odor interferes with outdoor activities	-50	56	22	-11	14	-7	66
Odor induces anger	-19	55	50	-3	14	-9	63
Odor interferes with falling asleep	-26	23	79	-3	5	-2	75
Odor disturbes sleep	-25	16	73	-3	11	-2	64
Odor induces headache	-29	30	66	-9	16	-10	65
Odor induces nausea	-17	35	59	-12	40	-12	70
Odor induces fits of coughing	-19	30	58	-7	14	-18	52
Odor interferes with reading and thinking	-18	52	57	-8	0	-4	63
Odor induces bad mood	-18	56	57	-8	4	-7	69
Odor interferes with recreation	-37	48	54	-12	0	-14	72
Odor induces vomiting	-10	38	52	-10	37	-23	63
Odor interferes with normal breathing	-44	42	48	-13	16	-11	66
Air in neighborhood "clean"	26	-6	-10	84	-8	2	80
Air in neighborhood "fresh"	27	-9	-7	83	-9	6	80
Contribution of factor (% of total variance)	22	15	14	5	6	5	67

Table 1: Factorial structure of odor items after principal components analysis and subsequent rotation according to the Varimax-criterion. C% = % Communality; N=7o4 (after 5).

bothered by odors. This factor has therefore been labelled "Generalized annoyance based on sensory experience". The second item-cluster (F$_2$) deals mainly with social and emotional effects of odor perception; it has therefore been labelled "Social-emotional annoyance reaction". The third item-cluster (F$_3$)contains primarily those items, ascribing somatic reactions to odor perception, and was, therefore, called "Somatic-vegetative annoyance". There is only very little overlap between these factors. The remaining three factors are of only minor importance and have been neglected in subsequent analyses. Invariance of this 3-dimensional structure of annoyance was shown by splitting the original sample at random into two subsamples; essentially the same

factor-structure emerged for both these samples. It was, therefore, decided, to combine the most salient and unequivocal items
for each of these factors, thus yielding seperate annoyance
scores for the three dimensions of annoyance.

RELIABILITY OF ANNOYANCE REACTIONS

Subsequent to the first Duesseldorf study in 1974 two follow-
up studies were conducted on small subsamples of the original
sample, in order to measure changes of annoyance after introduction of odor-abatement technologies at the different sources,
and to establish the stability of annoyance with time[10]. Test-
retest-coefficients for test- and control-areas are given in
table 2. These stability-coefficients are sufficiently high to
support the conclusion that in dealing with odor annoyance we
are obviously dealing with a markedly stable attitude, amenable
to scientific study.

VALIDITY OF ANNOYANCE SCORES

A first attempt to establish the validity of annoyance-
measures was made by testing the discriminating power of the
three annoyance-scores for test- and control-areas of the original Duesseldorf-sample. All three measures were found to discriminate significantly between polluted and odor-free areas
($p < 0.001$; $df = 1/702$), with F_1, F_2 and F_3 accounting for 50,
23 and 24% of total variance, respectively [5].

Subsequent studies, which have not yet been completed, are

RELIABILITY OF ANNOYANCE REACTIONS				
ANNOYANCE MEASURE	POLLUTED AREAS Duesseldorf n = 87		CONTROL AREAS Duesseldorf n = 37	
	1974/75	1974/76	1974/75	1974/76
Sensory Experience	.70	.58	.74	.59
Social Emotional Disturbance	.61	.59	.61	.59
Somatic Disturbance	.63	.60	.81	.71
	r_{tt} (p>.05) <.21		r_{tt} (p>.05) <.32	

Table 2: Test-retest-coefficients (r_{tt}) for three annoyance-
measures for one- and two-year intervals (from 10).

dealing with validity in a more refined manner. About 2ooo Ss
in the vicinity of 8 qualitatively different industrial plants
in the cities of Duisburg (460 000 inhabitants) and Cologne
(1 000 000 inhabitants) have been sampled at random from the
local census-files and are being interviewed with a slightly
modified questionnaire. Validity is being studied by relating
annoyance-scores to distance from the source, as well as by
correlating them with ambient odor-concentrations, measured by
means of the well established dilution to theshold-principle[9].

As for changes of annoyance with distance from the source
preliminary data will be given for a tar-oil plant in Duisburg,
emitting mainly hydrocarbons and sulphur compounds, and a manu-
facturing plant for insulation-material in Cologne, emitting
mainly phenolic compounds. The former may be qualified as an
area-source, the latter as a point-source. Change of annoyance
with distance is completely different for both these plants, as
is already apparent from looking at single items (figure 1).
Cumulated frequency has been plotted against degree of affirmative statement for two typical items representing factor III.
i.e. the somatic annoyance dimension. The precise wording of
these items was: "How often does it happen that odors induce
headache (or nausea) with you?" Ss had to answer using a 7
point ratingscale ranging from "never" to "permanently". Whereas for the insulation plant in Cologne the frequency curves are
regularly displaced to the left with increasing distance from
the source, which for practical purposes means the boundary of
the plant, this is not true for the taroil plant in Duisburg.
Other items show the same tendency.

If single items are now combined to yield annoyance scores
corresponding to the three annoyance-dimensions, the change with
distance gets even more clearcut and amenable to precise statistical treatment (figure 2). Degree of annoyance is plotted
against distance from the source. The solid lines represent the
situation in the vicinity of the tar-oil plant in Duisburg, whereas
the broken lines stand for odor-annoyance near the insulation-
plant. Decrease of annoyance with distance is significant for
the insulation-plant only ($p < 001$; df = 4/89).

The width of the shaded areas at the bottom of each graph

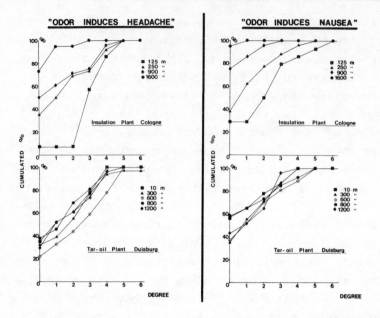

Figure 1: Frequency curves for two items of F_3 (somatic annoyance) in the vicinity of an insulation plant (upper part) and a tar-oil plant (below), broken down for distance from source.

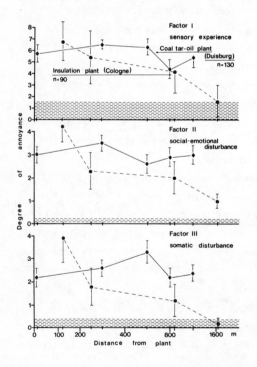

Figure 2: Change of annoyance with distance from plant-boundary for three annoyance-dimensions and two different plants.

represents the degree of annoyance as determined from the control-areas of the Duesseldorf-samples[5]. More data from control-areas will have to sampled, in order to be able to establish background-annoyance more precisely.

In looking at the decline of annoyance near the insulation plant (broken lines) more closely, it is obvious that a marked decrease of scores in the immediate vicinity, i.e. between about 100 and 300 m from the plant-boundaries, does occur only for factors II and III; Scheffé-comparisons[11] between the first two points were highly significant for both these factors,whereas for factor I they were not. This supports our hypothesis that social-emotional and somatic aspects of annoyance are in fact indicative of more severe degrees of disturbance than are sensory of stimulus-centered odor experiences. This, furthermore, illustrates the superiority of a multi -dimensional approach to odor-annoyance as opposed to one-dimensional odor-indexes[4].

Since the annoyance-situation near the two plants in Duisburg and Cologne with regard to distance was so markedly different (see fig. 2), it would be highly desirable to be able to relate these differences to quantitative odor exposure data. Preliminary information in this respect does exist, because a program of measuring ambient odor-concentrations in the vicinity of odor-emitting sources has been started in 1976. In this program we are using a mobile laboratory-unit equipped with olfactometers, which has been built in collaboration with the Karolinska Institute (Stockholm)[12].

In this routine program leeside measures are being made near different plants and odor-concentrations are determined according to the sensory dilution-to-threshold principle[9]. Two Ss are tested at a time, with one threshold determination taking about 2 minutes to be performed. The odor concentrations measured in this way are expressed as odor-units, i.e. as volume of odor-free air to volume of odorous air-sample at threshold. Median (50%) and extreme (95%) values were computed as characteristics of the degree of odor-pollution in a given area at a given point in time. These values for the two plants considered here are given in figure 3; they are based on a one-year measurement-program, which has not yet been completed.

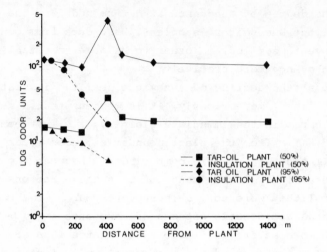

Figure 3: Median (50%) and extreme (95%) odor-concentrations, expressed as odor-units, in the vicinity of the tar-oil plant in Duisburg and the insulation plant in Cologne.

It was relatively easy to measure odor-concentrations of more than 10 (50%) or 100 (95%) odor-units beyond 1400m from the plant boundary of the tar-oil plant. This was not at all true for the insulation-plant in Cologne, even at distances beyond only 500m from the plant. We, thus, feel that the differences in decrease of odor-annoyance with distance for both these plants (see fig. 2) are clearly reflected in odor-concentrations near these plants.

CONCLUSIONS

Odor annoyance has been shown to be a multi-dimensional attitude, with sensory, social-emotional and somatic aspects. The composite scores derived for these main annoyance-dimensions have shown to be remarkably stable across time and have, furthermore, been shown to be related to quantitative odor exposure-data. We, thus, feel that odor control might eventually progress, if odor-annoyance data and odor-concentrations in ambient air will actually turn out to be related in a meaningful way, as is suggested by the data presented here.

REFERENCES

1. Copley International Corporation (1970)National Survey of the
    Odor Problem, Phase I.
    Publ.No. PB-194376, U.S. Dep. of Commerce, Springfield

2. Jonsson,E. and Soerenssen,S.(1967)
    Nord.Hyg.Tidskr. 47,21-34

3. Leonardos,G.(1974)
    J.Air.Poll.Control Ass. 24,456-468

4. Copley International Corporation (1973)National Survey of the
    Odor Problem, Phase III.
    Report No.EPA-650/5-73-001, Environmental Protection Agency,
    Research Triangle Park,N.C.

5. Kastka,J.(1976) in Umweltpsychologie (Kaminski,G.,ed.),
    pp.187-223,Klett,Stuttgart

6. Winneke,G. und Kastka,J.(1975) in Geruchsprobleme bei Tier-
    haltung und Tierkoerperbeseitigung
    VDI-Berichte Vol.226,pp.11-24,VDI-Verlag,Duesseldorf

7. Winneke,G. und Kastka,J.(1975)
    Prax.Pneumol. 29,393-399

8. Winneke,G. und Kastka,J.(1976)
    Zbl.Bakt.Hyg.,I.Abt.Orig.B.,162,41-50

9. Huey,N.A.,Broering,L.C.,Jutze,G.A., and Gruber,C.W.(1960)
    J.Air Poll.Control Ass.,10,441-446

10. Kastka,J. und Winneke,G.(1976)
    Paper presented at 6.Arbeitstagung d.DGfHM, Mainz

11. Winer,B.J.(1962) Statistical Principles in Experimental De-
    sign
    McGraw-Hill,New York

12. Lindvall,T.(1970)
    Nord.Hyg.Tidskr.,Suppl. 2

o. Footnote: The studies reported here were supported by "Mini-
    sterium des Innern", Bonn (F.R.G.), Project No.UB II 5-235-01

Abstracts of Poster Presentations

Odor intensity: Resolving power and the psychophysical function W. S.
Cain, (John B. Pierce Foundation and Yale University, 290 Congress Ave.,
New Haven, CT U.S.A.)

Subjects attempted to resolve small differences in the concentration of
odorous vapors. Success at this task was compared with predictions derived
from chromatographic analysis of fluctuations in stimulus magnitude. The
correlation between psychophysical performance and chromatographic predictions approached 0.9, thereby revealing that noise in the stimulus limits
olfaction's resolving power considerably. When fluctuations in the stimulus
were minimized, subjects could reliably resolve differences as small as 4%,
almost an order of magnitude below previous estimates. Such an outcome
implies that olfaction's resolving power rivals that of audition and vision.
Nevertheless, resolving power varies from one odorant to another. Whereas
resolution of butyl alcohol requires only a 4% difference in concentration,
resolution of amyl butyrate requires a 9% difference. Such variation
prompts attention to the question of whether resolution of small differences
in concentration relates to differences in the growth of perceived intensity as assessed by magnitude estimations of widely-spaced, and hence easily
discriminable, concentrations. That is, do odorants that permit relatively
easy discrimination also give rise to relatively steep psychophysical functions? Indeed, butyl alcohol hielded a much steeper function than amyl
butyrate. But amyl alcohol, for which resolution was relatively poor,
yielded a function almost as steep as butyl alcohol. The results support
the conclusion that resolving power and the growth of the psychophysical
function may be related, but only imperfectly.

An "air feed-back" olfactometer for single odours and mixtures P.Duyvesteyn,
(Psychological Laboratory, State University Utrecht, The Netherlands)

A programmable olfactometer has been designed for eight odours, six can be
switched on or off automatically and two can be changed by hand. In this
way, stimulation with any particular odour is possible. The output-flow is
about 50 ml/min. The olfactometer has 24 dilution steps, with a maximum
dilution of 10,000. It has been specifically developed for electrophysiological experiments on the frog, but it can be modified easily for use on
other animals and for psychophysical experiments. The olfactometer has been
designed for producing square-shaped odorous pulses with various pulse
lengths and different concentrations, for single odours and for mixtures. A
feed-back system has been developed to produce those pulses: odorous flow
(50 ml/min) to the preparation (stimulus situation) is attained by sucking
away the total moist air flow (110 ml/min); in the non-stimulus situation
the total odorous flow as well as part of the moist air flow (60 ml/min) is
sucked away. A three-way valve is used to alternate between stimulation and
non-stimulation. In this way, pressure changes on the preparation can be
avoided. For example, in case of acetone, the rise time of the odorous pulse
is less than 100 msec. The feed-back system is made out of small stainless
steel blocks, to which stainless steel capillaries (0.9 mm i.d.) are fixed
with gold solder. For the production of mixtures, a similar feed-back system
is used. This system ensures that the concentration of an odour in the
mixing situation is exactly the same as in the non-mixing one. In both cases
the dilution is identical, because the total amount of flow (odour or air)
does not change in the mixing chamber. An identical feed-back system is used
several times for making different concentration steps.

A new model for taste psychophysics: the role of pulsatile stimulation B. P. Halpern and H. L. Meiselman, (Dept. of Psychology and Sec. of Neurobiol. & Behav., Cornell Univ., Ithaca, NY, and Army Natick Labs, Natick, MA, U.S.A.)

Humans report no taste adaptation when 1, 2, or 3 sec flows of 100 to 500 mM NaCl or 2 sec flows of 2 mM Na-saccharin (NaSa) at 5 ml/sec across the antero-dorsal portion of their tongue alternate with 1, 2, or 3 sec flows of H_2O, 'artificial saliva', or no liquid, for 60 sec; the same participants report significant adaptation, with a 40%-50% decrease in estimated magnitude, for continuous NaCl or NaSa flows. Partial adaptation with continuous flow is ex-pected (Meiselman and Halpern, Physiol. & Behav., 11, 713-716, 1973; Meiselman and DuBose, Percep. & Psychophys., 19, 226-230, 1976). Since single human sips from a drinking glass have a duration of ca. 1 sec (Halpern, In: Olfaction and Taste-V, 47-52, 1975), the pulsatile NaCl or NaSa flows constitute 'artifi-cial sips', while the alternate H_2O or 'artificial saliva' flows simulate the pause and swallowing-produced tongue wipe which separates sips (Halpern and Nichols, The Physiologist, 18, 238, 1975; Halpern, In: Drinking Behavior, Weijnen and Mendelson, 1-92, 1977). Presentation of taste stimuli is artificial sips may yield psychophysical judgements which predict human taste judgements during natural liquid ingestion. This alternate-flow simulation of human drinking contrasts with the now traditional, continuous-flow presentation method. Since continuous flow produces substantial adaptation, while pulsatile flow, for our conditions, yields no decrease in judged intensity, different predictions, which constitute distinguishable models, are generated. A con-tinuous flow approach predicts that adaptation is a major variable in human judgements of ingested liquids, and states that measures such as cross-adap-tation are the method of choice for psychophysical evaluations of taste stim-uli. In contrast, the drinking simulation approach of pulsatile flow predicts that little adaptation occurs during normal liquid ingestion, and advocates the alternate pulse technique for understanding taste judgements (NSF BNS74-00878 support).

Classification and evaluation of annoyance reactions to environmental odors J.Kastka u. G.Winneke (Med.Inst.f.Lufthyg.,
4 Düsseldorf, Gurlittstr. 53, W.-Germany)

In order to find some rational and empirical basis for the
development of a threshold concept for tolerable and intole-
rable exposition to environmental odors a number of questio-
naired response-variables of 704 residents living in 9 areas
with different degree of odorous pollution were analyzed by
two different psychometric methods:
1. By the Principal-Components-Analysis in order to classify
annoyance-responses into main classes of annoyance reactions
and to measure the degree of annoyance on component-scales/1/.
2. The Thurstone-Succesive-Categories-Technique, by which the
degree of experienced annoyance in every area was scaled on a
psychological annoyance continuum, which was divided by scaled
normative standards of the residents in regions of tolerability
and intolerability of odor annoyance/2/The main results of the
combined analysis were:
1. With rising degree of odor exposition as defind by loca-
tions of the 9 areas with respect to odor emitting sources
the composition of odor annoyance extends from a simple sensory or "stimulus-centered" experience to a "subject-centered"
experience of threatened somatic integrity, impaired social
and recreational activities and unpleasant emotional states,
attached to odorous stimulation.
2. The lower level of odor annoyance, which is dominated by
so called "stimulus-centered" experiences is positioned within the tolerable region of the psychological annoyance continuum, while the higher degrees of annoyance, which are completed by the so called "subject centered" experiences, are positioned in the region of intolerability of annoyance. This association of changing composition of content of annoyance
with changing normative evaluation of odorous pollution effects - if proved by further research - could be used for
development of a threshold concept for exposition to environmental odors.

/1/ KASTKA,J.:Untersuchungen zur Belaestigungswirkung der Umweltbedingungen
    Verkehrslaerm und Industriegerueche,in:KAMINSKI,G.(Ed.):Umweltpsychologie,
    Perspektiven-Probleme-Praxis, Stuttgart:E.Klett-Verlag 1976, p187-223

/2/ KASTKA,J.:Zur inhaltlichen Bodeutung von Geruchsbelaestigung und ihrer
    Bewertung, in: AURANDT,K. et al(Eds.):Organische Luftverunreinigungen,
    Erkennen-Bewerten-Vermindern, Berlin: Pabel-Verlag 1977 (in press)

Effects of androstenol on sexual and other social attitudes M.Kirk-Smith and
D.A.Booth, (Department of Psychology, University of Birmingham, Birmingham
B15 2TT, England)

The boar pheromone, 5α-androst-16-en-3-ol, was tested in two sessions on 24
human subjects for effects on which human chemical communication could be based (Cowley et al., 1977). The subjects were instructed that the experiment
was to test the stress effect of a surgical mask worn throughout each session.
At one session (the first in half the subjects) the mask was impregnated with
androstenol and at the other it was clean. At each session subjects judged 16
human, four animal and four building photographs on 16 bipolar category scales
derived from Osgood's semantic differential. Eighteen analogue mood scales
were completed at the beginning and end of each session. Subjects' perceptions of the odour and beliefs about the experiment were determined at the end
of the second session.
By analysis of variance, both male and female subjects in the presence of androstenol rated photographs of women sexier**, more attractive**, and better**
- terms which correlated in factor analysis. All subjects rated all human
photographs as warmer* - a term which loaded as heavily as friendliness on the
most major factor in factor analysis. Certain photographs elicited the friendliness effect of androstenol more strongly than others. There were also effects of androstenol on judgments on an aggressive/defensive scale: women
rated all human photographs more defensive in the first half of the session;
men rated photographed women as more aggressive in the second half of the session. Such effects were not seen with animal or building photographs, although animals were judged rasher and buildings less sensitive in the presence
of androstenol.
Mood became more elated** at the start of the session in androstenol's presence. Mood also moved away from friendliness more** in the androstenol session.
Before the experimenter made reference to odour, subjects reported perceived
purposes of the experiment which were not to do with odour. Nevertheless, as
intended, subjects could discriminate odorized masks reliably, except for one
anosmic subject (whose data and those of his matched pair were excluded from
the above analyses).
Other putative pheromones and a food odour are being tested.
*p <0.05, **p <0.01 by Duncan's multiple range test.
Cowley, J.J., Johnson, A.L., and Brooksbank, B.W.L. (1977) Psychoendocrinol-
ogy 2, 159-172.

We thank Drs. D. Carroll and P. Davies for collaboration in the design of this
experiment and the N.I. Department of Education for studentship support. Androstenol pure by GLC and MP was kindly provided by Dr. B.W.L. Brooksbank.

Taste thresholds for bilaterally and unilaterally presented mixtures of sugar and salt Jan H.A. Kroeze, (Psychological Laboratory, University of Utrecht, The Netherlands)

Absolute thresholds for sucrose and NaCl of six subjects(3 male,3 female) were determined by the method of constant stimuli. The stimuli were presented by use of 1 ml - injectors in the left and right stimulation holes of a modified McBurney tongue box. A temporal two-alternative forced choice method was used. From the best fitting linear function in Log - Probit coordinates the threshold was determined for each subject. On the basis of the individual thresholds the following mixtures were prepared for each subject:Sucrose 80%/ NaCl 20%; Sucr.60%/NaCl 40%; Sucr.50%/NaCl 50%; Sucr.40%/NaCl 60%; Sucr.20%/ NaCl 80%. Each of these mixtures was presented under three laterality conditions:C-1 : mixtures presented to one half of the tongue; left and right were counterbalanced and each of the two subconditions obtained in this way contained 30 measurements per mixture. C-2: mixtures presented to both tongue halves simultaneously; each mixture was presented 30 times. C-3: The two components of the mixture were presented separately, one component to one tongue half and the other component to the opposite half.NaCl left and Sucr. right was counterbalanced by NaCl right and Sucr. left. In each of the counterbalanced subconditions the mixtures were presented 30 times each. To check stability of thresholds the pure solutions(100%/0% and 0%/100%) were also presented. Mixture detections were tested against the null hypo- thesis of independency of components.The expected frequencies under this null hypothesis were calculated according to a simple probability model: P(Sucr.) + P(NaCl) - P(Sucr.) x P(NaCl). The P-values to be substituted in the formula were determined from the threshold functions of the subjects. The results show a very significant enhancement effect in C-2(Chi-square analysis: P < .0001). This effect is not found in the conditions C-1 and C-3. Individual calculations show substantial differences between subjects, but these differences cannot cancel out the enhancement effect in C-2.

Temporal properties of taste: Evidence for basic tastes Donald H. McBurney,
Janneane F. Gent and Gary B. Levine,(University of Pittsburgh, Pgh., Pa.15260

Techniques of linear systems analysis were used to study the temporal properties of human taste. Concentration was varied as a sine function of time
in one condition and as a square wave in another. In both conditions, sensitivity to NaCl and sucrose was greatest at 0.1 Hertz and about 0.06 Hertz for
citric acid and quinine. The maximum sensitivity, 1.7% modulation for NaCl,
is much greater than that measured by classical techniques. Expressed as a
Weber fraction, sensitivity to NaCl was 3.4% compared to 9% in a previous
experiment. Sensitivity declined slowly at lower frequencies and was still
surprisingly great at 0.001 Hertz: 13% for NaCl. The tongue is insensitive
to temporal fluctuation above about 5 Hertz. Results at the low frequencies
imply that the tongue responds to rate, rather than amplitude, of concentration change. Sensitivity differed among representatives of the four taste
qualities. Similar sensitivities were found within qualities, except for
bitterness. The bitter quality is also unique in that cross adaptation does
not occur across all bitter compounds. The differences among, and the similarities within qualities argue for the validity of the four basic tastes.
These data are related to data collected by traditional methods, particularly
temporal summation and adaptation. For example, growth of sensation shows
different critical durations among qualities. Also, the high sensitivity to
very low frequencies explains the difficulty in demonstrating complete adaptation in taste. When care is taken to provide a constant stimulus by placing
a solution-soaked filter paper on the tongue, complete adaptation is found.
Control experiments showed that the adaptation observed was not the result of
solution loss.

A New Model For Taste Psychophysics: The Role Of Taste Adaptation. Herbert
L. Meiselman, Ph.D., (Army Natick R & D Command, Natick, MA U.S.A.) and Bruce
P. Halpern, Ph.D.*, (Cornell University, Ithaca, NY U.S.A.)

The taste literature asserts that most subjects show complete and relatively
rapid adaptation to moderate taste stimuli. However, in five separate studies
Meiselman and co-workers have shown that only between 1/3 and 2/3 of subjects
report complete adaptation to solutions of salt and sugar (Meiselman, 1968,
1972, 1975; Meiselman & DuBose, 1976; DuBose, Meiselman, Hunt & Waterman,
1977). Further, the consistency of subjects to be adaptors or nonadaptors
to varied stimuli was 73%.
    A number of variables have been found to affect the percentage of sub-
jects showing complete adaptation. (1) Fewer subjects show complete adaptation to quinine sulfate than to sucrose or sodium chloride. (2) In several
studies with salt, sugar, and quinine, a decreasing number of subjects show
complete adaptation with increasing stimulus concentration. (3) Different
response tasks produce different percentages of complete adaptation; a hand-
raise task in which subjects denote the disappearance of the stimulus by
raising their hand yields more adaptations than magnitude estimation or cross-
adaptation tasks. (4) Different stimulus presentation methods can affect
adaptation; in general, anterior dorsal tongue flow produces more adaptations
than sip, repeated sips, or whole mouth flow. (5) Suggestive instructions
do not appear to change the tendency to show complete adaptation. Current
method and theory in taste psychophysics must consider the probability that
taste adaptation is not complete for untrained subjects, and the tendency to
adapt or not to adapt is a reliable characteristic of individual subjects.

* The authors thank Cynthia DuBose and Deborah Hunt

<u>Towards shorter criterion free sensitivity measures</u> Michael O'Mahony

(Dept. Food Science and Technology, University of California, Davis, California 95616, U.S.A).

Richter and MacLean (1939) in defining the recognition and detection thresholds attempted to solve the problem, encountered in threshold measurement, of more than one taste quality for a stimulus at low concentrations. However, this two threshold model was shown to be inadequate when more than two taste changes were reported for NaCl (O'Mahony, 1973). Further studies (O'Mahony et al., 1976 a,b) with a range of taste stimuli, demonstrated that subjects could report up to eight taste changes at low concentrations, any one of which could be chosen as criteria for detection or recognition; furthermore there was little consistency in choice between subjects. Such results, along with reported changes of choice of criteria within subjects (O'Mahony et al. 1974) have led workers to consider criterion free signal detection measures of sensitivity (Green and Swets 1966). However, the length of such procedures have made workers in taste psychophysics reluctant to use such measures. This paper outlines a simple and short approach to a criterion free index, the R index (Brown, 1974) which may be adapted for sensitivity measurement.

Brown, J. (1974) Brit. J. Psychol., 65, 13-22.
Green, D. M., Swets, J. A. (1966) Signal Detection Theory and Psychophysics, Wiley, New York.
O'Mahony, M. (1973) Brit. J. Psychol., 64, 601-606.
O'Mahony, M., Ivory, H., King, E. (1974) Perception 3, 185-192.
O'Mahony, M., Kingsley, L., Harji, A., Davies, M. (1976a) Chemical Senses & Flavor 2, 177-188.
O'Mahony, M., Hobson, A., Garvey, J., Davies, M., Birt, C. (1976b) Perception 5, 147-154.
Richter, C. P., MacLean, A. (1939) Amer. J. Physiol., 126, 1-6.

Similarities between human and animal senses of smell J.R. Piggott and P.T. Osisiogu, (Food Science Dept., Univ. Strathclyde, Glasgow G1 1SD, UK)

Pinching and Døving (Brain Res. 82, 195, 1974) recorded that selective degeneration of mitral cells of the olfactory bulb occurred when rats were exposed to different odours for long periods. The degeneration patterns observed for different odorants implied that a mechanism for spatial coding of odour quality was operating. It was thought that it might be useful to compare the results of these experiments with those of human psychophysical characterisations of the same odorants. Firstly, samples of the majority of the original 44 odorants were supplied by K.B. Døving. An odour profiling technique was used for the characterisation, to attempt to reduce the effect of intensity variation and to generate the required similarity matrix from the minimum number of experimental trials. Thirteen members of the department served as assessors, and characterised 37 of the odorants from sniff-bottles. Secondly, Pinching and Døving's published degeneration patterns were described numerically, by dividing the olfactory bulb into 44 sectors and assigning a scale number to each sector showing degeneration. The data matrices, averaged over the panel in the case of the human assessors, were compared by applying a Procrustes rotation to fit the rat data to the human data. Correlation coefficients were calculated before and after rotation, and showed an increase from 0.05 to 0.63***. Each data set was then analysed by Principal Components. The component loadings matrix from the rat data was fitted to that from the human data, and correlation coefficients calculated. In this case, an increase from 0.03 to 0.42*** occurred. These results indicated that particular regions of the rat olfactory bulb appear to be associated with particular odour quality notes perceived by human assessors.

Application of Multidimensional Scaling to the Chemical Senses Susan S. Schiffman, (Department of Psychology, Duke University, Durham, NC)

Three different types of multidimensional scaling procedures were applied to experimental data to demonstrate the effect of age, weight, and disease state in gustation and olfaction. Multidimensional scaling (MDS) is a mathematical tool which allows us to represent spatially the similarities of odors and tastes by "maps". Experimental measures of similarity among chemical stimuli can be used by MDS to arrange the stimuli in a space so that those stimuli which taste (or smell) most similar are separated by the smallest distance in the resultant space or map; stimuli judged to be dissimilar are positioned distant from one another. The sets of similarity data presented illustrate three MDS methodologies: 1) the Guttman-Lingoes non-metric procedure (Guttman, L. Psychometrika, 1968, 33, 469 and Lingoes, J. C. Behavioral Science, 1965, 10, 183); 2) INDSCAL (Carroll, J. D. and Chang, J. J. Psychometrika, 1970, 35, 283-319); and 3) ALSCAL (Takane, Y., Young, F. W. and de Leeuw, J., Psychometrika, in press.) INDSCAL and ALSCAL are models which discriminate individuals from one another by providing weights for each subject on each of the dimensions of a common multidimensional space. Individual difference models were found to be very helpful in understanding the effect of age, weight, and disease state on taste and olfactory quality.

<u>Innate discriminative human facial expressions indicating hedonics of</u>
<u>taste and smell stimuli</u> Jacob E. Steiner, Ph.D. (Department of Oral
Biology, Hebrew University—Hadassah School of Dental Medicine, Jerusalem,
Israel)

Assessing the functional state of taste in adults of both sexes in normal
and pathological conditions, using a psychophysical testing procedure, it
was observed that suprathreshold sweet sour and bitter stimuli elicit
differential facial expressions. The features of the facial play appeared
with short latency and with a marked stereotypy in all examinees regardless of their cultural and educational background. It was assumed that
taste-induced facial play is an innate reflex. Examining neonate infants
in perinatal age, prior to any feeding experience, revealed the same
features. Later examining neonates with severe developmental malformations
of the brain revealed similar results. The reflex character of the response
and its low level control in the brain was ascertained. Food related odor
stimuli, presented to caucasian and negro infants in perinatal age, were
also found to be key stimuli unlocking similar facial expressions to those
elicited taste stimuli. Examination of a hydroanencephalic neonate support
the assumption that not only the response to taste, but also that to food
odor, is controlled without cortical involvement. Congenitally blind
adolescents, tested with identical stimulants, responded with identical
features of differential facial play. The nonverbal communicational tool,
pointing to the hedonics of taste and smell, is not only innate (non-
acquired) and operated at subcortical brain levels, but is maintained
without visual reinforcement. Congenitally deaf patients affected by
retinal degeneration (Usher's syndrome) responded to tastants and food
related odorants in the same features of differential facial play as did
neonate infants and blind adolescents. The reaction of the mentally
retarded, who is unable to acquire simple learning tasks, was identical.
Testing patients with craniofacial malformations showed that in the
distorted human face the taste and odor-induced facial play still carries
the communicational message pointing to hedonics of perceived stimuli.
Behavioral experiments on neonate rabbits and electrophysiological
investigation is adult cats and rabbits hints at the cross species nature
of the response. The elicitation of the gustofacial and nasofacial response
may serve as diagnostic aid in examining the function of the two major
chemical senses in man already at neonatal age.

Taste of monosodium L-glutamate and its psychophysical properties   S. Yamaguchi, (Central Research Laboratories, Ajinomoto Co., Inc., 1-1, Suzuki-cho, Kawasaki, Japan)

Many people in Japan believe that there is a 5th taste quality in addition to the 4 common tastes, since Dr.Ikeda discovered the taste of glutamates (1908). It is called *umami* in Japan and represented by monosodium glutamate (MSG). The fundamental psychophysical properties of MSG were systematically studied and the following results were obtained: (1)The stimulus-subjective intensity relationship of MSG was logarithmically linear as well as that of the other 4 common tastes, although the slope for MSG was somewhat smaller than the others. (2) The recognition threshold of MSG was 0.625 mM, almost the same as for NaCl. The effect of 5mM of MSG on the threshold of the other common tastes was not significant except that the value of sour taste was raised by buffer action of MSG. (3)Supraliminal levels of the 4 tastes were more or less supressed by higher levels of MSG. Conversely, *umami* was more or less supressed by the higher levels of the 4 tastes. However, among these combinations, *umami* and saltiness were least affected by each other. (4)MSG enhances no other common tastes in particular but its own *umami* by the synergistic effect with nucleotides, which belong to another type of *umami* substances. In general, the intensity of *umami* , p , of a given solution of *umami* substance mixture is expressed as $p = u + \gamma uv$, where u and v are the concentrations of amino acid type and nucleotide type *umami* substances calculated in terms of MSG and 5'-inosinate, respectively, according to their *umami* strength. p is the concentration calculated in terms of MSG. γ is a constant. (5)The above mentioned equation holds also in the 4 common taste solutions. (6)Furthermore, general mathematical definitions of the taste interactions including the synergistic effect were given.

As a conclusion, MSG is, at least, not an enhancer for the 4 common tastes. It is a taste substance which has its own taste, *umami*, and is characterized by its remarkable synergistic effect with nucleotides,

Concluding Remarks

A few impressions of the meeting

Lloyd M. Beidler

Department of Biological Science, The Florida State University, Tallahassee, FL 32306, USA

We are concluding several days of excellent communications between participants of many countries who are interested in some aspects of the chemical senses. This communication was of three forms. First, formal lectures by leading experts served to review and integrate recent advances of the field. Second, the poster sessions presented the results of very recent research, much of it still in progress. In many ways, the poster sessions were the most stimulating and informative. Third, informal discussions between individual participants allowed them to probe specific points in great detail. These discussions also allowed students and young investigators to meet senior researchers whose reports they had read but whom they had never met in person.

STIMULUS-RECEPTOR INTERACTION

What have we learned? Progress in our understanding of the chemical senses often appears to be slow. Why should this be? I believe it is due to the complexity of the most fundamental problem we face. The chemical stimulus is assumed to interact with certain molecular sites on the membrane of the receptor cell which eventually results in some type of response. In shorthand notation:

$$S + P \to \to \to R$$

We know almost nothing of the nature of the receptor sites, P. The exact 3-dimensional conformation of the stimulus S is seldom given. The response, R, whether behavioral or electrophysiological, is far removed from the time and place of the stimulus-receptor site interaction and many unknown and probably nonlinear events are interspersed between R and S-P. Many of the lectures and posters were concerned with these events. It is impossible for me to comment on all lectures and posters presented so I chose to present my personal view of what has been discussed here during the past several days concerning the above fundamental problem. Please do not assume that I chose papers or posters based upon their merit since there is not enough time for a complete and thorough review.

Cohn published in 1918 a very large book entitled <u>Taste of Organic Substances</u> in which he reported the tastes of thousands of different chemicals and tried to relate the nature of the chemicals to their tastes. There is a tremendous range of chemicals that produce a similar taste. For example, chloroform, beryllium chloride, sucrose, sodium saccharin and sodium cyclamate all have sweet tastes. If the chemist is to relate molecular properties to taste quality he must first be sure that all the molecules he wishes to study actually interact with the same receptor site. Many participants of this conference have indicated that several different receptor sites may be involved in the development of a sweet taste. Morita elegantly showed that at least two subsites are involved in sugar stimulation of insects and Hiji presented evidence for the same in mammals. The one may interact with glucose and the other with fructose. Caprio and Tucker showed that two or more different receptor sites are involved in amino acid stimulation of fish. Faurion et al. used behavioral methods to show that at least four different groups of sweet stimuli exist for humans. Continued study of this problem will enable the chemist to better predict molecular properties responsible for sweet taste.

Another complexity is that the response itself is difficult to control. Birch stressed the fact that not all sugars or their derivatives have a pure sweet taste. Furthermore, it is not clear what feature of sweet taste should be used for correlations with taste quality. For example, should thresholds be used or levels of equisweetness? If the latter, what level should be chosen? It is clear that students of taste psychophysics have much to contribute in this area. Bartoshuk related difficulties in the study of taste mixtures. Her methodology in this field could be used to study the mixed tastes of sugars that disturbs Birch, for example, and might be used to determine the amount of sweetness associated with such substances. Jakinovich used an ingenuous approach to measure the amount of bitterness in a bitter-sweet substance. He inhibited the sweet taste with gymnemic acid and then measured the remaining bitterness. Only close cooperation between chemists and psycophysicists will allow the correlation of molecular structure and taste function to proceed in a rational manner. It should be noted that Kaissling emphasized many times the difficulty of selecting response properties that could be used to better correlate with odor structure. Even though electrophysiological measurements are made closer to the stimulus-receptor site event than are behavioral measurements, many cellular and chemical processes are involved in both so that neither type of measurement is totally satisfactory.

Several lecturers and poster researchers utilized gross behavioral responses to study initial events in the chemoreceptor process. Many others were skeptical of such procedures and I agree that skepticism is in order. On the other hand, we should remember the history of visual science. It was a researcher who used a stopwatch to measure latencies in clam siphon retraction to light who revealed evidence for the kinetics of the photochemical reactions. Similarly, by merely asking subjects whether they could see a flash of light, a scientist developed the theory that only one quantum is necessary to excite one photoreceptor. In fact, one of his students received the Nobel prize for further development of our understanding of the visual photochemistry. We might conclude that originality and incisive insight are more important in receptor science than instrumental complexity.

One of the most promising areas of future chemoreception research is illustrated by the genetic studies of fruit fly olfaction started by Kikuchi. Such studies will aid us to appreciate the variety of receptor sites. Morita is even studying the chromosomal loci of the mutations he produced in fruit flies. He already has produced about 100 mutant strains in his studies of feeding responses to sugars. Eventually we may learn the basis of the large taste differences among individuals as described by Sato. The chemists should always be reminded of the large species differences to sweet stimuli.

In considering the above problems involved in defining the receptor sites and the responses, one might conclude that the stimulus itself is well defined. Such is not always true. Crosby has studied many dihydrochalcones and their analogs and showed that their hydrophobic nature and phenolic character could be related to their persistent taste. Others have also related specific molecular properties to taste quality. However, we have no model or theory good enough to be predictive. Part of the difficulty may be the lack of suitable stimulus definition. Precise definition by stating the positions of all electrons is only possible for two-body molecules such as that of hydrogen. This is of little help to us. However, physicists and chemists have shown that certain simplifications can be made concerning electron movements and that models based upon these assumptions can be very predictive for chemical reactions. A most useful model is that concerned with molecular orbitals and their interactions. Sophisticated analysis can result in the definition of a number of different conformations of a dipeptide, for example, that can exist in solution. Furthermore, the probability of the molecule being in any given conformation can be predicted. By comparing a number of similar molecules that produce a sweet taste, information concerning the 3-D features of a sweet receptor site can be obtained. In addition, the data Birch, Crosby and others have given us during the past two days will help define specific reactive sites in this 3-D picture. Inter-molecular hydrogen bonding can also be predicted and possibly related to the intensity of sweetness. We hope that when we again convene in 3 years from now, a much better understanding of the stimulus-receptor site inter-action will be discussed.

TASTE PROTEINS

No research on taste membrane proteins or lipids was presented at our meeting. Why? There appeared a flurry of papers on this subject a few years after the initial research of Dastoli and Price. Today the researchers are more cautious in their definition of a 'taste protein' and they set more vigorous standards. Much is yet to be known concerning macromolecules in a state of aggregation such as that which occurs in a membrane. If hydrogen bonding is important for sweetness, then the conformation of the macromole-cules that may make up the membrane receptor site is very important and may change when taken out of the membrane and placed into solution. Perhaps a more specific and sensitive interaction should be studied such as pheromone binding followed by covalent linkage. We hope our next meeting will include results of such studies.

NEURAL CODING

Over three decades ago, the first electrophysiological study of neural coding of taste qualities was performed by Pfaffmann. It overthrew the think-ing of the time since most single taste fibers responded to a wide variety of stimuli representing a number of taste qualities. Since then, many addi-tional studies were undertaken with many animal species. Today we have seen a number of leaders in taste research, notably Pfaffmann, Sato and Zotterman, agree that although a single fiber may respond to a variety of stimuli, the fiber responds best to those of but one of the four primary taste qualitites. The outstanding research of Marion Frank emphasizes this point. However, Schiffman stated today that human subjects cannot describe the sensation

elicited by certain substances on the basis of the four primary taste qualities. Boudreau, who uses a large battery of unusual chemicals, does not
classify taste fibers on the same basis as most other workers. Erickson discussed the concept of four primary taste qualities and indicated the uncer-
tainities in such a description and the relevance to electrophysiological
research. Thus, we have observed during the past few days lively disagreement concerning taste neural coding as well as the relevance of four primary
taste qualities.

How stable is the neural response? Can it change when the animal is
Most researchers in this field use the magnitude of neural response
during the first five seconds of taste stimulation or longer to obtain their
data for analysis. However, Dethier showed many years ago that insects can
make a behavioral decision in a very much shorter time and Halpern has demonstrated a similar event with rats. I conclude that we need to record from
a number of single taste fibers simultaneously in an awake animal with efferent control intact. This should be done over many days and in the condition
of the animal feeding normally. We hope that such data may be available at
our next meeting three years from now.

How stable is the neural response? Can it change when the animal is
under physiological stress? It is well known that sodium deficient animals
exhibit lower preference thresholds for NaCl. Bell showed us that Na-defi-
cient calves select a variety of sodium salts in preference to other salts.
Richter, who first studied this phenomenon, thought the preference was due to
an increased sensitivity of the salt taste receptors. Many researchers failed
to find evidence for this and the literature now clearly states that the
change in preference is due to structures more central than the receptors.
However, at this meeting Contreras had the temerity to challenge the classical interpretation and gave convincing evidence of receptor changes in
response to sodium deficiencies. The question now is posed for our next
meeting, can the taste receptors generally change their specific sensitivities

in response to other changes in their immediate environment?

TRANSDUCTION

In 1951 a model of taste transduction was introduced that was based upon stimulus adsorption to molecules of the receptor cell membrane. This was quantitatively described by a simple equation based upon the Langmuir adsorption isotherm. At this meeting additional events in transduction were reemphasized. Morita and Kaissling considered additional nonlinear events such as transmembrane conductance and new product transformations to produce equations that describe gustatory and olfactory transduction at variance with the simple adsorption isotherm. In addition, Mooser brought to our attention the possibility of allosteric mechanisms that may contribute to transduction. Since so little is actually known concerning the receptor membrane or the transduction events, it is remarkable that these quantitative models are as useful as they appear to be. This is not peculiar to chemoreceptors, as the same is true for all other receptor transduction events known at the present time.

Kurihara and De Simone and Price indicated the importance of the electrical properties of membranes and the application to chemoreceptor transduction. It is interesting to note that such electrical properties were known to biologists many, many years ago. Later colloidal chemists noted their importance and then physical chemists such as Debeye brought it to the attention of other chemists. Only recently are biologists rediscovering the importance of electric fields associated with membrane surfaces.

DEVELOPMENT AND TROPHISM

A study of chemoreceptors may lead to information that can be generalized to many other biological systems. Such is particularly true of the study of development and trophic influences associated with gustatory and olfactory receptors.

Christina Arvidson related her results of research on human taste buds.

At our next meeting we hope she will tell us whether properties of these taste buds are the same after regeneration as they were before. Bradley and Mistretta are contributing a great service to us in their studies of fetal development of taste. Of what importance is prenatal taste experience? Ferrell is following up these researches of fetal development by asking whether prenatal events can influence taste preference of young animals.

The morphological changes in human fetal tongues was studied by Ganchrow and similar changes in other animals by Mistretta and by Ferrell. Perhaps we will soon know whether such morphological changes can be related to behavioral changes known to occur in developing animals.

At our very first meeting in Stockholm in 1962, evidence was presented for the dynamic characteristics of taste receptors, particularly their short life span. At this meeting, both Farbman and Raderman-Little have revealed new information concerning the temperature dependence of the turnover rate and the difference in life span between light and dark cells of rat taste bud. An even greater contribution to biology is the finding that olfactory receptors also can be renewed. Barber has also shown us that vomeronasal receptors either turnover or else there is continued growth of the epithelium. There is now great interest in the rapid replacement of visual rod discs. Some relate this to the ability of the sensory system to maintain extremely high sensitivity.

Oakley brought us up to date concerning his excellent research on the influence of the taste nerves on the regeneration of taste buds. This is an age old problem of great significance. He reviewed his most recent attempts to relate axoplasmic transport to trophic properties. We wait with antici-pation the results of these investigations at our next meeting.

In summary, we have had a most successful meeting. We are appreciative of everything Professor Le Magnen and colleagues did to insure this. The community of chemoreceptor researchers is growing and international cooperation is most impressive. This series of symposia on olfaction and taste was originally started to interest students in the field. The number attending this meeting is a tribute to the success of the venture.

INDEXES

Author Index

Subject Index

List of Participants

ACHE, B.   –Department of Biological Sciences, Florida Atlan-
                 tic University, Boca Raton, Florida 33431, USA.

ADDA, J.   –Station de Recherches Laitieres, CNRZ, 78350 Jouy
                 en Josas, France.

ADDINK, A.   –Zoologisch Laboratorium der Rijksuniversiteit te
                 Leiden, Kaiserstraat 63, Leiden, The Netherlands.

ALTNER, H.   –Fachbereich Biologie Universität Regensburg, 8400
                 Regensburg, Germany.

ANDRES, K.   –Lehrstuhl Anat. II, Ruhr Universität, 2148 Bochum,
                 Germany.

ANGIOY, A.   –Instituto di Fisiologia Generale dell'Universita
                 di Cagliari, v.le Poetto 1, 09100 Cagliari, Italy.

ARVIDSON, K.   –Karolinska Institutet Histology, S 10401 Stockholm,
                 Sweden.

ARON, C.   –Institut d'Histologie, Faculté de Médecine, 67000
                 Strasbourg, France.

ASTIC, L.   –Laboratoire de Psychophysiologie, Université
                 Claude Bernard, 43 Bd du 11 novembre 1918, 69621
                 Villeurbanne, France.

ATEMA, J.   –Boston University Marine Program, Marine Biological
                 Laboratory, Woods Hole, Massachussets, 02543, USA.

AUGUSTUS, J.   –Zoologisch Laboratorium der Rijksuniversiteit te
                 Leiden, Kaiserstraat 63, Leiden, The Netherlands.

BARBER, P.   –National Institute for Medical Research, Labora-
                 tory of Neurobiology, London, NW7 1AA, UK.

BARREAU, C.   –Centre de Recherches Unilever, 10 Impasse Montjoie,
                 93210 La Plaine Saint Denis, France.

BARTOSHUK, L.   –Pierce Foundation, 290 Congress Ave., New Haven
                 Connecticut 06519, USA.

BEETS, M.   –Int. Flavors & Fragrances (Europe), PO Box 309,
                 Hilversum, The Netherlands.

BEHAN, M.   –Larvickse Allee 11, Room 507, Wageningen, The
                 Netherlands.

BEIDLER, L.   –Biological Science, Florida State University,
                 Tallahassee, Florida 32306, USA.

BELITZ, H.   –Institut fur Lebensmittelchemie der Technischen
                 Universitat, Lohstrasse 17, D – 8 000 München 2,
                 Germany.

BELL, F.   –Department of Medicine, Royal Veterinary College,
                 Hawkshead Lane, Brookmans Park, Nr Hatfield, Hert-
                 fordshire, AL9 7TA, U.K.

BERGLUND, B.   –Department Psychology, University of Stockholm,
                 Box 6706, S – 113 85 Stockholm, Sweden.

BERTMAR, G.   –Department Biology, Section of Ecological Zoology,
                 University of Umea, 901 87 Umea, Sweden.

BHATNAGAR, K.   –Department of Anatomy, University of Louisville
                 School of Medicine, Health Sciences Center, Louis-
                 ville, Kentucky 40201, USA.

BIRCH, G.   –National College of Food Technology, St. George's
                 Avenue, Weybridge, Surrey, KT13 ODE, UK.

BOECKH, J.   -Fachbereich Biologie, Universität Regensburg,
                D - 8400 Regensburg, Germany.
BOOTH, D.   -Department of Psychology, University of Birmingham,
                PO Box 363, Birmingham B 15 2TT, UK.
BOPPRE, M.   -Max Planck Institut für Verhaltensphysiologie,
                D 8131, Seewiesen/Obb., Germany.
BOUDREAU, J.   -Sensory Sciences Center, University of Texas, 6420
                Lamar Fleming, Houston, Texas 77030, USA.
BRADLEY, R.   -Department Oral Biology, School of Dentistry, Uni-
                versity of Michigan, Ann Arbor, Michigan 48109, USA.
BROCK, O.   -Biological Science, Unit 1, Florida State Univer-
                sity, Tallahassee, Florida 32306, USA.
BROWN, R.   -A.B.R.G. Department Zoology, South Park Road,
                Oxford OX1 3 PS, UK.
BROUWER, J.   -Unilever Research, PO Box 114, Vlaardingen, The
                Netherlands.
BUJAS, Z.   -Department Psychology, 41 000 Zagreb, Dure Salaja,
                3, Yugoslavia.
CAIN, W.   -J.B. Pierce Foundation Laboratory, 290 Congress
                Ave., New Haven, Connecticut 06519, USA.
CANCALON, P.   -Department Biological Science, Unit, Biology Unit 1
                Florida State University, Tallahassee 32306, USA.
CATTARELLI, M. -Psychophysiologie, Université Claude Bernard,
                69621 Villeurbanne, France.
CHANEL, J.   -Psychophysiologie, Université Claude Bernard,
                69621 Villeurbanne, France.
CHAPUT, M.   -Labo. Electrophysiologie, Faculté des Sciences,
                43 Bd du 11 Novembre 1918, 69621 Villeurbanne,
                France.
CLARK, A.   -Physics Department, Guy's Hospital Medical School,
                London Bridge SE 1, UK.
CONTRERAS, R.   -The Rockfeller University, 1230 York Avenue, New
                york, New York 10021, USA.
CRNJAR, R.   -Piazza Bibbiena 1, 20136 Milan, Italy.
CROSBY, G.   -Dynapol, 1454 Page Mill Road, Palo Alto, Califor-
                nia 94304, USA.
CZAPCZYNSKA, B. -Pollena Aroma, Ul. Klasykow 10, 03 115 Warszawa,
                Poland.
DAVAL, G.   -Université Paris VI - UER 61, 9 quai Saint-Bernard,
                75005 Paris, France.
DAVIS, E.   Stanford Research Institute, 333 Ravenswood Ave.,
                Menlo Park, California 94025, USA.
DEGOBERT, P.   -Institut Francais du Pétrole, 2-4 rue du Bois-Préau
                BP 18, 92502, Rueil Malmaison, France.
DENNIS, B.   -Department Physiology, University of Adelaide,
                Adelaide, South Australia.
DEN OTTER, C.   -Department Zoology, Groningen State University,
                Kerklaan 30, Haren, The Netherlands.
DENTON, D.   -Howard Florey Institute, University of Melbourne,
                Parkville 3052, Australia.
DESGRANGES, J. -Laboratoire d'Evolution, 105 Boulevard Raspail,
                75006 Paris, France.
DE SIMONE, J.   -Medical College of Virginia, Virginia Common-
                wealth University, MCV Station, Richmond, Virginia
                23298, USA.
DETHIER, V.   -Department Zoology, University of Massachusetts,
                Amherst, Massachussetts 01003, USA.

DICKENS, J.   -Universität Freiburg, Forstzoologisches Institut,
               Bertoldstr. 17, 78 Freiburg i. Br., Germany.
DODD, G.   -Department Molecular Sciences, University of War-
               wick, Coventry CV4 7 AL, U.K.
DOTY, R.   -University of Pennsylvania, 3500 Market Street,
               Philadelphia, Pennsylvania 19104, USA.
DØVING, K.   -Institute of Zoophysiology, University of Oslo,
               Blindern Post Box 1051, Oslo 3,
               Norway.
DRAVNIEKS, A. -I.T.T. Research Institute, 10 West 35th Street,
               Chicago, Illinois 60466, USA.
DUCHAMP, A.   -Laboratoire Electrophysiologie, Batiment 404,
               Université Lyon 1, 69621 Villeurbanne, France.
DUGAS du VILLARD, X. - Centre de Recherches Unilever, 10 Impasse
               Montjoie, 93210 La Plaine Saint-Denis, France.
DUVEAU, A.   -Electrophysiologie, Universite Claude Bernard, 43
               Bd du 11 Novembre 1918, 69621 Villeurbanne, France.
DUYVESTEYN, P. -Psychologisch Lab., Fyisch Lab., Princetonplein,
               De Uithof, Utrecht, The Netherlands.
DAGET, N.   -Société d'Assistance Technique pour les Produits
               Nestlé, BP 88, CH 18 14 La Tour du Peilz, Switzer-
               land.
ERICKSON, R.   -Duke University, Durham, North Carolina 27706, USA.
FARBMAN, A.   -Department Anatomy, Northwestern University, 303
               E. Chicago Avenue, Chicago, Illinois 60611, USA.
FAURION, A.   -Neurobiologie Sensorielle, EPHE - CEN FAR, BP N.6
               92260 Fontenay aux Roses, France.
FERRELL, M.   -Biological Sciences, Unit 1, Florida State Univer-
               sity, Tallahassee, Florida 32306, USA.
FRANK, M.   -The Rockfeller University, 1230 York Avenue, New
               York, 10021 New York, USA.
FRAZIER, J.   -Department Entomology, Mississipi State University,
               Mississipi Agricul. & Forestry Exp. Stn., Mississi-
               pi, Mississipi 39762, USA.
FREEMAN W.   -Department Physiol. Anat., University of Califor-
               nia, Berkeley, California 94720, USA.
GANCHROW, D.   -Department Oral Biology and Anatomy, The Hebrew
               University, Hadassah Dental Medical School, Jeru-
               salem, Israel.
GANCHROW, J.   -Department Oral Physiology, The Hebrew University,
               Hadassah Dental Medical School, Jerusalem, Israel.
GERVAIS, R.   -Electrophysiologie, Batiment 404, Universite
               Claude Bernard, Lyon 1, 69621 VILLEURBANNE, France.
GETCHELL, T.   -Department of Physiology, School of Medicine, Yale
               University, 333 Cedar Street, New Haven, Connecticut
               06510, USA.
GIACHETTI, I. -Neurobiologie Sensorielle, EPHE - CEN FAR, BP N.6,
               92260 Fontenay aux Roses, France.
GLASER, D.   -Anthropologisches Institut der Universität, 8001
               Zurich, Kunstlergasse 15, Switzerland.
GOLDBERG, S.   -Department Anatomy, MCV VCU, Medical College of
               Virginia, Richmond, Virginia 23298, USA.
GOMEZ, M.   -Department Anatomy, Bowman Gray School of Medicine,
               Winston Salem, North Carolina 27103, USA.
HALL, W.   -Institute of Animal Behavior, 101 Warren Street,
               Newark, New Jersey 07102, USA.

HALPERN, B.   -Department Psychology, Section of Neurobiology &
              Behavior, Uris Hall, Cornell University, Ithaca,
              New York 14853, USA.
HANSEN, K.   -University Regensburg, Zoologisches Institut, 8400
              Regensburg, Germany.
HARA, T.   -Freshwater Institute of the Department of the En-
              vironment, 501 University Crescent, Winnipeg, Mani-
              toba, R 3 T 2 N 6, Canada.
HARPER, R.   -Department of Food Science, University of Reading,
              London Road, Reading RG 15 AQ, UK.
HAUG, M.   -Laboratoire de Psychophysiologie, 7 rue de l'Uni-
              versité, 67000 Strasbourg, France.
HAZELBAUER, G. -Wallenberg Laboratory, University of Uppsala,
              Box 562, 751 22, Uppsala, Sweden.
HELLEKANT, G. -Department of Physiology, Veterinarhogskolan,
              S - 750 07, Uppsala 7, Sweden.
HIDAKA, I.   -Faculty of Fisheries, Mie Prefectural University,
              Tsu, Japan.
HIJI, Y.   -Department of Physiology, Miyasaki Medical College,
              Miyazaki 889-16, Japan.
HOLLEY, A.   -Electrophysiologie, Universite Claude Bernard,
              69621 Villeurbanne, France.
HORNUNG, D.   -Biology Department, St Lawrence University, Canton,
              New York 13617, USA.
HUTCHISON, L. -Department of Physiology, UCLA School of Medicine,
              Los Angeles, California 90024, USA.
ICHIOKA, M.   -Department of Physiology, Faculty of Dentistry,
              Tokyo Medical & Dental University, N.5-45, 1-Chome,
              Yushima, Bunkyo-Ku, Tokyo, Japan.
ITO, H.   -Department of Physiology, Kumamoto University Medi-
              cal School, Honjo 2-2-1, Kumamoto 860, Japan.
JAHAN-PARWAR, B. -Worcester Foundation for Experimental Biology,
              222 Maple Avenue, Shrewsbury, Massachussetts 01545,
              USA.
JAKINOVICH, W. -Proctor & Gamble Company, Miami Valley Lab.,
              Cincinnati, Ohio 45239, USA.
JOUNELA-ERIKSSON, P. -Research Laboratories of the State Alcohol
              Monopoly (ALKO), Box 350, SF - 00101 Helsinki 10,
              Finland.
KAFKA, W.   -Max Planck Institut Verhaltensphysiologie, D - 8131
              Seewiesen, Germany.
KAISSLING, K. -Max Planck Institut für Verhaltensphysiologie -
              8131, Seewiesen, Germany.
KASTKA, J.   -Medizinisches Institut fur Hufthygiene und Silikose-
              forschung an der Universität Düsseldorf, 4, Düssel-
              dorf, Gurlittstr.53, Germany.
KAUER, J.   -Department of Neurosurgery, Yale University School
              of Medicine, 333 Cedar Street, New Haven, Connecti-
              cut 06510, USA.
KAWAMURA, Y. -Department of Oral Physiology, Dental School,
              Osaka University, 32 Joancho, Kitaku, Osaka, Japan
KERJASCHKI, D. -Department Pathology, EM Unit, Inst. Micromorph.
              & Electronmicroscopy, A - 1090, Vienna, Schwarzspa-
              nierstr. 13, Austria.
KENNEDY, J.   -Unilever Research, Colworth House, Sharnbrook
              Bedford, MK 44 1L Q, UK.

KERR, D.   -Department of physiology and pharmacology,
                  University of Adelaide, Adelaide,
                  South Australia, 5001.
KEVERNE, E.   -Department Anatomy, Downing Site, University of
                  Cambridge, Cambridge CB 2 D DY, UK.
KIKUCHI, T.   -Department Biological Science, Tohoku University,
                  Kawauchi, Sendai, 980, Japan.
KIRK-SMITH, M.   -Department of Psychology, University of Birming-
                  ham, PO Box 363, Birmingham B15 2TT, UK.
KIYOHARA, S.   -Department of Biological Science, The Florida State
                  University, Tallahassee, Florida 32306, USA.
KLEIN, U.   -Max Planck Institut für Verhaltensphysiologie,
                  8131, Seewiesen, Germany.
KOBAL, G.   -Institut für Physiologie und Biokybernetik,
                  Universitätstrasse 17, D - 8520 Erlangen, Germany.
KOELEGA, H.   -Psychological Laboratory, University of Utrecht,
                  Varkenmarkt 2, Utrecht, The Netherlands.
KOGURE, S.   -Department Physiology, School of Medicine, Gunma
                  University, 39-22 - 3 Chome, Showa Machi, Maebashi,
                  Gunma, Japan.
KOSTER, E.   -Psychological Laboratory, Varkenmarkt 2, Utrecht,
                  The Netherlands.
de KRAMER,   -Zoologisch Laboratorium der Rijksuniversiteit te
                  Leiden, Kaiserstraat 63, Leiden, The Netherlands.
KROEZE, J.   -Psychology Laboratory, University of Utrecht,
                  Jacobstraat 14, Utrecht, The Netherlands.
KURIHARA, K.   -Faculty of Pharmaceutical Sciences, Hokkaido Uni-
                  versity, N 12 - W 6, Sapporo, Hokkaido, Japan.
LAFFORT, P.   -Physiologie de la Chimioreception, CNRS, Groupe
                  de Laboratoires du CNRS, 91190, Gif sur Yvette,
                  France.
LARUE-ACHAGIOTIS, C. -Laboratoire Neurophysiologie Sensorielle
                  et Comportementale, Collège de France, 11 Place
                  Marcelin-Berthelot, 75231 Paris Cedex 05, France.
LEE, C.   -National College of Food Technology, St George's
                  Avenue, Weybridge, Surrey, KT 13 ODE, UK.
LE MAGNEN, J.   -Laboratoire de Neurophysiologie Sensorielle et
                  Comportementale, 11 Place Marcelin-Berthelot,
                  75231 Paris Cedex 05, France.
LEVETEAU, J.   -Bt B, 4 Place Jussieu, Université Paris VI, UER 61,
                  75230 Paris Cedex 05, France.
LINDVALL, T.   -The National Swedish Environment, Protection Board,
                  Department of Environmental Hygiene Fack, S - 104 01
                  Stockholm, Sweden.
LISCIA, A.   -Instituto di Fisiologia Generale dell'Universita
                  di Cagliari, v. le Poetto, 1, 09100 Cagliari, Italy.
LITTLE, E.   -Department of Biological Science, Florida State
                  University, Tallahassee, Florida 32306, USA.
LUDVIGSON, H.   -Department Psychology, Texas Christian University,
                  Fort Worth, Texas 76129, USA.
MAC BURNEY, D.   -University of Pittsburgh, 420 Langley Hall,
                  Pittsburgh, Pennsylvania 15260, USA.
MAC LEOD, P.   -Laboratoire de Neurobiologie Sensorielle, EPHE BP 6
                  CEN FAR, 92260 Fontenay aux Roses, France.
MACRIDES, F.   -Worcester Foundation for Exptl Biology, 222 Maple
                  Avenue, Shrewsbury, Massachussetts 01645, USA.

MANKIN, R.   -700 S.W. 23 Rd Drive University of Florida, PO Box
                14565, Gainesville, Florida 32604, USA.
MARSHALL, D.   -Anatomy Laboratory, Department Animal Biology,
                University of Pennsylvania, Philadelphia,
                Pennsylvania 19104, USA.
MATULIONIS, D. -Department of Anatomy, University of Kentucky,
                MN220 Medical Center, Lexington, Kentucky 40506,
                USA.
MASSON, C.   -Laboratoire de Neurobiologie Sensorielle, EPHE,
                BP 6, 92260 Fontenay aux Roses, France.
MEISAMI, E.   -Institute of Biochemistry & Biophysics, University
                of Tehran, PO Box 14-1700, Tehran, Iran.
MARCSTRÖM, A.   -Institute of Zoophysiology, University of Uppsa-
                la, Box 560, S 751 22, Uppsala,
                Sweden.
MEISELMAN, H.   -Food Sciences Laboratory, US Army Natick R & D
                Command, Natick, Massachussets 01760, USA.
MENCO, B.   -Psychologisch Lab., Varkenmarkt 2, Utrecht, The
                Netherlands.
MEREDITH, M.   - Rockefeller University, 1230 York Avenue, New York,
                New York 10021, USA.
MICHELL, A.   -Physiology Department, Royal Veterinary College,
                Royal College St, London NW1 OTU, UK.
MILLER, I.   -Department of Anatomy, Bowman Gray School of Medi-
                cine of Wake Forest University, Winston Salem,
                North Carolina 27103, USA.
MISTRETTA, C.   -Department of Oral Biology, School of Dentistry,
                University of Michigan, Ann Arbor, Michigan 48109,
                USA.
MORI, K.   -Department Physiology, School of Medicine, Gunma
                University, 39-22-3 Chome Showa Machi, Maebashi,
                Gunma, Japan.
MORIMOTO, K.   -Department of Physiology, Kumamoto, University
                Medical School, Honjo 2-2-1, Kumamoto, 860, Japan.
MORITA, H.   -Department of Biology, Faculty of Science, Kyushu
                University 33, Fukuoka 812, Japan.
MOSKOWITZ, H.   -MPI Sensory Testing Inc., 770 Lexington Avenue,
                New York, New York 10021, USA.
MOTOKIZAWA, F. -Department Physiology, Nara Medical College,
                Kashihara, Nara 634, Japan.
MOULTON, D.   -Monell Center, University of Pennsylvania, 3500
                Market Street, Philadelphia, Pennsylvania 19104,
                USA.
MOZELL, M.   -Physiology Department, Upstate Medical Center,
                Syracuse, New York 13210, USA.
MUSTAPARTA, H. -Institute of Biology, Odense University, Niels
                Bohrs Alle 75, 5000 Odense, Denmark.
NOMURA, H.   -Department Physiology, Matsumoto Dental College,
                1780 Hirooka-gobara, Shiojiri 399-07, Japan.
NORGREN, R.   The Rockefeller University, 1230 York Avenue, New
                York, New York 10021, USA.
NOWLIS, G.   -The Rockefeller University, 1230 York Avenue, New
                York, New York 10021, USA.
OAKLEY, B.   -Department Zoology, University of Michigan, Natu-
                ral Sciences Building, Ann Arbor, Michigan 48109.
                USA.

OGAWA, H.   -Department of Physiology, Kumamoto University
                 Medical School, Kumamoto 860, Japan.
OHLOFF, G.   -Firmenich S.A., Route de l'Aire, BP 239, 1211 -
                 Geneve 8, Switzerland.
O'MAHONY, M.   -Department Food Science & Technology, University of
                 California, Davis, California 95616, USA.
ONODA, N.   -Department Physiology, Gunma University, 39-22-
                 3 Chome, Showamachi, Maebashi, Japan.
OTTOSON, D.   -Department Physiology II, Karolinska Institutet,
                 S - 104 01, Stockholm, Sweden.
PAGER, J.   -Laboratoire de Psychophysiologie, Université Claude
                 Bernard, 69621 Villeurbanne, France.
PATTE, F.   -Physiologie de la Chimioreception, Groupe de
                 Laboratoires du CNRS, 91190 Gif sur Yvette, France.
PAYNE, T.   -Department of Entomology, Texas A & M University,
                 College Station, Texas 77843, USA.
PELOSI, P.   -Instituto di Industrie Agrarie, via S. Michele
                 degli Scalzi 4, 56100 Pisa, Italy.
PFAFFMANN, C. -Rockfeller University, 1230 York Avenue, New York,
                 New York 10021, USA.
PIETRA, P.   -Instituto di Fisiologia Generale dell'Universita
                 di Cagliari, v. le Poetto 1, Cagliari 09100, Italy.
PIGGOTT, J.   -Department of Food Science, University of Strath-
                 clyde, 131 Albion st, Glasgow G1 1SD, UK.
PLATTIG, K.   -Institut für Physiologie und Biokybernetik, Univer-
                 sitätsstr.17, D- 8520 Erlangen, Germany.
POLAK, E.   -Laboratoire de Neurobiologie Sensorielle, EPHE -
                 CEN FAR, BP N.6, 92260 Fontenay aux Roses, France.
PRICE, J.   -Department Anatomy & Neurobiology, Washington Uni-
                 versity School of Medicine, 660 S. Euclid Avenue,
                 St Louis, Missouri 63110, USA.
PRICE, S.   Department of Physiology, Medical College of Virgi-
                 nia, Virginia Commonwealth University, Richmond,
                 Virginia 23298, USA.
PUNTER, P.   -Psychological Laboratory, Varkenmarkt 2, Utrecht,
                 The Netherlands.
RADERMAN-LITTLE, R. -Biological Sciences, Unit 1, Florida State
                 University, Tallahassee, Florida 32306, USA.
RAUSCH, L.   -Department of Physiology, University of California,
                 UCLA School of Medicine, Los Angeles, California
                 90024, USA.
REVIAL M.   -Laboratoire d'Electrophysiologie, Batiment 404,
                 Université Lyon 1, 69621, Villeurbanne, France.
RYAN, M.   -Department Zoology, University College, Dublin 4,
                 Ireland.
SASS, H.   -Zoologisches Institut der Universität Regensburg,
                 D- 8400 Regensburg, Germany.
SATO, M.   -Tokyo Metropolitan Institute for Neurosciences,
                 2-6 Musashidai, Fuchu City, Tokyo 183, Japan.
SAWYER, M.   -Department Food Science, University of Reading,
                 London Road, Reading, RG1 5AQ, UK.
SAYLE, B.   -Unilever Research Port Sunlight Laboratory, Unile-
                 ver Ltd, Port Sunlight, Wirral, Merseyside L62 4 XN,
                 UK.
SCHIFFMANN, S. -Psychology Department, Duke University, Durham,
                 North Carolina 27706, USA.

SCHILLING, A. -4, avenue du Petit Chateau,
91800 Brunoy, France.
SCHNEIDER, D. -Max Planck Institut für Verhaltensphysiologie,
8131 Seeviesen, Germany.
SCOTT, J.   -Department of Anatomy, Emory University, Atlanta,
Georgia 30322, USA.
SCOTT, T.   -University of Delaware, 220 Wolf Hall, Newark,
Delaware 19711, USA.
SHAFA, F.   -Institute of Biochemistry and Biophysics, Universi-
ty of Tehran, PO Box 14- 1700, Tehran, Iran.
SHEPHERD, G. -Yale University Medical School, 333 Cedar Street,
New Haven, Connecticut 06510, USA.
SHIBUYA, T.   -Institute of Biological Sciences, University of
Tsukuba, Sakura-Mura, Ibaraki 300 31, Japan.
SLY, J.   -Department of Medicine, Royal Veterinary College,
Hawkshead Road, Brookmans Park, Nr Hatfield,
Hertfordshire AL9 7TA, UK.
SMITH, D.   -Department Psychology, University of Wyoming, Box
3415, Univ. Station, Laramie, Wyoming 82071, USA.
STEINER, J.   -Department Oral Biology, School of Dental Medicine,
PO Box 1172, Jerusalem, Israel.
STEINHOLZ, G. -Institute of Zoophysiology, University of Uppsa-
la, Box 560, S 751 22, Uppsala,
Sweden.
SUNDT, E.   -Firmenich et Cie, 1211 Genève 8,
Switzerland.
TAKAGI, S.   -Department Physiology, School of Medicine, Gunma
University, Showa-machi 3, Maebashi-city, Gunma ken
311, Japan.
THOMMESEN, G. -Inst. of Zoophysiol. , University of Oslo,
Postbox 1051, Blindern, Oslo 3, Norway.
TJALLINGII, W. - Agricultural University, Haarweg 10, Wageningen,
The Netherlands.
TRINDLE, D.   -The Proctor and Gamble Company, PO Box 39175,
Cincinnati, Ohio 45247, USA.
TRUCHITANI, C. -Sensory Sciences Center, University of Texas,
6420 Lamar Fleming, Houston, Texas 77030, USA.
TUCKER, D.   -Department Biological Science, Florida State Uni-
versity, Tallahassee, Florida 32306, USA.
UZIEL, A.   -Laboratoire d'Explorations Neuro-Sensorielles,
Clinique ORL - Hopital St Charles, 34059
Montpellier, France.
VAN DER PERS, J. -Department Zoology, Groningen State University,
Kerklaan 30, Haren, The Netherlands.
VAN DER STARRE, H. -Zoologisch Laboratorium, 63 Kaiserstraat,
Leiden, The Netherlands.
VAN DER WOLK, - Zoologisch Laboratorium, 63 Kaiserstraat, Leiden,
The Netherlands.
VAN DER WEL, H. -Unilever Research, PO Box 114, Vlaardingen,
The Netherlands.
VAN DRONGELEN, W. -Land Bouwhogeschool, Haarweg 10, Wageningen,
The Netherlands.
VERNET-MAURY, E. -Laboratoire de Psychophysiologie, Lyon 1,
43, Boulevard du 11 Novembre 1918, 69621 Villeur-
banne, France.
VERRIER, M.   -Université Paris VI - UER 61, 9 quai St Bernard,
75005 Paris, France.

VON SYDOW, E. -SIK - The Swedish Food Institute, 400 21 Goteborg,
        Sweden.
WALDOW, U.   -Institut für Zoologie, Fachbereich Biologie, Uni-
        versität Regensburg, Universitätsstr. 31, D- 8400
        Regensburg, Germany.
WALKER, J.   -Department of Psychology, Florida State University,
        Tallahassee, Florida 32306, USA.
WEISINGER, R. - Howard Institute of Experimental Physiology &
        Medicine, University of Melbourne, Parkville 3052,
        Australia.
WENZEL, B.   -Department Physiology, School of Medicine, Univer-
        sity of California, Los Angeles, California 90024,
        USA.
WIECZOREK, H. -Fachbereich Biologie der Universitat, D- 8400
        Regensburg, Germany.
WILLIAMS, A. -Cider & Fruit Juices Section, University of Bristol
        Long Ashton, Bristol BS18 9AG, UK.
WINNEKE, G.   -Medizinisches Institut für Lufthygiene und Sili-
        koseforschung an der Universität, D- 4000 Düssel-
        dorf, Germany.
WYSOCKI, C.   -Department Psychology, Florida State University,
        Tallahassee, Florida 32306, USA.
YAMAGUCHI, S. -Central Research Laboratories, 1-1 Suzuki-cho,
        Kawasaki-ku, Kawasaki, Japan.
YAMAMOTO, T. -Department of Oral Physiology, Dental School,
        Osaka University, 32 Joancho, Kitaku, Osaka 530,
        Japan.
YAMASHITA, S. -Biological Institute, Liberal Arts College,
        Kagoshima University, Kohrimoto 1-21-30, Kagoshima
        890, Japan.
YARITA, H.   -Department Physiology, School of Medicine, Gunma
        University, 39-22, 3-chome, Showa-machi, Maebashi,
        Gunma, Japan.
ZACK, C.   -Max Planck Institut für Verhaltensphysiologie,
        8131 Seewiesen, Germany.
ZIPPEL, H.   -Physiologisches Inst. der Universität, Lehrstuhl
        II, Humboldtallee 7, 3400 Göttingen,
        Germany.
ZOETEMAN, B. -National Institute for Water Supply, PO Box 150,
        Leidschendam, The Netherlands.
ZOTTERMAN, Y. -Wenner-Gren Center, Sveavagen 166, 113 46
        Stockholm, Sweden.